BELOW-REPLACEMENT FERTILITY IN INDUSTRIAL SOCIETIES

BELOW-REPLACEMENT FERTILITY IN INDUSTRIAL SOCIETIES
CAUSES, CONSEQUENCES, POLICIES

Kingsley Davis
Mikhail S. Bernstam
Rita Ricardo-Campbell
Editors

Based on papers presented at a seminar held at the
Hoover Institution, Stanford University, November 1985

POPULATION AND DEVELOPMENT REVIEW
A Supplement to Volume 12   1986

CAMBRIDGE UNIVERSITY PRESS
Cambridge
London   New York   New Rochelle
Melbourne   Sydney

CAMBRIDGE UNIVERSITY PRESS
Cambridge, New York, Melbourne, Madrid, Cape Town, Singapore, São Paulo

Cambridge University Press
The Edinburgh Building, Cambridge CB2 2RU, UK

Published in the United States of America by Cambridge University Press, New York

www.cambridge.org
Information on this title: www.cambridge.org/9780521343244

© The Population Council, Inc. 1987
All rights reserved.

First published 1987
This digitally printed first paperback version 2006

A catalogue record for this publication is available from the British Library

Library of Congress Cataloguing in Publication data
Main entry under title:
Below-replacement fertility in industrial societies.
  "Based on papers presented at a seminar held at the Hoover Institution, Stanford University, November 1985."
  Originally published: New York, N.Y. : Population Council, © 1987.
  "Population and development review, a supplement to volume 12, 1986."
  Includes bibliographical references.
  1. Fertility, Human—Congresses. I. Davis, Kingsley, 1908— . II. Bernstam, Mikhail S. III. Ricardo-Campbell, Rita. IV. Hoover Institution on War, Revolution and Peace. V. Population and development review. Vol. 12 (Supplement)
  [HB901.B45   1987b]   304.6′32   87-6371

ISBN-13 978-0-521-34324-4 hardback
ISBN-10 0-521-34324-0 hardback

ISBN-13 978-0-521-67336-5 paperback
ISBN-10 0-521-67336-4 paperback

Contents

Preface	ix
Trends	
The Unprecedented Shortage of Births in Europe	3
Jean Bourgeois-Pichat	
The Decline of Fertility in Non-European Industrialized Countries	26
Samuel H. Preston	
Low Fertility in Evolutionary Perspective	48
Kingsley Davis	
Models	
Altruism and the Economic Theory of Fertility	69
Gary S. Becker Robert J. Barro	
Comment: Paul A. David	77
The Value and Allocation of Time in High-Income Countries: Implications for Fertility	87
T. Paul Schultz	

Comment: Ronald D. Lee ... 108

Competitive Human Markets, Interfamily Transfers, and Below-Replacement Fertility ... 111
Mikhail S. Bernstam

Interpretation

The Family That Does Not Reproduce Itself ... 139
Nathan Keyfitz

Perspective on Nuptiality and Fertility ... 155
Charles F. Westoff

Comment: Shigemi Kono ... 171

Changing Values and Falling Birth Rates ... 176
Samuel H. Preston

Comment: Harriet B. Presser ... 196

Consequences

Demographic Effects of Below-Replacement Fertility and Their Social Implications ... 203
Ansley J. Coale

Economic Growth with Below-Replacement Fertility ... 217
Geoffrey McNicoll

Comment: Ester Boserup ... 238
Comment: Thomas Gale Moore ... 243
Comment: Carmel U. Chiswick ... 244

Population Dynamics with Immigration and Low Fertility ... 248
Thomas J. Espenshade

Immigration as a Counter to Below-Replacement Fertility in the United States ... 262
David M. Heer

Comment: Barry R. Chiswick ... 269

Policies

Social Security in Aging
Societies   273
    Carolyn L. Weaver
    Comment: Thomas Gale Moore   295

US Social Security Under
Low Fertility   296
    Rita Ricardo-Campbell
    Comment: Annelise Anderson   313

Recent Pronatalist Policies
in Western Europe   318
    C. Alison McIntosh

Pronatalist Policies
in Low-Fertility Countries:
Patterns, Performance,
and Prospects   335
    Paul Demeny

Authors   359

Preface

It may seem audacious to try to determine the causes and consequences of the recent scarcity of births in industrial countries. Not only is the scarcity new and complex in its origins, but its ultimate duration and many of its consequences lie in the future, a time that social scientists find baffling. For instance, the experts did not anticipate the baby boom (which lasted for 18 years in the United States) and did not foresee the present low fertility (which in the United States has been below replacement for 15 years). How, then, can we now expect social scientists to judge the future course and consequences of very low fertility?

The answer is that, audacious or not, the task cannot be evaded. Like any other major social change, the prolonged reproductive weakness of the industrial countries raises questions that call for an answer, no matter how difficult. The phenomenon has to be analyzed and explained, placed in a context with other changes and with things that do not change. It has to be "understood."

Why is it that while the advanced countries are failing to replace themselves, the rest of the world continues to reproduce at a prodigious rate? Does the resulting hiatus in population growth create an irresistible migratory pressure? How "aged" will industrial societies become and what social and economic backlashes will this bring about?

Impressed by the profundity and yet slight public awareness of such questions, the Hoover Institution at Stanford University decided to hold a three-day conference on nonreplacement fertility in industrial societies. The conference took place at Hoover's Stauffer Auditorium, on 7–9 November 1985, with 18 main speakers, 16 commentators, several discussants at large, and numerous spectators. The conference was not primarily concerned with documenting or measuring the fertility trends in industrial countries but rather with assessing the causes and consequences of those trends.

The present book is an outgrowth but not a product of the conference. With only one exception (Espenshade), all of the articles were originally presented as papers at the conference; but all have been revised, some drastically. The book is therefore a scholarly symposium in its own right.

The volume starts with two articles that describe in some detail the below-replacement fertility now characterizing the industrial countries. The rest of the volume then takes these data for granted and interprets them from different perspectives. The third article considers present low fertility in long-run human perspective, and the articles in the section on Models describe formal economic reasoning in terms of which an explanation might be found. The next section—on Interpretation—presents analyses that are less formal but more empirical, and drawn from various disciplines. The section entitled Consequences then deals with the major consequences of continued below-replacement fertility, including the impact on the age structure, economic growth, and immigration. Finally, the last section analyzes policies designed either to raise the birth rate or to solve problems of social security and public welfare created by low fertility.

By its very nature and persistence, we believe that below-replacement fertility is a profound development in industrial societies, and that, as such, it needs more scholarly attention than it has received. The present book, it is hoped, will increase that attention. We wish to thank the Hoover Institution for its willingness to sponsor and fund the conference. We are also grateful to the Alfred P. Sloane Foundation for help in defraying some of the conference costs and to the Draeger Foundation for its contribution toward publication costs. We also wish to thank our various authors for their tolerance and patience in responding to editorial intrusions. Particular credit goes to Ethel Churchill and her editorial colleagues at the Population Council for their final editing and handling of the manuscript. Among those at Hoover whose managerial skills helped to save us from chaos were Christina Rosas-Maxemin, John P. Holland, and Nancy Hinsen (at the time of the conference) and Valerie Wetter (in connection with manuscript preparation).

The Hoover Institution
Stanford University

Kingsley Davis
Mikhail S. Bernstam
Rita Ricardo-Campbell

TRENDS

The Unprecedented Shortage of Births in Europe

Jean Bourgeois-Pichat

The unprecedented decline of fertility in Europe during the last 20 years has provoked a stream of descriptive analysis in an effort to assess underlying causes as well as to detect any signs of an upswing in births. Any prospective demographic assessment of this situation must build on the most recent raw data, rather than rely solely on more refined measures that take time to appear in published compendia.

The analysis to follow, drawing on preliminary data for 1983 and in some cases 1984, suggests that even the few upswings in births that appear in measures of the total fertility rate have been of short duration. The decline in nuptiality and the rise in divorce, two common phenomena in the industrialized countries, have led to a decline in the population of married women and, by extension, to lower fertility throughout Europe. To the extent that some marriages are contracted owing to prenuptial pregnancy ("dependent marriages"), we will argue, the decline of nuptiality in Europe may be the result of the fertility decline and not the reverse, as is often assumed.

The article explores trends in nuptiality, including the changing patterns of marital composition and the growing prevalence of illegitimate fertility. The latter will be seen to result from the steep decline in legitimate births and the sharply growing population of single women. The number of illegitimate births as a proportion of all births is expected to continue to increase even if the fertility rate remains unchanged. Inasmuch as a sizable part of the decline in nuptiality is due to the gradual disappearance of dependent marriages—attributable in part to more effective practice of contraception—levels of marriage will probably remain at a low level in the future.

The total population

In six countries of Europe the total population is declining: Austria, Belgium, Denmark, West Germany, Hungary, and Iceland. In all but West Germany and Hungary the decline is as yet very small.

In Central Europe deaths exceed births in a large and growing area. This area includes the following countries:

Country	Population as of 1 January 1983 (thousands)
Austria	7,551.0
Belgium	9,853.0
Denmark	5,112.1
West Germany	61,307.0
Hungary	10,679.0
Italy (North-Central)	36,506.3[a]
Total	131,008.4

[a]Population as of 31 October 1984.
SOURCES: For Belgium, Denmark, and West Germany: EUROSTAT, *Demographic Situation 1985*. For Austria and Hungary: A. Monnier, "La conjoncture démographique—l'Europe et les pays développés d'outre-mer," *Population* (July–October 1985). For Italy (North Central): *Rapporto sulla Situazione Demografica in Italia*. June 1985. Consiglio Nazionale delle Ricerche, Istituto di Ricerche Sulla Popolazione.

The total fertility rate

Total fertility rates are given in Table 1 for 34 industrialized countries in Europe and elsewhere. The total fertility rate is the number of children a woman would have if she lived through the childbearing years and gave birth at prevailing age-specific fertility rates. The United States, with a total fertility rate of 1.79 per woman in 1983, is close to the average of the industrialized countries. With the low mortality prevalent in the developed countries, the replacement level of the total fertility rate is a little below 2.1 children per woman. A population whose fertility remains indefinitely below this level will eventually decline. Only five countries in Table 1 were above the replacement level in 1983: Poland, Ireland, Northern Ireland, the Soviet Union, and Israel. This means that all the other countries are already embarked on what may be a long-term declining population trend. The fertility decline started around 1965, almost simultaneously in every country, and took everybody by surprise. Some countries, particularly in Eastern Europe, have tried to reverse the decline by adopting pronatalist policies. These measures generally seem to succeed for a while, but after some years the decline starts again. This decline has not been steady, even in countries that did not adopt specific policies to counteract it. Some reversals have occurred, suggesting that fertility could go up again,

TABLE 1 Total fertility rates in selected industrialized countries, 1965–84

Country	1965	1970	1975	1978	1979	1980	1981	1982	1983	1984
Eastern Europe										
Bulgaria	2.03	2.18	2.23	2.15	2.15	2.05	2.01	2.02	2.00	NA
Czechoslovakia	2.37	2.07	2.43	2.36	2.33	2.16	2.10	2.10	2.08	2.07
East Germany	2.48	2.19	1.54	1.90	1.90	1.94	1.85	1.85	1.79	NA
Hungary	1.82	1.96	2.35	2.07	2.01	1.91	1.88	1.79	1.72	1.73
Poland	2.52	2.20	2.27	2.20	2.25	2.26	2.22	2.31	2.40	NA
Romania	1.91	2.89	2.60	2.52	2.48	2.43	2.35	2.19	2.00	NA
Northern Europe										
Denmark	2.61	1.95	1.92	1.67	1.60	1.55	1.44	1.43	1.38	1.40
Finland	2.47	1.83	1.68	1.64	1.64	1.63	1.64	1.72	1.74	1.70
Iceland	3.71	2.81	2.65	2.35	2.49	2.48	2.33	2.26	NA	NA
Ireland	4.03	3.87	3.41	3.24	3.23	3.23	3.08	2.96	2.74	NA
Norway	2.93	2.50	1.98	1.77	1.75	1.72	1.70	1.71	1.65	1.65
Sweden	2.42	1.92	1.77	1.60	1.66	1.68	1.63	1.62	1.61	1.65
United Kingdom	2.83	2.44	1.82	1.77	1.88	1.92	1.84	1.78	1.77	NA
England and Wales	2.85	2.42	1.78	1.73	1.84	1.88	1.80	1.76	1.76	1.76
Scotland	3.00	2.57	1.91	1.75	1.85	1.84	1.86	1.73	1.70	1.68
Northern Ireland	NA	3.13	2.63	2.58	2.74	2.72	2.55	2.47	2.42	NA
Southern Europe										
Greece	2.32	2.43	2.33	2.29	2.29	2.21	2.09	2.02	1.94	NA
Italy	2.55	2.37	2.19	1.85	1.74	1.66	1.57	1.57	1.53	NA
Portugal	3.07	2.62	2.59	2.28	2.17	2.12	2.04	2.02	1.96	NA
Spain	2.97	2.87	2.80	2.53	2.31	2.16	1.99	1.87	NA	NA
Yugoslavia	2.71	2.29	2.27	2.15	2.12	2.13	2.06	NA	NA	NA
Western Europe										
Austria	2.68	2.30	1.83	1.60	1.60	1.65	1.67	1.66	1.56	1.52
Belgium	2.60	2.24	1.73	1.69	1.69	1.68	1.66	1.60	1.56	NA
France	2.84	2.47	1.93	1.82	1.86	1.95	1.95	1.91	1.79	1.81
West Germany	2.50	2.01	1.45	1.38	1.38	1.45	1.43	1.41	1.33	1.29
Netherlands	3.04	2.58	1.66	1.58	1.56	1.60	1.56	1.49	1.47	1.49
Switzerland	2.01	2.10	1.61	1.50	1.52	1.55	1.54	1.55	1.51	1.52
Soviet Union[a]	2.46	2.39	2.41	2.32	2.28	2.26	2.25	2.29	2.37	2.41
Australia	2.97	2.85	2.14	1.95	1.90	1.89	1.93	1.93	1.93	NA
Canada	3.15	2.33	1.90	1.75	1.75	1.73	1.70	1.69	1.67	NA
Israel	3.19	3.97	3.67	3.26	3.21	3.14	3.12	3.12	3.14	NA
Japan	2.14	2.13	1.89	1.77	1.74	1.73	1.75	1.75	1.80	1.81
New Zealand	3.53	3.17	2.36	2.10	2.10	2.03	1.95	1.95	1.92	NA
United States	2.93	2.48	1.77	1.76	1.81	1.84	1.82	1.83	1.79	1.82

NA = not available.
[a]Average rates calculated on 1978–79 for the rate shown for 1979.
SOURCES: A. Monnier, "La conjoncture démographique—l'Europe et les pays développés d'outre-mer," published annually since 1979 in *Population* (July–October). For the most recent years, the national statistical yearbooks have also been used.

but these have been of short duration. Gradually the various countries reached lower and lower fertility levels—levels that 20 years ago would have been considered unbelievable.

In 1983 the North-Central region of Italy, with some 36.5 million inhabitants, had the lowest total fertility rate ever observed in a large population.

The total fertility rates of Central Europe, where deaths exceeded births, are as follows for 1983:

Country	Total fertility rate (per woman)
Austria	1.56
Belgium	1.56
Denmark	1.38
West Germany	1.32
Hungary	1.72
Italy (North-Central)	1.28

SOURCES: Same as table on p. 4.

The most recent data, for 1984, seem to signal a new reversal. Some increases in the total fertility rate have been observed, to be documented later in this article, and where the decline has continued it has been less steep.

Taken together with trends in other regions of the world, however, the low and declining fertility rates in Europe presage major shifts in the distribution of population. If China is set aside, the world can be divided into three parts: the developed countries with fertility below the replacement level (1.18 billion); those developing countries where fertility started to decline 20 years ago and that now have low mortality and high but declining fertility (1.70 billion); and those developing countries where mortality is declining while no decline in fertility has so far been detected (892 million). These last countries are in the midst of the so-called demographic explosion.

The United Nations Population Division has developed a model of future population trends in which the fertility of all countries will reach the replacement level some time during the twenty-first century and remain at that level. The population of all countries would eventually reach a constant level under this model. Using the model, the World Bank has determined the constant level for each country. Using these data to calculate the constant level of the three country groupings we have just defined produces the following results: the population of the developed countries would be multiplied by 1.25, the developing countries experiencing declining fertility by 2.5, and the third group by 5.5. For the Soviet Union the World Bank gives 377 million as the level of stability; for the United States, 292 million; and for Europe excluding the Soviet Union, 553 million.

Total fertility rate versus completed cohort fertility

The total fertility rate is obtained by summing the age-specific fertility rates for a given calendar year. If these rates were those observed in an actual cohort of women, their sum would represent the completed fertility of women of this cohort living through the reproductive span. When the sum is calculated with the rates observed during a calendar year, 35 birth cohorts are involved (i.e., for women aged 15–50). It is therefore difficult to interpret the significance of a change in the total fertility rate: A decrease or increase may be transitory and not have any influence on the completed cohort fertility. If a steady decrease (or increase) is observed, it is probable that it will affect cohort fertility, but it is difficult to decide whether a change is transitory or permanent in character. This explains why most demographers supplement the analysis of the total fertility rate with an analysis of completed cohort fertility.

When the period age-specific fertility rates are calculated by single-year age groups, it is easy to allocate each rate to a given birth cohort. However, some countries continue to publish age-specific fertility rates only by five-year age groups. The same practice is followed by international publications even for countries publishing their own rates annually. It is therefore necessary to allocate period rates for the five-year age groups to single-year birth cohorts. I have used a well-established procedure to calculate the completed fertility of 13 cohorts born from 1876 to 1936 in Denmark. The cohorts born after 1936 have not yet finished bearing children, and even for the 1936 cohort there is uncertainty because the rate for the period 1981–85 is not yet completely known. It is possible, however, to extend the series beyond 1936 by making some hypotheses about the missing rates. For instance, the completed fertility for the 1941 cohort can be estimated as 2.20 per woman, that for the 1946 cohort as 2.04, and that for the 1951 cohort as 1.86.

Finally, it is possible to graph the trend of completed fertility for the cohorts born from 1871 to 1951 (see Figure 1). If the timing of the arrival of

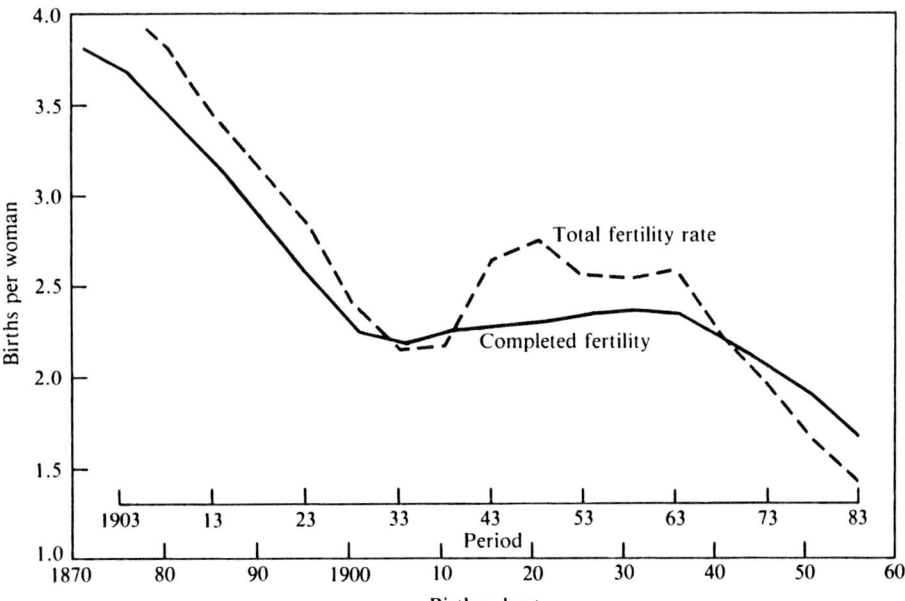

FIGURE 1 Denmark: Total fertility rates, 1908–83, and completed fertility for cohorts born from 1871 to 1951

SOURCES: *Statistik Årbog Danmark* (Statistical Yearbook of Denmark), successive issues.

births in each cohort did not vary, the mean age of the mother at birth of her children would remain constant. Let us denote the mean age as a_m. Thus the curve of the total fertility rate displaced by a_m on the left would coincide almost exactly with the curve of completed fertility. In reality the timing of arrival of births is not constant, but, in spite of the variation, the mean age of women at birth of their children does not vary much around 28 years. In Figure 1 the total fertility rate has been displaced on the left by 28 years. The gaps between the two curves give an idea of the importance of the variation in timing of births.

For Denmark we are fortunate to have a long series of age-specific fertility rates. Most such series are much shorter. This is particularly the case for Eastern Europe, where it is relatively easy to obtain a series starting just after World War II but difficult to extend the series back into the past, due mainly to border changes. Yet even with a series starting as late as 1946–50 some interesting results can be obtained. As an example, take Hungary. Strictly speaking it is only possible to reconstruct the completed fertility for the cohorts born in 1931 and 1936. But in making some plausible assumptions about the missing rates, as we did for Denmark, we can estimate the completed fertility for the cohort born in 1926 and the cohorts born in 1941, 1945, and 1951. Tentatively we include a result for the cohort born in 1956. Figure 2, which

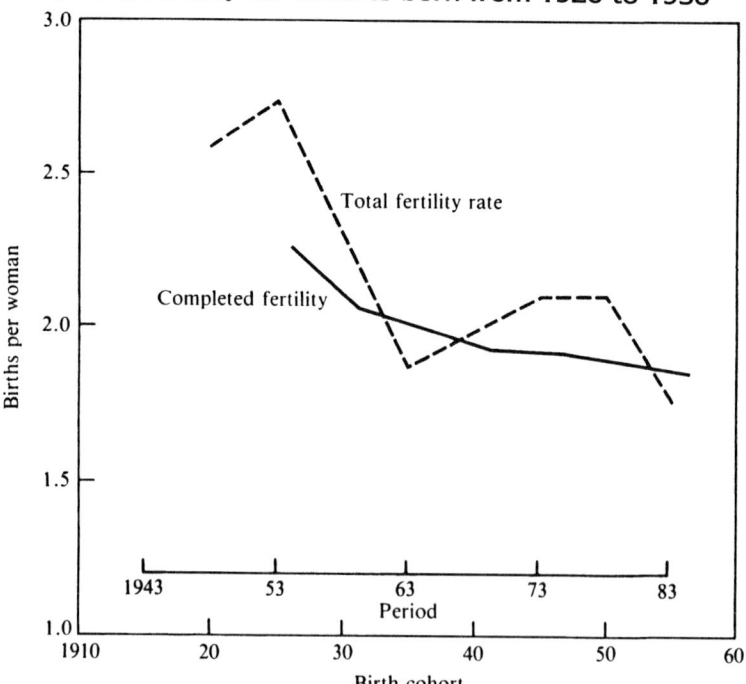

FIGURE 2 Hungary: Total fertility rates, 1948—83, and completed fertility for cohorts born from 1926 to 1956

SOURCE: *Demográfiai Évkönyv* (Demographic Yearbook), Küzponti Statisztikai Hivatal (Central Bureau of Statistics), Budapest, successive issues.

FIGURE 3 Completed fertility by cohort in eight countries in Northern and Western Europe and in the United States

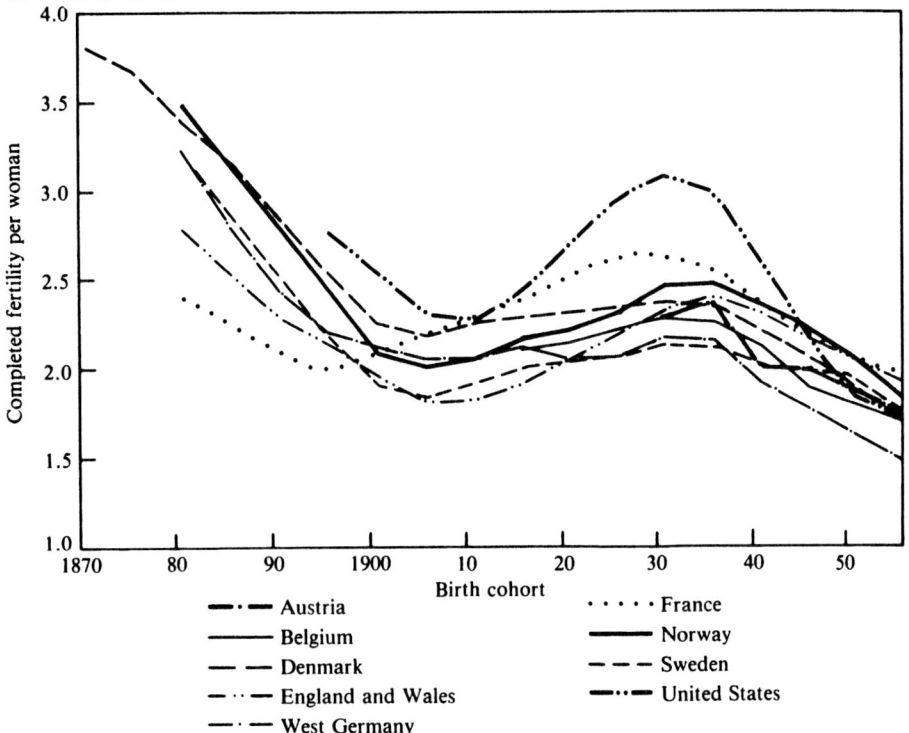

SOURCES: Completed fertility calculated by using the age-specific fertility rates published in successive statistical yearbooks of each country and successive issues of the United Nations *Demographic Yearbook*. For the United States, the rates are taken from Robert L. Heuser, *Fertility Tables for Birth Cohorts by Color: United States, 1917-1973* (Rockville, Maryland: National Center for Health Statistics, 1976). After 1973 the rates for white women have been estimated from the rates published in the UN *Demographic Yearbook* for the entire population.

is similar to Figure 1 for Denmark, is highly interesting, as one can see clearly from the curve representing the total fertility rate the results of the government efforts to halt the fertility decline. These efforts changed the timing of births but not the completed family size. From 1961–65 to 1971–75 the total fertility rate per woman rose from 1.84 to 2.10, that is, an increase of 14 percent; but this increase did not last. Very soon the total fertility rate started to decline again. The trend in completed fertility showed hardly any change.[1]

Figures 3 and 4 show the great similarity among countries in the course of fertility change. The curves have the same shape, and the turning points occur among cohorts born at roughly the same time. France is an exception. There, the minimum completed fertility was reached for the cohort born around 1895, whereas in other countries the minimum was reached by the cohort born around 1905. In 1941, when Pierre Depoid published his study of net reproduction in Europe,[2] he stopped at the cohort born in 1900. At that time France

FIGURE 4 Completed fertility by cohort in Finland, Ireland, the Netherlands, and Switzerland

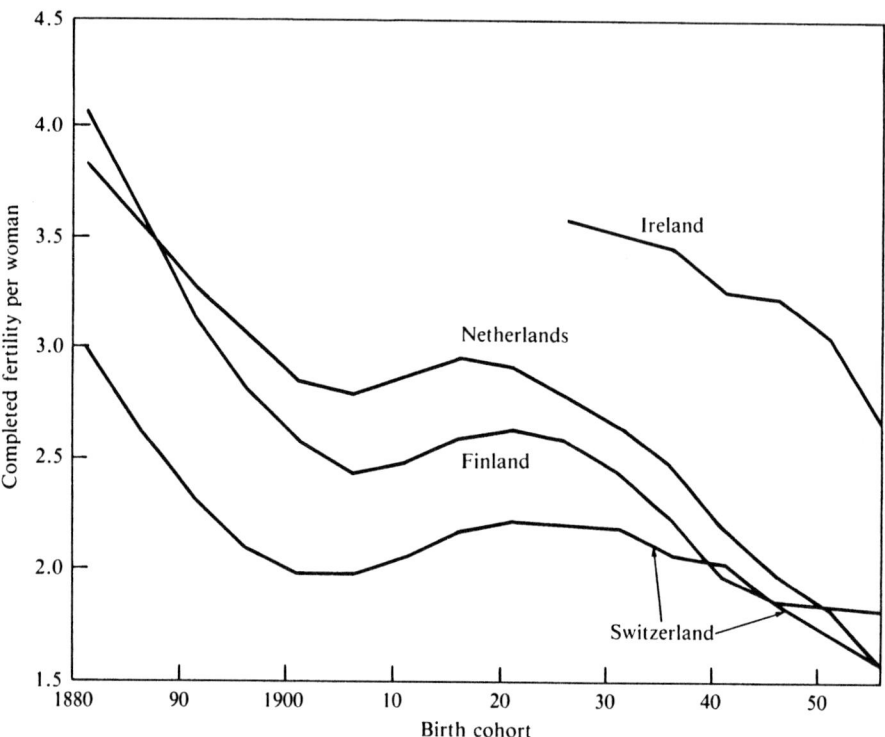

SOURCES: Completed fertility calculated from the age-specific fertility rates published in successive statistical yearbooks of each country and successive issues of the United Nations *Demographic Yearbook*.

was the only country showing an upturn in completed fertility; all other European countries had declining fertility. Depoid mentioned this upturn in France, but he could not guess that it was the first sign of the baby boom that would start a few years later everywhere in the developed world.

Although the shape of the curves is similar, the turning points are located at different levels in different countries. Table 2 gives these levels for the baby boom and Table 3 for the baby bust. Let us start with the baby boom; in absolute terms the greatest difference between the maximum and minimum levels of fertility was recorded in the United States (.82 births per woman, that is, a difference of about one child per woman). France followed (.64 per woman), then England and Wales (.57) and Norway (.47). The baby boom was more modest in some other countries. In West Germany the gain was only .14 births per woman. In relative terms France and the United States were close to each other, recording fertility increases of 32.5 percent and 36.3 percent. But the increase was spread over 34 cohorts in France, as against only 22 cohorts in the United States.

TABLE 2 The baby boom in selected European countries and the United States

Country	Dates of cohort turning points			Completed fertility at the turning points (per woman)		Difference	
	Minimum fertility level	Maximum fertility level	Time elapsed (years)	Minimum	Maximum	Absolute (births)	Relative (percent)
Northern Europe							
Denmark	1906	1931	25	2.18	2.37	0.19	8.7
England and Wales	1908	1936	28	1.81	2.38	0.57	31.5
Finland	1907	1921	14	2.40	2.63	0.23	9.5
Ireland	NA	1920	NA	NA	3.60	NA	NA
Norway	1907	1934	27	2.01	2.48	0.47	23.4
Sweden	1905	1935	30	1.84	2.13	0.29	15.8
Southern Europe							
Italy	1926	1931	5	2.28	2.28	0.00	0.0
Portugal	1926	1931	5	2.86	2.87	0.01	0.3
Spain	1920	1936	16	2.51	2.70	0.19	7.6
Western Europe							
Austria	NA	1935	NA	NA	2.36	NA	NA
Belgium	NA	1932	NA	NA	2.27	NA	NA
France	1896	1930	34	1.97	2.61	0.64	32.5
West Germany	1906	1933	27	2.06	2.20	0.14	6.4
Netherlands	1906	1917	11	2.79	2.96	0.17	6.1
Switzerland	1903	1921	18	1.98	2.23	0.25	12.6
United States (white)	1911	1932	22	2.26	3.08	0.82	36.3

NA = not available.
SOURCES: For Northern Europe, Western Europe, and the United States, the minima and maxima are taken from Figures 3 and 4. For Southern Europe, they are taken from similar figures not shown here.

TABLE 3 The baby bust in selected European countries and the United States

Country	Maximum-fertility cohort	Number of years between maximum-fertility cohort and 1956	Completed fertility		Difference	
			For the maximum-fertility cohort	For the 1956 cohort	Absolute (births)	Relative (percent)
Northern Europe						
Denmark	1931	25	2.37	1.60	0.77	32
England and Wales	1936	20	2.38	1.92	0.46	19
Finland	1921	35	2.14	1.82	0.32	15
Ireland	1920	36	3.60	2.65	0.95	26
Norway	1934	22	2.48	1.84	0.64	26
Sweden	1935	21	2.13	1.76	0.37	17
Southern Europe						
Italy	1930	26	2.28	1.64	0.64	28
Portugal	1931	25	2.87	1.94	0.93	32
Spain	1935	21	2.70	1.90	0.80	30
Western Europe						
Austria	1935	21	2.36	1.72	0.64	27
Belgium	1932	24	2.27	1.69	0.58	26
France	1930	26	2.61	1.97	0.64	25
West Germany	1933	23	2.20	1.48	0.72	33
Netherlands	1917	39	2.96	1.58	1.38	47
Switzerland	1925	31	2.23	1.57	0.66	30
United States (white)	1932	24	3.08	1.71	1.37	44

SOURCES: See Table 2.

As for the baby bust, there are also differences among countries as can be seen in Table 3. Before commenting on this table, we must remember that the baby bust is still in progress in most industrialized countries. The 1956 cohort is used here as a provisional limit. In absolute terms the greatest fertility decline occurred in the Netherlands (1.38 births per woman), followed by the United States (1.37), Ireland (.95), Portugal (.93), Spain (.80), Denmark (.77), and West Germany (.72). The smallest declines occurred in England and Wales (.46), Sweden (.37), and Finland (.32). In relative terms the United States and the Netherlands experienced far greater declines than the other countries (44 and 47 percent), but the decline is spread over 39 cohorts in the Netherlands, as against only 24 cohorts in the United States. The smallest relative declines took place in England and Wales (19 percent), Sweden (17 percent), and Finland (15 percent).

In Eastern Europe only the end of the baby bust can be traced, because the earliest available vital statistics permit the reconstruction only of cohorts born from 1920 to 1956. Three countries at the end of the baby bust deviate from the general trend: Finland, East Germany, and Poland. In all three the fertility decline seems to have reached a turning point. Do these deviations from the general trend signal a general upturn, much as the trend in France did in 1941 when Pierre Depoid published his study? To try to answer this question, we return to the period fertility for the last 15 years, and we include the seven Soviet Republics in which an increase has recently been observed (Table 4). These Republics, all on the western side of the Soviet Union, are known for their resemblance to European demographic behavior. It is also known that the Soviet Union adopted a new pronatalist policy in 1981.

TABLE 4 Recent increases in fertility in Eastern Europe, including selected Soviet Republics

Country or Republic	Population (millions)[a]	Total fertility rate per woman	
		Minimum	Recent[b]
East Germany	16.7 (1984)	1.54 (1974)	1.95 (1980)
Finland	4.9 (1984)	1.50 (1973)	1.74 (1983)
Poland	37.1 (1985)	2.20 (1978)	2.40 (1983)
Russia	137.5	1.89 (1979–80)	2.08
Byelorussia	9.6	2.02 (1980–81)	2.14
Estonia	1.5	2.01 (1979–80)	2.13
Georgia	5.0	2.24 (1982–83)	2.28
Latvia	2.5	1.86 (1978–79)	2.10
Lithuania	3.4	1.97 (1981–82)	2.09
Moldavia	3.9	2.38 (1978–79)	2.67
Ukrania	49.8	1.94 (1980–81)	2.10

[a]As of 1979 unless otherwise noted.
[b]1983–84 unless otherwise noted.
SOURCES: East Germany: *Statistical Yearbook* (various issues); Finland: *Yearbook of Population Research in Finland;* Poland: *Rocznik Demograficzny* (Demographic Yearbooks of Poland); USSR: *Vestnik Statistiki* (monthly Review of Statistics).

We can immediately eliminate East Germany as a harbinger of a new trend because it is known to have adopted an official pronatalist policy in 1975 to halt the steep decline in fertility. As Table 4 suggests, the policy was temporarily effective, but after 1980 fertility resumed its decline. (In 1983 the total fertility rate was 1.81.)

As for the Soviet Union, it is too early to say whether, in time, the effect of the 1981 policy will fade and the decline will resume, as happened in East Germany.

There remain the cases of Poland and Finland. In Poland, preliminary results seem to indicate that fertility in 1984 was lower than in 1983; but this decline could not wipe out the increase observed from 1978 to 1983. The case of Finland is more puzzling. The total fertility rate bottomed out in 1973. The rise over the next decade, at least for certain age groups, was substantial—52.3 percent for the age group 30–34 years and 53 percent for the age group 35–39. A phenomenon spread over ten years can hardly be termed ephemeral. Nor has population policy in Finland changed much over the last 15 years. It therefore seems plausible to regard the increase of fertility in that country since 1974 as a sign of a possible upturn a few years from now in the fertility of the developed countries. Tenuous as this conclusion is, further doubt is cast by the finding of an apparent decline in Finland's total fertility rate, from 1.74 in 1983 to 1.70 in 1984.

Trends in nuptiality

Two well-known trends in the industrialized countries—the decline in nuptiality and the increase in divorce—have a similar effect on the marital structure of the population. They lead to a decline in the proportion of married women. In terms of childbearing, this means that more and more women are choosing illegitimate fertility. Table 5 shows the proportion of all births that are illegitimate in European countries for which rates are available. There is great diversity among countries. In Sweden in 1983, 44 percent of births were illegitimate, compared with only 5.4 percent in Switzerland and 1.6 percent in Greece. It is intrinsically interesting to discover that in Sweden in 1983 there were almost the same number of legitimate and illegitimate births, but it would be even more interesting to know how such a situation came about. Why is the proportion of illegitimate births so high in Sweden and so low in Switzerland? This is the question we will now try to answer. To do so, we first go back to the decline of nuptiality.

Fertility is generally held to be a dependent variable of nuptiality: when nuptiality declines, if everything else remains the same, fertility also declines. In a recent document published in the 1985 *Yearbook of Population Research* in Finland, the Swedish demographer Erland Hofsten, in commenting on the recent report of the Norwegian Population Commission, writes as follows:

> Among a great part of the population in Scandinavia nuptiality has been the dependent variable. It is when it is discovered that the woman is pregnant that

TABLE 5 Illegitimate births per 100 live births in Europe, 1956–60 to 1983

Country	1956–60	1961–65	1966–70	1971–75	1976–80	1980	1981	1982	1983
Eastern Europe									
Bulgaria	7.6	8.5	9.5	9.8	10.1	10.9	10.3	11.4	11.3
Czechoslovakia	5.1	4.7	5.5	5.0	5.1	5.7	5.7	5.8	NA
East Germany	12.5	9.9	12.6	15.9	18.3	22.9	25.6	29.3	NA
Hungary	6.0	5.3	5.1	5.8	6.3	7.1	7.4	7.7	8.3
Poland	5.1	4.2	4.8	4.8	4.8	4.7	4.6	4.6	NA
Northern Europe									
Denmark	7.2	8.8	10.9	16.9	28.3	33.2	35.7	38.3	40.0
Finland	NA	NA	5.3	7.8	11.7	13.1	13.3	NA	NA
Iceland	25.2	25.7	29.7	33.0	36.6	39.7	41.2	44.6	NA
Ireland	1.7	1.9	2.5	3.2	4.2	5.0	5.4	6.1	6.8
Norway	3.6	4.0	5.7	9.1	12.4	14.5	16.1	17.6	NA
Sweden	10.4	12.7	16.0	27.8	36.2	39.7	41.2	43.0	43.7
United Kingdom	4.7	6.6	8.0	8.5	10.2	11.5	12.5	14.1	15.4
Southern Europe									
Greece	1.4	1.2	1.1	1.2	1.4	1.5	1.6	1.5	1.6
Italy	2.7	2.2	2.1	2.6	3.7	4.1	4.3	4.6	4.8
Portugal	10.4	8.7	7.6	7.2	7.9	9.2	9.5	10.0	10.7
Spain	2.9	2.0	1.5	1.6	2.5	2.9	NA	NA	NA
Yugoslavia	NA	NA	8.4	7.8	8.1	8.6	8.3	NA	NA
Western Europe									
Austria	13.3	11.7	12.0	13.5	15.4	17.8	19.5	21.6	22.4
Belgium	2.1	2.2	2.6	3.1	3.5	4.1	4.5	5.2	NA
France	6.2	5.9	6.3	8.0	9.7	11.6	12.7	14.2	NA
West Germany	6.9	5.3	4.9	6.1	6.9	7.6	7.9	8.5	8.8
Luxemburg	3.1	3.3	3.4	4.2	5.0	6.0	7.1	6.2	6.3
Netherlands	1.3	1.6	2.1	2.0	3.2	4.1	4.7	5.9	7.0
Switzerland	3.8	4.1	3.8	3.7	4.2	4.7	5.2	5.5	5.4

NA = not available.
NOTE: Rates not available for all years shown for the following countries: Romania, England and Wales, Scotland, Northern Ireland, Albania, and the Soviet Union.
SOURCES: Various issues of the United Nations *Demographic Yearbook*. For the most recent years the national statistical yearbooks or national demographic yearbooks have been used.

the young couple make the decision to marry. . . . The commission explained the reduced number of births during the 1970's with the declining number of marriages. To my mind the relation may very well be the opposite.

Dependent and independent marriages

A marriage will be considered to be "dependent" if a child was conceived before the wedding. The other marriages will be called "independent"; they are the independent variables of the classical interpretation of nuptiality. The dependent marriages depend at least partly on fertility. When fertility declines through increased practice of contraception, the dependent marriages will also decline. It follows that part of the decline of nuptiality in Europe may be the result of the fertility decline shown in Table 1 and not the reverse, as is usually assumed.

Only a few countries publish data permitting the estimation of premarital conceptions. The basic tool is a table giving births by number of months married during the first year of marriage. Births occurring before eight months of marriage can be taken as an estimate of premarital pregnancies. Such tables are published by Denmark, England and Wales, France, West Germany, Sweden, and Switzerland. In the Netherlands a similar table is published, but only for births occurring 0–6 months since marriage. Most other countries give the birth by year of marriage duration (duration 0–11 months for the first year), and some give the births occurring the same year as the year of marriage—data that are difficult to use.

Figure 5 shows a certain similarity between dependent and independent marriages in France, West Germany, and Switzerland. The two curves have, at first sight, similar shapes. This similarity relates to the first aspect of dependent marriages, namely that they follow the overall trend in nuptiality. But the second aspect appears as soon as we try to describe in quantitative terms the similarity of the two curves.

If the dependent marriages were ordinary marriages, that is, marriages influenced only by the behavior of the population toward nuptiality, the ratio of dependent to independent marriages would remain constant. This is not the case, because dependent marriages are influenced by the fertility trend. In a period of fertility decline, dependent marriages also decline, and this decline is added to the variation caused by the trend in nuptiality. We will now try to measure the two effects.

Let us take West Germany as a specific example. Figure 6 gives the trend, and Table 6 the data. Let us look at the year 1968. In that year, some

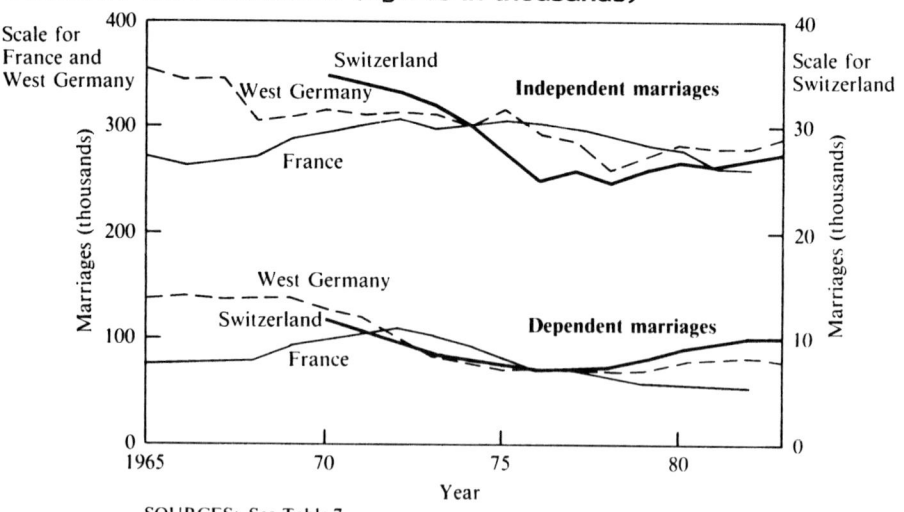

FIGURE 5 Dependent and independent marriages in France, West Germany, and Switzerland (figures in thousands)

SOURCES: See Table 7

FIGURE 6 The decline in the annual number of marriages in West Germany, 1965–83

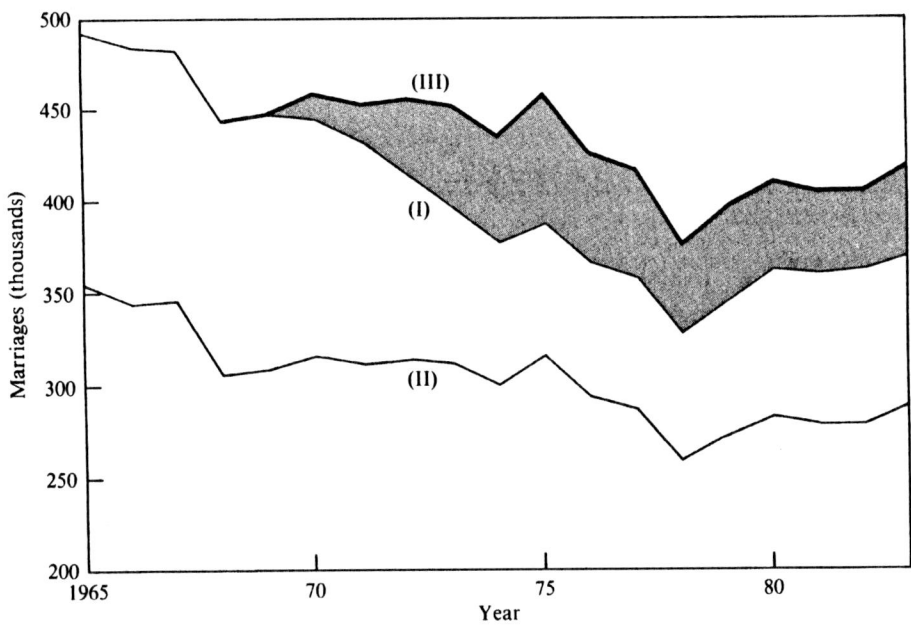

(I)   = Marriages.
(II) = Independent marriages.
(III) = Marriages at the 1968 level of dependent marriages.

SOURCE: See Table 7.

444,000 marriages were registered, out of which 138,000 were dependent marriages and 306,000 were independent marriages. The ratio of dependent to independent marriages was 0.45 to 1.

The "true" trend in nuptiality in West Germany is shown by curve II, representing the course of independent marriages. If dependent marriages had remained at their 1968 level, we could calculate the true level of total nuptiality by multiplying curve II by 1.45. This hypothetical trend is represented by curve III on the graph. But the actual curve of marriage is curve I. It is below curve III because dependent marriages did not stay at their 1968 level. Due to increasing use of contraception, more and more marital conceptions were prevented and fewer and fewer dependent marriages were contracted. The shaded area in the figure represents the effects of these prevented conceptions on the trend in nuptiality.

From 1968 to 1983 the decline in the number of marriages due to the "true" trend in nuptiality in West Germany would have been 444,000 minus 420,000 = 24,000. But because of the effect of contraception on the number of dependent marriages, the actual decline in the total number of marriages

TABLE 6 The decline in the annual number of marriages in West Germany, 1965–83

Year (1)	Total number of marriages (thousands) (2)	Dependent marriages[a] (thousands) (3)	Independent marriages[b] (thousands) (4)	Ratio of independent to dependent marriages (5)	Births during first year of marriage (thousands) (6)	Ratio of births during first year of marriage to dependent marriages (7)	Hypothetical number of dependent marriages at the 1968 level[c] (thousands) (8)	Hypothetical total nuptiality at the 1968 level of dependent marriages[d] (thousands) (9)
1965	492	138	354	2.39	215	0.64		
1966	485	140	345	1.41	215	0.65		
1967	483	137	346	1.40	208	0.66		
1968	444	138	306	1.45	203	0.68	138	444
1969	447	138	309	1.45	193	0.71	139	448
1970	445	128	316	1.41	177	0.72	142	458
1971	432	120	312	1.38	166	0.72	141	453
1972	415	101	314	1.32	141	0.71	141	446
1973	395	83	312	1.27	118	0.70	140	452
1974	377	78	300	1.26	110	0.70	135	435
1975	387	71	316	1.22	100	0.70	142	458
1976	366	72	294	1.24	100	0.72	132	426
1977	358	71	287	1.25	97	0.73	129	416
1978	328	69	259	1.27	95	0.73	117	375
1979	245	72	273	1.26	96	0.74	123	396
1980	362	79	283	1.28	107	0.74	127	411
1981	359	81	279	1.29	109	0.74	126	405
1982	362	83	279	1.30	108	0.76	126	405
1983	370	80	290	1.28	104	0.77	130	420

[a] The number of dependent marriages is equal to the number of births occurring at less than 8 months' duration of marriage (0–7 months). Strictly speaking a portion of the marriages allocated to a particular year were celebrated in the preceding year, and therefore the total should be allocated between the two years. In this table, however, all marriages have been allocated to the later year.
[b] Column (2) minus column (3).
[c] Column (4) multiplied by 0.45, which is the ratio of dependent to independent marriages in 1968.
[d] Column (4) plus column (8) or column (4) multiplied by 1.45, which is the ratio of independent to dependent marriages in 1968.
SOURCES: *Bevölking und Erwerbstätigheit*, Reche 2. *Bevölkerungs bewegung* (vital statistics); *Statistisches Bundesant Wiesbaden* (successive issues).

was 444,000 minus 370,000 = 74,000. The effect of contraception was therefore equal to 74,000 minus 24,000 = 50,000, that is, 67.6 percent of the total. I have made similar calculations for the other countries for which data on premarital conceptions exist (see Table 7).

The entry for Switzerland deserves an explanation. In that country dependent marriages follow the trend in independent marriages closely. Not differentially affected by contraceptive knowledge, the dependent marriages behave as do other marriages and hence do not affect the total birth rate disproportionately.

Hungary also appears in Table 7, although that country does not publish data permitting the estimation of premarital conceptions. It publishes data only on births occurring less than one year after marriage. Since these births started to decline in 1976, we may infer that dependent marriages started to decline at the same time. Hungary is among the countries in which nuptiality changed very little until recently, but since 1980 the country has experienced declining nuptiality. It was tempting to try to determine the effect of this decline on dependent marriages. To estimate these marriages, we multiplied the births of one-year duration by 0.625—the average ratio of dependent marriages to births occurring at less than one year of marriage observed in France during 1970–83. This procedure is not very satisfactory, and we have to interpret the results with caution. They suggest that in Hungary dependent marriages explain only

TABLE 7 Percent of the decline in all marriages (dependent and independent) explained by the decline in dependent marriages

Country	Period of decline	Percent explained by decline in dependent marriages
Denmark	1972–83	93.2
England and Wales	1971–83	40.7
France	1972–82	36.9
West Germany	1968–83	67.6
Hungary	1976–83	17.5
Netherlands	1967–82	27.6
Sweden	1965–83	34.0
Switzerland	1965–83	Negligible

SOURCES: Denmark: *Denmarks Statistik Befolkingens bevaegelser* (vital statistics), successive issues; England and Wales: Office of Population Censuses and Surveys, *England and Wales—Birth Statistics*. A publication of the Government Statistical Service, successive issues; France: *La situation démographique—Les collections de l'INSEE*, Série D, successive issues; West Germany: See Table 6; Hungary: See Figure 2; Netherlands: *Maandstatistiek van de bevolking*, Centraal Bureau voor de Statistiek, successive issues; Sweden: *Population Changes, Part 3*, official statistics of Sweden, successive issues; Switzerland: Office Fédéral de la Statistique, Berne, *Mouvement de la population en Suisse*, successive issues.

a small part of the decrease in marriages from 1976 to 1981, but nevertheless the phenomenon observed in other countries has at least started in Hungary.

This analysis at least partly confirms the interpretation offered by Hofsten. It is interesting to note that the decline in nuptiality measured by independent marriages is not so sharp as that measured by the fall in total marriages. The dependent marriages are probably lost forever, and consequently nuptiality will never again reach the high level that prevailed before 1965.

The existence of dependent marriages may also explain the simultaneity of nuptiality decline in so many countries in Europe. This decline was at least in part the consequence of more effective practice of contraception, a behavioral change that spread rapidly across all borders.

Changes in marital composition

The decline in nuptiality produced sizable increases in the proportion of women remaining single, particularly in Western Europe. For four countries with a high proportion of never-married women aged 20–24, the percentages increased as follows:

	1970	1980	1981	1982
Denmark	44.7	72.5	75.3	78.3
West Germany	41.6	60.1	62.7	
Netherlands	46.4	55.9	58.4	61.2
Norway	46.2	61.9	64.6	

Elsewhere in Europe nuptiality did not vary greatly, as illustrated by the following percentages of never-married women 20–24:

	1970	1980	1981
Czechoslovakia	34.9	33.3	
Hungary	32.3	30.1	30.9
Poland	40.7	45.9	

To study the phenomenon of changing marital composition more intensively, we will use the example of Denmark. As our objective is to throw some light on the relation of illegitimate births to legitimate births, we will abandon as an index the proportion of women never-married and consider the proportion of currently married women and its complement, the proportion of nonmarried women, which includes widows and divorcées. Three factors are responsible for the changes in the proportion of currently married women in Denmark from 1950 to 1983. These are:

1 The variation in nuptiality—not only the decline during the past 20 years but also the increase prior to 1965.

2 The increase in divorce, which tends to shrink the proportion of currently married women.

3 The decline in mortality, which, by diminishing the proportion of widows, tends to inflate the proportion of currently married women.

The effect of mortality decline is very small. The effect of rising divorce is more important, particularly above 30 years of age. Let us examine the marital composition of Danish women aged 45–49 in 1970 and 1984:

	Percent		Difference
	1970	1984	
Married or separated	82.5	79.8	−2.7
Single	7.0	4.9	−2.1
Widowed	4.2	3.8	−0.4
Divorced	6.3	11.5	+5.2
Total	100.0	100.0	0.0

For divorced women and widows, we find what we expected. The increase in divorce is responsible for a large increase in the proportion of women who are divorced, while the decline in mortality only slightly lowers the proportion of women widowed. The effect of nuptiality change is to reduce both the proportion married and the proportion single. The 45–49-year-old women belong to cohorts married before 1965, during a time of increasing nuptiality. Consequently the proportion of single women is lower in 1984 than in 1970. The increase in nuptiality before 1965 counteracts the effect of the increase in divorce. The story is quite different for younger women. Let us take the women aged 25–29 in 1970 and 1984:

	Percent		Difference
	1970	1984	
Married or separated	82.3	48.9	−32.4
Single	13.8	44.7	+30.9
Widowed	0.3	0.2	−0.1
Divorced	3.6	5.3	+1.7
Total	100.0	100.0	0.0

Again we find that the rise in divorce increased the proportion of divorcées. The effect of the decline of mortality is again very low. The most substantial difference occurs in the proportion of single women. This time it is the fall of nuptiality after 1965 that is at work. It increases the proportion of single women by some 30 percentage points. For the 25–29 age group the change in nuptiality and the change in divorce act in the same direction. But of course the contrast between the 25–29-year-olds and the 45–49-year-olds is transitory. When cohorts of women who married during the last 20 years reach the end of the reproductive period, the effect of the increase in nuptiality observed before 1965 will have been replaced by the effect of the decline in nuptiality observed during the last 20 years. For women now at the beginning of the reproductive period, we do not know what will happen. An increase in nuptiality in future years is conceivable; if it occurs, there will again be opposing patterns between the two age groups, but in reverse. However, we have seen that a sizable part of the decline in nuptiality was due to the gradual disappearance of dependent marriages. This part is therefore lost forever, and nuptiality will probably stay at a low level in the future.

For the group 15–49 years as a whole, there has been a slow decline in the number of currently married women and a large increase in the number of currently nonmarried women. The proportion of nonmarried women rose from 33.2 percent in 1970 to 48.0 percent in 1984.

Legitimate and illegitimate fertility in Denmark

With Danish data it is easy to calculate the legitimate and illegitimate general fertility rates, that is, the fertility rates for the age group 15–49 years as a whole. The results at five-year intervals from 1960 to 1980 and for 1983 are given in Table 8. One sees clearly the steady decline in legitimate fertility since 1965. The illegitimate rate increased slowly from 1960 to 1970, then rapidly from 1970 to 1975, and thereafter remained more or less stable. In 1983 illegitimate and legitimate fertility were similar.

We can now understand why the proportion of illegitimate births among total births increased so sharply in Denmark. First, a constantly decreasing legitimate fertility rate has been applied to a sharply decreasing population of married women. The result has been a steep decline in the number of legitimate births. Second, a slightly increasing illegitimate fertility rate has been applied to a sharply growing population of single women. The result has been a marked increase in illegitimate births, as delineated in Table 9. The two phenomena act in concert to increase the proportion of all births that are illegitimate. The ratio rose from .10 to 1 in 1966 to .41 to 1 in 1984. This movement will not stop in the near future, since the fall in nuptiality is not yet fully reflected in the marital composition of 15–49-year-old women.

Denmark is not an exceptional case. That country's change in patterns of marriage has also occurred in other countries as well. Four other countries—

TABLE 8 Denmark: Legitimate and illegitimate fertility for women 15–49 years old, 1960–83

Year	Fertility rate per woman	
	Legitimate	Illegitimate
1960	0.097	0.016
1965	0.105	0.021
1970	0.082	0.020
1975	0.077	0.036
1980	0.055	0.036
1983	0.046	0.035

SOURCE: See Table 7.

TABLE 9 Denmark: Legitimate and illegitimate fertility for women 15–49 years old in 1966, 1974, and 1984

	Legitimate fertility			Illegitimate fertility			
Year	Currently married women (thousands)	Legitimate fertility rate (per woman)	Legitimate births (thousands)	Currently non-married women (thousands)	Illegitimate fertility rate (per woman)	Illegitimate births (thousands)	Ratio of illegitimate births to all births
1966	751	0.106	79	382	0.023	9	0.10
1974	743	0.078	58	429	0.031	13	0.19
1984	663	0.046	30	597	0.034	21	0.41

SOURCE: See Table 6.

FIGURE 7 Percent of currently nonmarried women, aged 15–49 years, in Denmark, France, East Germany, Hungary, and Sweden

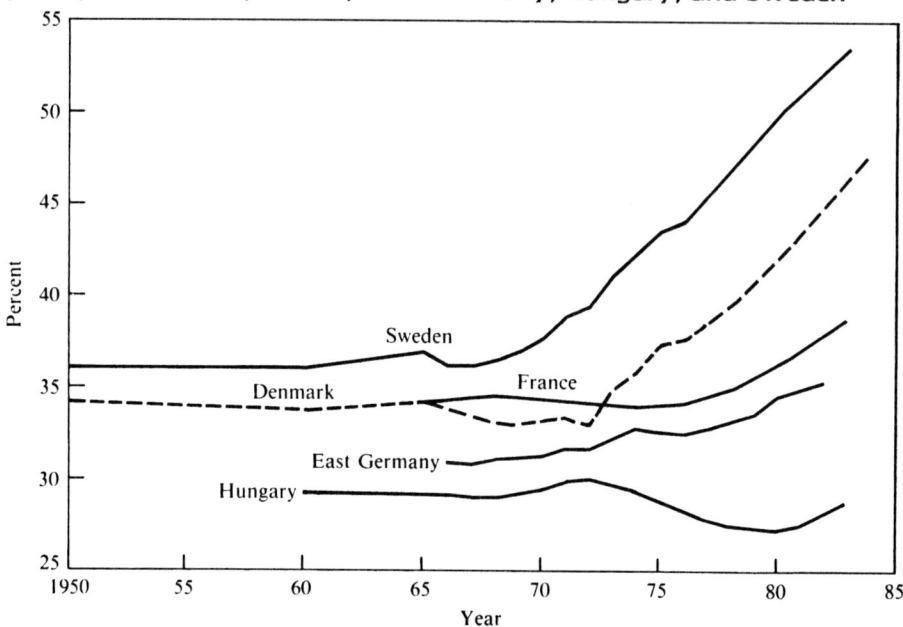

SOURCES: Percentages calculated from the age composition of the female population by marital status published in successive issues of the UN *Demographic Yearbook*. For the most recent years national statistical yearbooks were used.

Sweden, France, East Germany, and Hungary—illustrate what is happening generally throughout Europe. Sweden was the first country in Europe to experience nuptiality decline. It therefore led all other countries in modifying the marital composition of women of reproductive age. In the West, Denmark was second followed by France. The decline in East Germany began earlier than in France but at a slower pace. Hungary is more typical of Eastern Europe: an increase in the proportion of currently nonmarried women is just beginning. The evolution of the five countries is summarized in Figure 7. All the curves representing the proportion of nonmarried women are rising and will continue to do so. It is expected that the ratio of illegitimate births to total births will continue to increase even if the fertility rate remains unchanged.

Concluding remarks

As stated at the beginning, my purpose was not to seek an explanation of below-replacement fertility in industrialized countries during the last 20 years, but rather to provide and examine the data that any such theory must take into account. The general conclusion that can be drawn from the data assembled here is that Europe and more generally the industrialized countries seem to be in the midst of a complex process of evolution that casts doubt on the basic principles accepted until recently by a large majority of scholars. The old consensus seems to be on the verge of collapsing, and disastrous demographic consequences seem possible. The fate of the human species—or at least of certain national populations—is at stake in this process. Well before the close of this century, the population "implosion" may replace the population explosion of today as the main subject of concern.

Notes

1 Figures and supporting data similar to those given here for Denmark and Hungary can be obtained for all European countries (except the USSR) and for the United States from the author upon request.

2 Pierre Depoid, *Reproduction nette en Europe depuis l'origine des statistiques de l'Etat Civil*. Etude démographique No. 1. Statistiques Générales de la France.

The Decline of Fertility in Non-European Industrialized Countries

Samuel H. Preston

This article presents a quantitative description of change in fertility and the proximate determinants thereof, derived from primary and secondary sources, for non-European industrialized countries since World War II. Table 1 presents annual period total fertility rates since 1945 in each of the countries considered. These rates are graphed in Figure 1.

Good correspondence exists in the general shape of the graphs among all English-speaking countries, with a hill-shaped pattern evident in all. The descent from the peak is fastest in the United States and Canada and, for an extended period, slowest in New Zealand. Japan, on the other hand, experienced an earlier rapid decline between 1947 and 1961, followed by a long plateau with a slightly declining slope. A peak fertility of 3.5–4.2 children per woman in the English-speaking countries was reached somewhere between 1957 and 1961. Whatever the initial starting point and pattern during the first 30 years of these series, it is evident that all five countries had reached a common range of 1.7–2.0 children per woman by the early 1980s.

These trends are not related in any immediately obvious way to national economic performance. For example, economic growth was extraordinarily rapid in Japan in both the 1950s and 1960s; the former decade produced a very rapid fall in fertility and the latter, a slight rise. There is even less correspondence between international levels of fertility and levels of real income. Japan had below-replacement fertility in 1960 at a per capita real income that was only one-fifth of the US level of 1980, and only 28 percent of its own 1980 income. New Zealand has yet to reach the income level of the United States in 1960, but has a total fertility rate that is 47 percent lower.

The absence of simple mechanistic relations with fertility is shared by other development indicators. For example, the below-replacement fertility of Japan in 1962 was achieved with a labor force participation rate in paid employment outside the home for married women of only 12.6 percent, compared

TABLE 1   Total fertility rates in selected industrialized countries

Year	Australia	Canada[a]	Japan	New Zealand	United States[b]
1945	2.74	3.00	—	2.91	2.42
1946	2.98	3.36	—	3.25	2.86
1947	3.06	3.59	4.54	3.45	3.18
1948	2.98	3.44	4.40	3.38	3.03
1949	3.07	3.37	4.32	3.33	3.04
1950	3.06	3.37	3.65	3.38	3.03
1951	3.06	3.42	3.26	3.36	3.20
1952	3.18	3.56	2.98	3.52	3.29
1953	3.19	3.64	2.69	3.48	3.35
1954	3.19	3.74	2.48	3.60	3.46
1955	3.27	3.75	2.37	3.72	3.50
1956	3.33	3.77	2.22	3.77	3.61
1957	3.42	3.84	2.04	3.88	3.68
1958	3.42	3.80	2.11	3.96	3.63
1959	3.44	3.85	2.04	4.00	3.64
1960	3.45	3.81	2.00	4.03	3.61
1961	3.54	3.75	1.96	4.16	3.56
1962	3.42	3.68	1.98	4.11	3.42
1963	3.33	3.61	2.00	3.99	3.30
1964	3.15	3.46	2.05	3.73	3.17
1965	2.98	3.11	2.14	3.33	2.88
1966	2.88	2.75	1.58	3.44	2.67
1967	2.85	2.53	2.23	3.35	2.53
1968	2.89	2.39	2.13	3.33	2.43
1969	2.89	2.33	2.13	3.27	2.43
1970	2.86	2.26	2.13	3.16	2.48
1971	2.95	2.14	2.16	3.18	2.27
1972	2.74	1.98	2.14	3.00	2.01
1973	2.48	1.89	2.14	2.77	1.88
1974	2.40	1.84	2.05	2.58	1.84
1975	2.22	1.82	1.91	2.37	1.77
1976	2.14	1.80	1.85	2.26	1.74
1977	2.04	1.81	1.80	2.21	1.79
1978	1.98	1.76	1.79	2.07	1.76
1979	1.94	1.76	1.77	2.12	1.81
1980	1.92	1.75	1.75	2.03	1.84
1981	1.94	1.70	1.74	2.01	1.82
1982	1.94	1.69	1.77	1.95	1.83
1983	—	—	1.80	1.92	—

[a] Does not include Newfoundland.
[b] Prior to 1959, does not include Alaska; prior to 1960 does not include Hawaii.
SOURCES: Australia: Bureau of Statistics, *Australian Demographic Statistics Quarterly*, November 1983 (for 1971–82); earlier years from United Nations, *Demographic Yearbook*, various years; and OECD, *Demographic Development in OECD Countries*, Paris 1979, as reported in Romaniuk, 1984.
Canada: Romaniuk, 1984.
Japan: "Population reproduction rates for all Japan: 1983," *The Journal of Population Problems* (Tokyo), No. 173 (January 1985): 74–81.
New Zealand: New Zealand Department of Statistics, *Population and Migration Statistics, 1983–84*, Part A, Wellington (for 1971–82); 1983 from *Vital Statistics of New Zealand*, 1983. Earlier years from United Nations, *Demographic Yearbook*, various issues; and OECD, *Demographic Development in OECD Countries*, Paris, 1979, as reported in Romaniuk, 1984.
United States: US National Center for Health Statistics, 1984a; Heuser, 1976 (before 1970).

FIGURE 1 Total fertility rates in selected industrialized countries

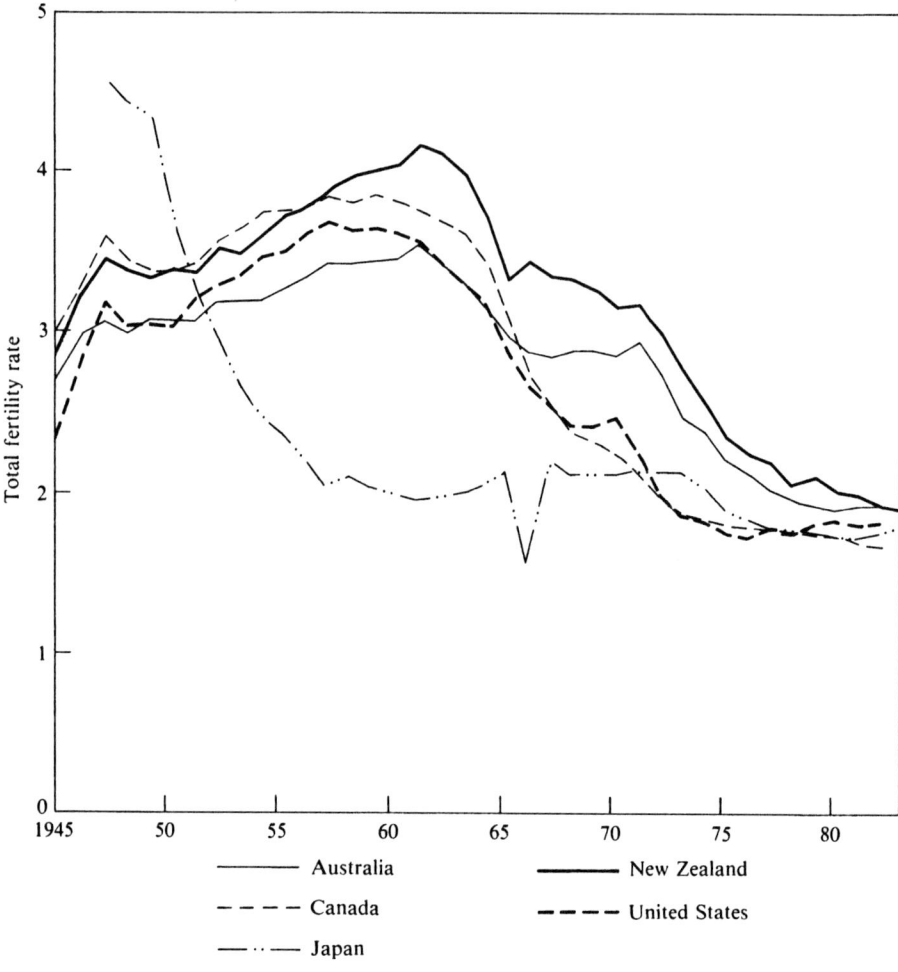

NOTES: Data for Canada do not include Newfoundland. For the United States, data prior to 1959 do not include Alaska; data prior to 1960 do not include Hawaii.
SOURCES: See Table 1.

with a level of 50–51 percent in the United States or Australia in 1980 (Mincer, 1984: Table 1). Women in Australia had an average of 4.0 years less schooling than American women in 1970 (1984: Table 4), although these countries had similar fertility profiles throughout the postwar period. Obviously, one cannot expect to find any simple mechanical formula that would satisfactorily account for postwar fertility trends in and differences among these countries.

While fertility rates have been below the replacement level for a decade or so in most of these countries, no recent cohorts of married women who have completed childbearing have had below-replacement fertility, as shown in Table 2. The data in this table, of course, are for women who bore children

TABLE 2 Average family size among older women in recent censuses or surveys

	Age group	Mean number of children ever born
Canada, 1981, ever-married women	35–39	2.33
	40–44	2.84
Japan, 1984, currently married women	35–39	2.17
	40–44	2.28
	45–49	2.25
New Zealand, 1981, women	35–39	2.66
	40–44	3.03
	45–49	3.28
United States, 1983, women	35–39	2.147
	40–44	2.688
	45–49	2.996

SOURCES: Canada: Romaniuk, 1984: Table 4.1.
Japan: Population Problems Research Council, 1984: Table III-8.
New Zealand: Department of Statistics, New Zealand Census of Population and Dwellings, 1981, Vol. 2: Ages, Marital Status, and Fertility: Table 20. Refers to females usually resident in New Zealand.
United States: US Bureau of the Census, 1983: Table 9.

under the high rates of the 1950s and 1960s as well as the low rates of the 1970s and 1980s. Japanese rates were low throughout this period, so that their mean completed family size is the lowest. Results from the 1981 Australian census were still unavailable at the time this was written.

The comparison of period and cohort rates raises the issue of appropriate fertility measures. Thanks primarily to the work of Norman Ryder, a now-standard approach to period fertility measures is to decompose them into timing and volume components. Unfortunately, space does not permit us to pursue this distinction. Period fertility measures have unquestionably been more variable than cohort measures in the English-speaking countries in the past half-century (see, e.g., Thornton and Freedman, 1983; Romaniuk, 1984). This pattern suggests that cohort-specific influences may have been important in period fertility. But this conclusion is not inevitable, since cohort rates would also be less variable if they simply represented averages over period-specific influences. A review of age-period-cohort fertility analyses by John Hobcraft et al. (1982) finds a domination of period effects over cohort effects. Rates for all ages tend to rise and fall together. I believe that period fertility measures are meaningful indicators of the volume of fertility implied by a period's conditions, although these measures are doubtless confounded in many circumstances by timing components.

Changes in marriage and marriage-related behavior

Because fertility rates are much higher among married women than among the unmarried in each of the countries, the frequency of marriage is a "determinant" of fertility levels, at least in a formal arithmetic sense. The convenient analytic relation becomes less useful when the event of marriage often follows conception, when nonmarital fertility rates are rapidly changing, when childbearing is the major purpose of marriage, or when nuptiality and marital fertility present alternative responses to the same set of forces.

The postwar period has seen major changes in the rate of entry into first marriage in each of the countries considered. In the English-speaking countries, the decade of the 1950s was one of increased first marriage rates. As shown in Table 3, the proportion never-married at ages 20–24 declined by 9–12 percentage points in Australia, New Zealand, and Canada, and by 4 points in the United States. Less dramatic declines occurred at other reproductive ages. The United States began the period with substantially earlier marriage than the other countries and maintained this position until the 1980s; in 1960, 71.6 percent of American women aged 20–24 had already married.

Beginning in the 1960s in the United States and Canada and in the 1970s in Australia and New Zealand, marriage trends reversed themselves. The reversal was most marked in the United States, where by 1984 the proportions never-married at ages 20–24, 25–29, and 30–34 were double their values in 1960. Clearly, the boom-and-bust cycle of fertility in these countries was matched by a boom-and-bust cycle of first marriage.

The degree to which the marriage changes were "responsible" for changes in fertility has been the subject of several inquiries. But it is clear from Table 3 that changes in the proportions never-married cannot account for a very large fraction of the recent fertility decline. The total fertility rate declined by an average of 52 percent, peak-to-trough, in these countries. The proportions *ever*-married (the relevant index) changed by only a few percent above age 30 and by 3–16 percent at ages 25–29. Even at ages 20–24, the proportion ever-married declined by less than 25 percent in all countries except the United States, where it declined by 40 percent between 1960 and 1984 (but only by 30 percent between 1960 and 1980, by which time the total fertility rate decline had ended). Only at ages 15–19, which account for a very small fraction of the total fertility rate, were changes in the ever-married proportions as large as the proportionate decline in the total fertility rate. Using standardization procedures, Anatole Romaniuk (1984) attributes 10 percent of the decline in Canada's total fertility rate between 1961 and 1981 to changing marital proportions (including first marriage as well as marital disruption), and Andrew Cherlin (1981) attributes 16 percent of the US decline between 1961 and 1975 to this source. Increases in marriage probably played a larger role in the earlier and milder increase in the total fertility rate. In Australia, L.T. Ruzicka and C. Choi (1983) calculate that 63 percent of the rise in fertility

TABLE 3 Proportion of women never-married, by age group in selected industrialized countries

	Age group						
	15–19	20–24	25–29	30–34	35–39	40–44	45–49
Australia							
1947	94.4	51.4	21.0	13.8	12.6	12.9	12.6
1961	93.0	39.5	12.4	7.7	6.5	6.6	7.4
1971	91.2	35.7	11.6	6.5	5.0	4.8	4.9
1976	92.7	40.1	13.1	7.0	5.1	4.5	4.6
1981	95.7	54.5	19.1	8.4	5.4	4.4	4.1
Canada							
1951	92.1	48.5	20.7	13.8	12.4	12.3	11.7
1961	91.3	40.5	15.4	10.5	9.2	8.9	9.5
1971	92.5	43.5	15.4	9.1	7.3	6.9	7.0
1980	95.6	55.2	20.2	9.6	6.9	5.9	5.7
Japan							
1950	96.6	55.3	15.2	5.7	3.0	2.0	1.5
1960	98.6	68.3	21.6	9.4	5.5	3.2	2.1
1970	97.8	71.6	18.1	7.2	5.8	5.3	4.0
1975	98.6	69.2	20.9	7.7	5.3	5.0	4.9
1980	99.0	77.7	24.0	9.1	5.5	4.4	4.4
New Zealand							
1951	93.7	49.2	18.9	12.4	10.9	11.3	11.8
1961	91.6	40.5	12.5	8.1	7.3	7.5	8.3
1966	90.3	38.9	11.8	6.9	6.0	6.2	6.7
1976	89.6	37.4	11.8	6.2	4.7	4.4	4.7
1981	93.4	49.3	15.7	8.0	5.0	4.3	4.7
United States							
1950	82.9	32.3	13.3	9.3	8.3	7.9	7.7
1960	83.9	28.4	10.5	6.9	6.1	6.1	6.5
1970	90.3	35.8	10.5	6.2	5.4	4.9	4.9
1980	91.2	50.2	20.9	9.5	6.2	4.8	4.7
1984	93.4	56.9	25.9	13.3	7.5	5.4	4.6

SOURCES: Australia: Carmichael, 1984.
Canada and New Zealand: United Nations, *Demographic Yearbook*, 1979 (Historical Supplement) and 1982.
Japan: United Nations, 1984; and Japan, Institute of Population Problems, 1985.
United States: United Nations, *Demographic Yearbook*, 1979 (Historical Supplement); US Bureau of the Census, 1984a.

between the birth cohorts of 1901–06 and 1931–36 was a result of increases in age-specific proportions married.

As in the case of fertility, Japan's time trend in marriage differs from those of the English-speaking countries. Proportions ever-married declined sharply between 1950 and 1960, the decade when fertility also declined very quickly. Little change was evident between 1960 and 1975, after which the proportion ever-married at ages 20–24 again declined rapidly. By the early 1980s only half as high a fraction of 20–24-year-old women had married in Japan as in the English-speaking countries. Although the fertility decline during the 1950s was much faster than could be accounted for by marriage changes alone, the smaller decline since 1974 seems largely attributable to changing marriage behavior. Shigemi Kono (1984) provides for Japan the most detailed analysis of the interrelations between changes in marriage and in fertility available for any of the countries under discussion. Using fertility simulation, he concludes that, had first marriage remained at the level observed for the 1930–34 birth cohort rather than declined, the period total fertility rate would have averaged 2.0 for the period 1975–79 rather than 1.82, thereby eliminating slightly more than half of the fertility decline between the early 1970s and late 1970s. In a more conventional decomposition, Kono (1982) attributes 58 percent of the total fertility rate decline between 1970 and 1980 in Japan to changing proportions married, but only 15 percent of the larger fertility decline between 1950 and 1960.

The importance of marriage behavior in Japan is enhanced because that country maintains the largest differential between marital and nonmarital fertility of any of those under review. Marital fertility rates remain very high below age 30, as shown by the following age-specific fertility rates for married Japanese women (per 1000):

Age group	1930	1970	1980
15–19	306	246	384
20–24	334	346	352
25–29	284	259	243
30–34	240	95	83
35–39	183	22	14
40–44	84	3	2
45–49	10	0	0

SOURCE: Japan, Institute of Population Problems, 1985.

Marital fertility rates below age 30 are nearly as high in 1980 as in 1930; the 1980 marital total fertility rate is 5.39. These figures imply very rapid childbearing in the early years of marriage in Japan, a suggestion confirmed by Philip Morgan et al. (1984). Of the Japanese marriage cohort of 1961–70, three-quarters had a first birth within the first two years of marriage. Furthermore, later marriage cohorts had children slightly faster than earlier cohorts. No educational differentials in the pace of first birth attainment were evident. Makoto Atoh (1985) reports that the Mainichi (nationally representative) survey of family planning in 1984 found that only 21 percent of Japanese married women had initiated contraception before the first birth and only an additional 25 percent before the second birth. The sum of these proportions has actually declined from the level of 50–55 percent observed between 1967 and 1979. The United States stands in sharp contrast: the timing of the first birth within marriage is slower, and the likelihood of an early marital birth is declining over time and is strongly negatively influenced by a woman's education (Morgan et al., 1984). A declining pace of childbearing within marriage has also been noted in Canada since the 1951–60 marriage cohorts (Romaniuk, 1984: 29) and in Australia, for wives not premaritally pregnant, since 1961 (Ruzicka and Caldwell, 1982: 210).

Proportions ever-married at a particular age are products of a cohort's entire history of entry into first marriage, and for older cohorts this history is lengthy. From two observations separated by five years, it is possible to compute the proportions ever-married in a synthetic cohort that would be subject at each age to cohort-specific attrition rates from the single population observed during the period (Agarwala, 1962). The procedure assumes no differences in age-specific mortality between the single and total population. This procedure can be applied to data in Table 3 for four of the five countries, with the following results (US data for 1979 are used—US Bureau of the Census, 1980: Table 1):

Period attrition rates from single population as recorded in	Percent of women never-married at ages 45–49 in synthetic cohort	Average number of years lived in single state below age 50 in synthetic cohort
Australia, 1976–81	10.4	26.6
Japan, 1975–80	6.2	26.9
New Zealand, 1976–81	10.8	25.7
United States, 1979–84	11.6	27.2

The proportions never-married are substantially higher than those recently observed for actual cohorts of 45–49-year-old women. But they are not historically unprecedented except in Japan, where fewer than 2 percent of 45–49-year-old women were single in each census from 1920 to 1960 (United Nations, 1984: 64). In all four countries shown, females can expect to spend a majority of their years below 50 in the single state.

During the period when entry into marriage was being delayed, exit from marriage accelerated. Table 4 shows that divorce rates in each country followed a U-shaped pattern during the postwar period. A period of low and basically stable rates stretched from 1955 to 1963 in the United States, 1950–62 in Canada, 1954–63 in Australia, 1955–67 in New Zealand, and 1956–66 in Japan. Although at their postwar trough, US rates between 1955 and 1963 were about three times higher than those in Australia, New Zealand, and Japan, and about six times higher than those in Canada. Legal changes facilitating divorce affected the trends in all countries, although these are probably best viewed as reflections of society's changing attitudes regarding the institution of marriage, rather than as a purely exogenous factor. Divorce laws were liberalized in 1968 in Canada (Dumas, 1985), in 1975 in Australia (Josephian, 1984), and throughout the 1970s in the United States on a state-specific basis to the point where nearly all states allowed unilateral divorce by 1980 (Thornton and Freedman, 1982). The US divorce rate in the late 1970s was such that about 50–52 percent of marriages would end in divorce if such rates were to continue (Weed, 1980; Preston, 1983). There is a determinate relation between

TABLE 4 Divorce rates (per 1000 population) in selected industrialized countries

	Australia	Canada	Japan	New Zealand	United States
1947	1.15	.65	1.02	1.24	3.37
1948	.93	.54	.99	1.07	2.79
1949	.83	.45	1.01	1.01	2.67
1950	.90	.39	1.01	.85	2.55
1951	.86	.38	.97	.81	2.48
1952	.82	.39	.92	.84	2.52
1953	.90	.41	.86	.75	2.47
1954	.72	.39	.87	.73	2.35
1955	.73	.38	.84	.69	2.30
1956	.68	.37	.80	.66	2.28
1957	.65	.40	.79	.62	2.24
1958	.70	.37	.80	.76	2.12
1959	.73	.37	.78	.70	2.24
1960	.65	.39	.74	.69	2.18
1961	.64	.36	.74	.72	2.26
1962	.68	.36	.75	.71	2.22
1963	.67	.40	.73	.75	2.26
1964	.72	.45	.74	.73	2.34
1965	.78	.46	.79	.69	2.46
1966	.80	.51	.80	.77	2.54
1967	.88	.55	.84	.75	2.63
1968	.93	.55	.87	.79	2.91
1969	1.04	1.24	.89	1.08	3.15
1970	1.18	1.37	.93	1.11	3.45
1971	1.51	1.37	.99	1.17	3.72
1972	2.41	1.48	1.02	1.19	4.02
1973	2.14	1.66	1.04	1.22	4.32
1974	2.29	2.01	1.04	1.47	4.57
1975	2.43	2.23	1.07	1.54	4.75
1976	2.56	2.35	1.11	1.24	4.94
1977	2.61	2.38	1.14	1.72	4.95
1978	2.90	2.43	1.15	1.85	5.08
1979	2.80	2.51	1.17	1.96	5.25
1980	2.99	2.59	1.22	2.08	5.19
1981	2.92	2.78	1.32	2.75	5.30
1982	2.9	—	1.39	3.92	5.08
1983	—	—	1.51	—	5.04
1984	—	—	1.51	—	4.89

SOURCES: Australia: United Nations, *Demographic Yearbook*, 1958, 1968, 1982; Josephian, 1984.
Canada and New Zealand: United Nations, *Demographic Yearbook*, 1958, 1968, 1982.
Japan: United Nations, 1984: Table 72; and Japan, Institute of Population Problems, 1985: Table 3.
United States: United Nations, *Demographic Yearbook*, 1958, 1968, 1982; and US National Center for Health Statistics, 1984b and 1985.

the divorce rate and the probability that a marriage will end in divorce, one that depends on demographic conditions, especially the growth rate of the population (Preston, 1983). These conditions are not too dissimilar in the countries under review, so multiplying the period divorce rate by a factor of 10, which is the appropriate multiplying factor in the United States, probably provides a reasonable (but rough) rule of thumb to estimate the period probability that a marriage will end in divorce.

In the English-speaking countries, the divorce rates in the early 1980s were higher than they had ever been, with the exception of a short period immediately following World War II. In Japan, however, the divorce rate was much higher in the past, with levels above 2.5 per thousand recorded in every year between 1883 (the beginning of the statistical series) and 1897 (United Nations, 1984: 71). These high rates have been attributed to conflict between wives and the husband's parents, conflict that weakened as intergenerational ties have been loosened. Divorce rates were typically higher in rural areas, where more traditional values probably persisted (Whitaker, 1974). The earlier decline was also probably related to divorce by mutual consent (required by the Civil Code but not always enforced) replacing unilateral repudiation (United Nations, 1984). In this instance, forces of modernization led Japan to legal changes and changes in divorce rates that were opposite to those witnessed more recently in English-speaking countries.

The exceptional nature of Japanese developments is underscored by trends in the fraction of births that occur out of wedlock (Table 5). Never very high in Japan, this fraction declined during the postwar period to the point where fewer than 1 percent of recent births have occurred to unmarried women. The trend in the English-speaking countries has been forcefully upward: 14–21 percent of recent births in these countries occur out of wedlock. Japan and the English-speaking countries begin the period at similar levels but end at radically different ones. A high fraction of the out-of-wedlock births in the United States and New Zealand occur to disadvantaged ethnic minorities: 51 percent to blacks in the United States in 1981 (US Bureau of the Census, 1984b: 86) and 30 percent to Maoris in New Zealand during the 1970s (Pool and Sceats, 1981: 104). In both groups, about half of all births are out of wedlock. In both countries, however, the dominant majority also had sizable proportions of out-of-wedlock births: 12 percent in the United States in 1982 and 16 percent in New Zealand in 1978. While proportions of US births occurring out of wedlock are quite high compared with several European countries, they are in line with those countries having the greatest cultural/historical similarities.

Trends in the proportion of out-of-wedlock births reflect trends in the proportion of reproductive-age women living in marital unions and trends in rates of childbearing among the married and unmarried. The rise in the extra-nuptial fraction since 1970 in the English-speaking countries is largely attributable to increasing fractions living outside of marital unions. Rates of childbearing among unmarried persons have risen somewhat in the United States since 1970, masking quite divergent trends between blacks and whites. In 1982, the total fertility rate for unmarried white women was 0.70, up from 0.39 in 1970, and for unmarried black women, 1.77, down from 2.22 in 1970 (compiled from US National Center for Health Statistics, 1984: 31–32).

In New Zealand, the fertility rate among the unmarried dropped during the 1970s, but the rate among the married and the proportions in marital unions fell even faster, causing a sharp rise in the proportion of out-of-wedlock births (Pool and Sceats, 1981: 104). In Canada, the rate of childbearing for unmarried

TABLE 5 Percent of births out of wedlock in selected industrialized countries

	Australia	Canada	Japan	New Zealand[a]	United States
1949	4.1	3.9	2.7	3.8	3.7
1950	3.8	3.9	2.5	4.0	4.0
1951	3.9	3.8	2.2	4.3	3.9
1952	3.9	3.8	2.0	4.5	3.9
1953	4.0	3.8	1.9	4.3	4.1
1954	4.0	3.9	1.7	4.3	4.4
1955	4.1	3.8	1.7	4.5	4.5
1956	4.2	3.9	1.6	4.6	4.6
1957	4.2	4.0	1.5	4.9	4.7
1958	4.6	4.0	1.4	5.0	5.0
1959	4.7	4.2	1.3	5.1	5.2
1960	4.8	4.3	1.2	5.3	5.3
1961	5.1	4.5	1.2	5.8	5.6
1962	5.4	4.8	1.1	8.0	5.9
1963	5.7	5.3	1.1	8.8	6.3
1964	6.5	5.9	1.0	9.9	6.8
1965	7.0	6.7	1.0	10.9	5.4
1966	7.4	7.6	1.1	11.6	8.4
1967	7.7	8.3	0.9	12.7	9.0
1968	8.0	9.0	1.0	13.0	9.7
1969	7.8	9.2	0.9	13.0	10.0
1970	8.3	9.6	0.9	13.3	10.7
1971	9.3	9.0	0.9	14.3	11.3
1972	9.8	9.0	0.9	14.7	12.4
1973	9.8	9.0	0.8	15.2	13.0
1974	9.5	9.0	0.8	15.8	13.2
1975	10.2	10.1	0.8	16.6	14.2
1976	10.1	10.5	0.8	17.4	14.8
1977	10.3	11.3	0.8	18.9	15.5
1978	11.0	11.7	0.8	20.1	16.3
1979	11.7	12.2	0.8	20.9	17.1
1980	12.5	13.2	0.8	—	18.4
1981	13.2	14.2	—	—	18.9
1982	13.7	15.5	—	—	—

[a]Before 1962, data exclude Maori population.
SOURCES: For all countries: United Nations, *Demographic Yearbook*, 1959, 1965, 1969, 1975, 1981.
Australia: Ruzicka, 1984.
Canada: Romaniuk, 1984: Table 2.7.
United States: US Bureau of the Census, 1985.

women in 1980–82 was about the same as in 1964–70, although it declined and then rose in the intervening years (Romaniuk, 1984: 36). In Australia, the pregnancy rate for unmarried persons reached a postwar peak in 1971 and declined rapidly during the 1970s, although the fraction of such conceptions that were later "resolved" by a marriage declined sharply also (Ruzicka, 1984). The net result, however, is that rates of nonmarital fertility in Australia declined at all ages between 1971 and 1981 (Ruzicka, Table 3). Clearly, the figures in Table 5 can be a misleading indicator of trends in fertility among unmarried women, which are generally downward.

There is clearly a good deal of consistency between postwar trends in fertility, marriage, and divorce in these countries. In the English-speaking countries, inverted-U–shaped trends in fertility and rates of entry into first marriage are echoed in U-shaped trends in divorce rates. The simultaneity of major movements in these series is not principally a product of necessary arithmetic relations between marriage and fertility, but rather suggests that the two series are responding to the same set of factors. Trends in illegitimacy, which are often lumped together with these other trends in the popular eye, are not nearly so coherent with them in general appearance. Furthermore, compositional factors—especially declining proportions currently married—seem largely responsible for recent major movements in the proportion of births occurring out of wedlock.

As in the English-speaking countries, rates of fertility and of entry into first marriage tend to move together in Japan. Both series declined sharply in the 1950s, in contrast to the rise-and-fall pattern observed in the English-speaking countries. However, these changes occurred at a time when divorce rates were also falling. Since around 1973, however, Japanese trends assume the more familiar anglophone pattern, with fertility and first marriage falling (in a related manner) and divorce rising. What is perhaps most strikingly different about Japan is the degree to which marriage remains a specialized institution: extramarital fertility is exceedingly low; marital fertility in the early years of marriage is quite high; and divorce is still rare and less frequent than a century ago. The specialized nature of marriage in Japan is almost certainly related to the high degree of sexual division of labor within marriage. Japan has the lowest labor force participation rates for married women—26.0 percent in 1980—of any industrialized country (Mincer, 1984: Table 1), and Japanese males work longer hours in the market and fewer in the home than males in other industrialized countries (Morgan et al., 1984).

Family size orientation

It is difficult to find comparable time series measures of family size attitudes—desires, ideals, expectations—in the various countries under review. Regardless of the measure used, however, the data show two distinct tendencies: an increasing convergence toward the two-child family, and a decline in the average number of children sought or expected. Table 6 illustrates these tendencies with time series data for Japan and the United States.

Married women in both countries (and in the other countries under review as well) continue to have fertility aspirations and/or expectations that imply above-replacement fertility levels. The family size distributions have become concentrated at two children, but combined proportions are larger at outcomes above two than below. The preference for a three-child family remains strong in Japan, although as a mode of the "ideal" this outcome was eclipsed in time series data by the proportion choosing two in 1974. The average "ideal" family size for oneself is almost exactly half way between the average desired

TABLE 6 Time series of family size attitudes in the United States and Japan (percent distribution)

United States: Expected number of lifetime births

Number of children	Married couples aged 18–39 in 1960[a]	Married women aged 18–39 in 1971[b]	Married women aged 18–34 in 1983[c]	All women aged 18–34 in 1983[c]
0	4	4	5	(11)
1	7	7	13	(14)
2	25	38	50	(47)
3	27	26	22	(20)
4	20	14	7	(7)
5	8	}11	}3	}(3)
6+	9			
Mean	3.2	2.79	2.24	2.08

Japan: Ideal number of children[d]

	Married women below age 50 in 1969	Married women below age 50 in 1984	Married women aged 25–29 in 1984
0	0.7	1.4	(1.4)
1	2.3	3.2	(4.0)
2	31.5	43.0	(42.0)
3	47.4	40.7	(44.2)
4	11.1	7.3	(6.0)
5	2.5	}1.6	}(1.4)
6+	0.4		
No answer	(4.0)	(2.7)	(0.6)
Mean	2.77	2.55	2.54

SOURCES: [a]Freedman and Bumpass, 1966.
[b]US Bureau of the Census, 1972.
[c]US Bureau of the Census, 1983.
[d]Population Problems Research Council, 1984: Tables I-1 and I-2. The question asked was, "What is the ideal number of children you wish to have?"

number of children (actual births plus desired additional births) and the number considered "ideal" for a Japanese couple:

Age group	Mean desired number of children, 1984	Mean ideal number of children for self, 1984	Mean ideal number of children for a Japanese couple, 1984
25–29	2.40	2.54	2.68
30–34	2.29	2.53	2.79
40–44	2.28	2.58	2.86
45–49	2.29	2.60	2.85

SOURCES: Population Problems Research Council, 1984: Tables III-2, III-20, and III-21.

This large disparity between ideals and desires/achievements suggests that many Japanese couples feel strongly constrained from acting out their wish to have more children.

In the United States, it is clear that family size expectations have collapsed around two. Very few married women expect to remain childless (5 percent), but the proportion increases to 11 percent when unmarried women aged 18–34 are included, 20 percent of whom expect to remain childless (US Bureau of the Census, 1983: Table 8). These expectations may be on the low side, according to extrapolations of recent cohort experience by David Bloom and Anne Pebley (1982). They project that 20–30 percent of the cohort born between 1950 and 1954 will remain childless, although only 11 percent of this cohort actually *expected* to remain childless as of 1983. Projected childlessness in Canada for younger cohorts reaches 16 percent (Romaniuk, 1984: 33) and in Australia, 22 percent (Caldwell, 1981: 49). Judith Blake (1979) is skeptical of the US projections, pointing to opinion polls indicating that childlessness is viewed as a seriously disadvantaged status in American society. In this regard, it might be noteworthy that very high levels of "completed" childlessness are about to be achieved by a large group of American women. In 1983, 23.2 percent of female college graduates aged 35–44 were childless (US Bureau of the Census, 1983: Table 10).

Although similar in some respects, Japan and the United States are quite different in the size of social class differentials in fertility expectations. The differentials are much wider in the United States than in Japan with regard to all standard socioeconomic variables according to which these expectations have been tabulated. The following data with respect to women's education are illustrative:

Educational attainment	Average number of births desired by married women below age 50: Japan, 1984	Average number of births expected by married women aged 18–34: United States, 1983
Less than high school	2.34	2.57
High school graduate	2.27	2.20
Some college	2.27	2.21
College graduate	2.36	2.08

SOURCES: US Bureau of the Census, 1983: Table 4; Population Problems Research Council, 1984: Table III-20.

The Japanese data also show very little class variation on questions of ideal family size. Some of this difference in the size of differentials may reflect the low labor force participation rates of Japanese wives relative to American wives.

New Zealand has never conducted a national fertility survey, and Canada took its first one in 1984, with few results available at this writing. Time series

TABLE 7 Trends in distribution of types of contraception used in selected industrialized countries

Australia[a]	1950–54	1960–63	1970–71	Melbourne, 1977
Abstinence	1	2	1	—
Periodic abstinence (rhythm)	18	19	14	7
Withdrawal	20	21	19	7
Condom	19	16	9	2
Spermicides	13	5	2	—
Douching	2	1	1	—
Diaphragm	19	15	5	1
Gräfenberg ring	6	6	2	—
IUD	—	—	8	15
Pill	—	14	38	33
Sterilization	—	—	—	34
Other; not specified	2	1	1	1
Total	100	100	100	100

Canada	Married women aged 18–45 in Toronto, 1968 (includes multiple use)	Married women in Canada using contraception, 1976
Rhythm	9.0	6.1
Withdrawal	8.8	3.4
Condom	16.7	6.0
Spermicides	3.4	2.5
Douching	3.5	—
Diaphragm	9.5	2.2
IUD	3.1	6.0
Pill	43.2	39.2
Sterilization	9.8	30.5
Total	107.0	100.0

Japan	Married women using contraception, 1954	Married women using contraception, 1974
Rhythm	30.9	8
Withdrawal	—	4
Condom	39.0	76
Spermicides	12.3	—
Diaphragm	5.1	2
IUD	—	5
Pill	—	2
Other	12.6	3
Total	99.9	100

data on family size attitudes are clearly not available in these countries. It is reasonable to expect, however, that trends would be similar to those in the United States.

TABLE 7 (continued)

United States	Married women aged 15–44 practicing contraception, 1965	Married women aged 15–44 practicing contraception, 1982
Rhythm	10.8	4.7
Withdrawal	5.7	1.7
Condom	22.0	14.4
Foam	3.3	2.9
Douching	5.0	0.2
Diaphragm	9.9	6.7
IUD	1.2	7.1
Pill	23.9	19.8
Sterilization	12.4	41.0
Other	5.8	1.5
Total	100.0	100.0

aQuestions about sterilization practice were not asked in the national survey because of its infrequency; in 1971, however, 4 percent of women in the Melbourne survey were sterilized.
SOURCES: Australia: Caldwell, 1982. Data for 1950–54, 1960–63, and 1970–71 are from a 1971 national survey of married women practicing contraception. Data for 1977 pertain to women under age 37 in that year who were followed up from a 1971 survey of Melbourne.
Canada: Romaniuk, 1984: Table 3.1.
Japan: Taeuber, 1958: 275; Atoh, 1981: Table 3, using data from the Japanese Fertility Survey (WFS) of 1974.
United States: Pratt el al., 1984.

Contraception and abortion

All countries with the pertinent data have seen a rise in the proportion of married couples practicing contraception and a switch by the contracepting population toward more efficient methods. In Australia, the proportion of 33–37-year-old married women practicing contraception grew from 59 percent in 1945–49 to 74 percent in 1970–71; and at ages 23–27, from 68 to 86 percent (Caldwell, 1982: Table 142). In Japan, the fraction of married couples below age 50 practicing contraception grew from 21.7 percent in 1952 to 35 percent in 1954 (Taeuber, 1958: 274) and reached 66.7 percent in 1974 (World Fertility Survey, 1979: Table 10). Fifty-five percent of US married women under age 45 were practicing contraception in 1965 (Ryder and Westoff, 1971: Table V-19) and 67 percent in 1982 (Pratt et al., 1984: Table 7). In Canada and New Zealand, the time trend of contraceptive use cannot be tracked in the absence of national surveys, although both countries conducted biomedically oriented contraceptive surveys in 1976.

The movement to more effective contraception among users is shown in Table 7. In Australia, Canada, and the United States, more than two-thirds of married women practicing contraception in the latest survey were using the most efficient methods: the IUD, the pill, and sterilization. Unpublished data from the Canadian Fertility Survey of 1984 show that the prevalence of sterilization at ages 18–49 has risen dramatically to the point where 54 percent of contraceptive users below age 50 were protected by sterilization (Lapierre-Adamcyk et al., 1985). Scattered regional data from New Zealand also suggest very high sterilization fractions by the late 1970s, in the neighborhood of 35–40 percent of contraceptive users (Pool and Sceats, 1981). Pill and Depo-Provera use is also high.

Japan again proves to be the exception. Only 7 percent of contraceptors were using the most efficient methods in 1974. No fewer than 76 percent of Japanese couples were using the condom, a method known for a century. Another 12 percent were relying on periodic abstinence and withdrawal. Such figures obviously argue against the notion that widespread use of modern methods of contraception is necessary to maintain below-replacement fertility. A 1979 survey in which couples were allowed to report more than one method showed an even higher fraction of contraceptors (82.0 percent) using the condom, 8.4 percent using IUDs, 3.2 percent the pill, and 4.0 percent sterilization (Atoh, 1985: Table 10).

The relatively inefficient contraceptive methods used in Japan are able to restrain fertility to such an extent at least partly because of widespread resort to abortion. Irene Taeuber (1958) inferred that the use of abortion was frequent in Japan even before World War II, despite its legal prohibition. It became legalized with the Eugenic Protection Law of 1948, which was subsequently liberalized on several occasions (Atoh, 1985). The number of abortions reported by physicians was 246,000 in 1949, rising quickly to 1.17 million in 1955 and showing a persistent downward trend since that date to 568,000 in 1983 (Atoh, 1985: Table 11). At its peak in 1957, the ratio of abortions to live births was .72, but the ratio had declined to .38 by 1983. While attitude surveys showed increasing acceptance of the general practice of abortion during the period, women having abortions expressed increasing guilt and regret. The fraction saying that their principal reaction to their first abortion was "guilt" or "feeling sorry for the aborted fetus" rose from 60 percent in 1963 to 78 percent in 1984, while the fraction saying they "did not care" declined from 19 percent to 6 percent (Atoh, 1985: Table 14). The frequent resort to abortion in the 1950s and 1960s undoubtedly explains how such low fertility levels could be achieved with "inefficient" contraception.

The other countries under review also had legal changes facilitating abortion during the postwar period: the Contraception, Sterilization, and Abortion Act of 1977 in New Zealand (Pool and Sceats, 1981); amendments to the Criminal Code in Canada in 1969 permitting hospital abortion when continued pregnancy would endanger the life or health of the pregnant woman, followed by administrative relaxation in 1977 (Beaujot, 1978); the Criminal Law Consolidation Act Amendment Act of 1969 in South Australia, allowing abortion for physical or mental reasons, followed by a more relaxed enforcement of existing laws in other states (Caldwell, 1982); and a US Supreme Court decision in 1973 (*Roe* v. *Wade*) that declared state laws forbidding all elective abortions to be unconstitutional.

Abortion has become an important method of birth control in all of these countries. The ratio of legal abortions to live births increased from .24 in 1973 to .43 in 1981 in the United States (US Bureau of the Census, 1985: Table 100); from .034 in 1970 to .073 in 1978 among married women and from .361 to 1.30 among unmarried women in South Australia (statistics are inadequate in other states) (Caldwell, 1982); from .086 in 1971 to .178 in 1982 in Canada (Romaniuk, 1984: Table 3.13); and from an unknown level to .071 in 1978 in New Zealand (Pool and Sceats, 1981: Table 8.2). The recorded level in New Zealand is one of the lowest among industrialized countries, but the data system is poor and it is known that a sizable number of women have gone to Australia for abortions.

The movement to more efficient contraception and to increased use of abortion has undoubtedly played a role in fertility reductions since the 1960s in the English-speaking countries and since the 1940s in Japan. But it is quite difficult to estimate the relative importance of this factor because it interacts in complex ways with family size preferences. A major attempt to estimate its importance has been made for the United States. Recent births are retrospectively classified into wanted births, mistimed births (wanted at some future date but not at the time of birth), and unwanted births. The distribution of births within the previous five years in national surveys of 1965, 1973, and 1982 are as follows:

	Percent wanted	Percent mistimed	Percent unwanted
1965	34.8	44.7	20.5
1973	63.2	23.8	13.0
1982	70.7	22.5	6.8

SOURCE: Pratt et al., 1984: Table 14.

Depending on how one treats the mistimed births, one can ascribe nearly all or only a minority of the fertility decline between 1961–65 and 1978–82 to improved birth control practice. Let us assume that all mistimed births would, in fact, have eventually occurred. The mean total fertility rates for the three periods are 3.27, 2.21, and 1.81. If the proportion unwanted were evenly distributed by age, the total fertility rates without unwanted births would have been 2.60, 1.92, and 1.69. The decline between 1961–65 and 1978–82 would have been .91 children, rather than the recorded 1.46. In this fashion, 38 percent of the recorded fertility decline between 1961–65 and 1978–82 could be ascribed to the reduction in rates of bearing unwanted children. The fraction should be larger if some of the mistimed births would never have been born. Likewise, 42 percent (.17/.40) of the fertility decline between 1969–73 and 1978–82 could be ascribed to the declining incidence of unwanted fertility. This is also the proportion computed by Pratt et al. (1984) based on total fertility rates for 1973 and 1982 alone.

Such decompositions are fraught with danger. Obviously, the availability of more efficient contraception can change family size preferences (e.g., by allowing a woman to plan and conduct a career), while the intensity of family size preferences can influence the success of birth control practice (Westoff et al., 1963). But as a first approximation, attributing some 40 percent of US fertility decline in the past two decades to improved birth control practice seems better than throwing up one's hands in despair.

In a complex and useful comparative study, Atoh (1981) compares rates of unwanted childbearing in the US 1970 National Fertility Survey to those in the Japanese Fertility Survey (WFS) of 1974. He concludes that the incidence of higher order unwanted births was much lower in Japan. Part of the explanation is higher contraceptive efficacy (despite the more traditional methods used), and part is the greater use of abortion by noncontraceptors wanting no more children. But the main explanation is the greater use of abortion by contraceptors to terminate unwanted pregnancies.

Summary

In this article we have described the major quantitative features of postwar change in fertility and certain of its proximate determinants in the United States, Canada, Australia, New Zealand, and Japan. The English-speaking countries have similar time trends in fertility, with total fertility rates first rising to a level above 3.5 and then falling below 2.0. The trends in fertility were echoed by trends in first marriage, which rose and then fell in each of the countries, and in divorce rates, which fell and then rose. Fertility rates for unmarried women have also typically fallen in the past decades (US whites are an exception); nevertheless, proportions of births that are out of wedlock have risen rapidly because of declining proportions of women in marital unions and declining marital fertility. The recent fall in fertility is related to declining proportions married, increased use of contraception and abortion, and a reduction in family size desires.

Japan's fertility rate fell much earlier than rates in English-speaking countries, as did its rate of entry into first marriage. Relative to the English-speaking countries, Japan is most distinct in its extensive use of less efficient means of contraception and in its maintenance of a marital monopoly on childbearing. Less than 1 percent of recent births in Japan occur out of wedlock, and childbearing is very rapid in the early years of marriage. Divorce rates, now rising after a long period of decline, are still less than half of those in the English-speaking countries. In a later article in this volume, I attempt to sketch an explanation of the trends and international differentials that I have described.

Note

The author is grateful to Katherine Condon for research assistance and to Shigemi Kono for supplying Japanese materials.

References

Agarwala, S.N. 1962. *Age at Marriage in India*. Allahabad: Kitab Mahal (W.D.) Pvt. Ltd.

Atoh, Makoto. 1981. "Comparative analysis of unplanned births between Japan and the United States, focusing on the effectiveness of fertility control measures," in *IUSSP International Population Conference, Manila 1981*. Liège: IUSSP, pp. 775–796.

———. 1985. "Changes in fertility and fertility control behavior in Japan," in *Basic Readings on Population and Family Planning in Japan*, ed. Minoru Muramatsu and Tameyoshi Katagiri. Tokyo: Japanese Organization for International Cooperation in Family Planning, Inc. (JOICFP), pp. 40–60.

Beaujot, Roderic P. 1978. "Canada's population: Growth and dualism," *Population Bulletin* 33, no. 2.

Blake, Judith. 1979. "Is zero preferred? American attitudes towards childlessness in the 1970's," *Journal of Marriage and the Family* 41: 245–257.

Bloom, David E., and Anne R. Pebley. 1982. "Voluntary childlessness: A review of the evidence and implications," *Population Research and Policy Review* 1: 203–224.

Caldwell, John C. 1981. "An explanation of the continued fertility decline in the West: Stages, succession and crisis." Canberra: Department of Demography, Australian National University.

———. 1982. "Fertility control," in *Population of Australia*, ESCAP Country Monograph Series No. 9, Vol. 1, United Nations, Economic and Social Commission for Asia and the Pacific. New York.

———, and Lado T. Ruzicka. 1978. "The Australian fertility transition: An analysis," *Population and Development Review* 4, no. 1 (March): 81–103.

Carmichael, Gordon. 1984. "The transition to marriage: Trends in age at first marriage and proportions marrying in Australia," in Australian Family Research Conference, *Proceedings*, Vol. 1. Melbourne: Institute of Family Studies, pp. 99–175.

Cherlin, Andrew J. 1981. *Marriage, Divorce, Remarriage*. Cambridge, Mass.: Harvard University Press.

Dumas, Andre. 1985. *Current Demographic Analysis: Report on the Demographic Situation in Canada 1983*. Ottawa: Statistics Canada.

Freedman, Ronald, and Larry Bumpass. 1966. "Fertility expectations in the United States, 1962–64," *Population Index* 32, no. 2 (April): 181–197.

Heuser, Robert L. 1976. *Fertility Tables for Birth Cohorts by Color*. Rockville, Md.: US National Center for Health Statistics.

Hobcraft, John, Jane Menken, and Samuel Preston. 1982. "Age, period, and cohort effects in demography: A review," *Population Index* 48, no. 1: 4–43.

Japan, Institute of Population Problems. 1985. *Selected Demographic Indicators of Japan*. Tokyo: Ministry of Health and Welfare.

Josephian, Virginia. 1984. "Divorce in Australia 1971–1981: An examination of period analysis," in Australian Family Research Conference, *Proceedings*, Vol. 1. Melbourne: Institute of Family Studies, pp. 295–316.

Kono, Shigemi. 1982. "Determinants and consequences of low fertility in low-fertility countries," in *Third Asian and Pacific Population Conference (Colombo, September 1982)*. United Nations, Economic and Social Commission for Asia and the Pacific, Asian Population Studies Series No. 58. New York, pp. 61–74.

———. 1984. "A biodemographic analysis of the Japanese fertility via microsimulation," *Journal of Population Studies* No. 7 (May): 24–32.

Lapierre-Adamcyk, Evelyne, T. R. Balakrishnan, and Karol J. Krotki. 1985. "Sterilization as a means of contraception in Canada: Preliminary results of the 1984 survey," presented at the General Conference for the International Union for the Scientific Study of Population, Florence, Italy.

Mincer, Jacob. 1984. "Inter-country comparisons of labor force trends and of related developments: An overview," *NBER Working Paper Series*, Working Paper No. 1438. Cambridge, Mass.: National Bureau of Economic Research.

Morgan, S. Philip, Ronald R. Rindfuss, and Allan Parnell. 1984. "Modern fertility patterns: Contrasts between the United States and Japan," *Population and Development Review* 10, no. 1 (March): 19–40.

Pool, Ian, and Janet Sceats. 1981. *Fertility and Family Formation in New Zealand: An Examination of Data Collection and Analyses*. Wellington: Ministry of Works and Development.

Population Problems Research Council, The Mainichi Newspapers. 1984. *Summary of Seventeenth National Survey on Family Planning*. Tokyo.

Pratt, William F., William D. Mosher, Christine A. Bachrach, and Marjorie C. Horn. 1984. "Understanding U.S. fertility: Findings from the National Survey of Family Growth, Cycle III," *Population Bulletin* 39, no. 5.

Preston, Samuel H. 1983. "Estimation of certain measures in family demography based upon generalized stable population relations," presented to an IUSSP Conference on Family Demography Methods and Their Application, held at New York.

Romaniuk, Anatole. 1984. *Current Demographic Analysis: Fertility in Canada: From Babyboom to Baby-bust*. Ottawa: Statistics Canada.

Ruzicka, L.T. 1984. "The early stages of the family life cycle in Australia: Demographic changes since the 1960s," in Australian Family Research Conference, *Proceedings*, Vol. 1, *Family Formation, Structure, Values*. Melbourne: Institute of Family Studies, pp. 176–200.

———, and John C. Caldwell. 1982. "Fertility," in *Population of Australia*, ESCAP Country Monograph Series No. 9, Vol. 1, United Nations, Economic and Social Commission for Asia and the Pacific. New York.

———, and C. Choi. 1983. "Trends in marriage and fertility," in Australia Bureau of Statistics, *Commonwealth Year Book*. Canberra: Government Printing Office.

Ryder, Norman, and Charles F. Westoff. 1971. *Reproduction in the United States 1965*. Princeton, N.J.: Princeton University Press.

Taeuber, Irene B. 1958. *The Population of Japan*. Princeton, N.J.: Princeton University Press.

Thornton, Arland, and Deborah Freedman. 1982. "Changing attitudes toward marriage and single life," *Family Planning Perspectives* 14, no. 6: 297–303.

———, and Deborah Freedman. 1983. "The changing American family," *Population Bulletin* 38, no. 4.

United Nations, Economic and Social Commission for Asia and the Pacific. 1984. *Population of Japan*, ESCAP Country Monograph Series No. 11. New York.

United States Bureau of the Census. 1972. *Current Population Reports* P-20, no. 232 (February).

——— Bureau of the Census. 1980. *Current Population Reports* P-20, no. 349 (August).

——— Bureau of the Census. 1983. "Fertility of American women: June 1983," *Current Population Reports* P-20, no. 395 (November).

——— Bureau of the Census. 1984a. "Population characteristics," *Current Population Reports* P-20, no. 391 (August).

——— Bureau of the Census. 1984b. *Statistical Abstract of the United States*. Washington, D.C.: US Government Printing Office.

——— Bureau of the Census. 1985. *Statistical Abstract of the United States*. Washington, D.C.: US Government Printing Office.

———, National Center for Health Statistics. 1984a. "Advance report of final natality statistics, 1982," *Monthly Vital Statistics Report* 33, no. 6 (8 September).

———, National Center for Health Statistics. 1984b. *Monthly Vital Statistics Report* 32, no. 13 (21 September).

———, National Center for Health Statistics. 1985. *Monthly Vital Statistics Report* 33, no. 12 (26 March).

Weed, James A. 1980. ''National estimates of marriage dissolution and survivorship,'' in *Vital and Health Statistics* Series 3, no. 9. National Center for Health Statistics. Washington, D.C.: US Government Printing Office.

Westoff, Charles F., Robert G. Potter, Jr., and Philip C. Sagi. 1963. *The Third Child: A Study in the Prediction of Fertility*. Princeton, N.J.: Princeton University Press.

Whitaker, Donald P. 1974. *Area Handbook for Japan*, third ed. Washington, D.C.: Foreign Area Studies, The American University.

World Fertility Survey. 1979. *The 1974 Japan National Fertility Survey: A Summary of Findings*, No. 14. Voorburg, the Netherlands: International Statistical Institute.

Low Fertility in Evolutionary Perspective

Kingsley Davis

Looked at in the long-run perspective of human evolution, the below-replacement fertility now characterizing most of the industrial countries is anomalous. Never before in recorded history—not in the Great Depression, not in the eighteenth and nineteenth centuries, and not in ancient times—has fertility been so low for whole societies as it is now in the industrial world. And never has it been so low during the millions of years of hominid evolution.[1]

Low fertility in hunting and gathering societies

But in another sense, the low fertility of today in advanced countries is less anomalous than the high fertility that characterized these countries at the inception of the industrial revolution and that characterizes most of the less developed countries today. The total fertility rate (TFR) of the white population of the United States in 1800 has been estimated as 7.04 births per woman (Coale and Zelnik, 1963, p. 36). This is more than four times the TFR (1.65) for 1976. The TFR for Jordan in 1979 was 8.34 (United Nations, *Demographic Yearbook,* 1983, p. 323). Although such high fertility rates characterize modern agrarian populations, they are evidently not the norm in human evolution. Instead, for millions of years extending back in prehistoric times, a special feature of hominid groups was their moderate fertility.

The evidence for this is indirect and varied, but taken together it is persuasive. First, over the long haul, the hominids had virtually zero population growth, and all of the hominid species eventually became extinct except modern man, *Homo sapiens sapiens.* Second, on the biological side, the human reproductive system became vulnerable to an extraordinary number of pathologies, and it lost two pronatalist traits—sexual promiscuity and oestrus, the second of which in most mammals binds copulation closely to ovulation. Third, according to field observation, our closest kin in the animal world, the subhuman primates, exhibit low fertility. Jane Goodall (1971, p. 12) found that female chimpanzees in the Gombe Reserve gave birth "about once every three and a half to five years." In another chimpanzee group (the pygmy chimpanzee) Michael Chiglieri (1984, p. 61) reported only two births in 17 months of observation, yielding an annual birth rate of 31 per thousand animals. Even gorillas, which mature at about seven years, have birth intervals of about four years (Schaller, 1964, p. 333). Fourth, reproduction among recently observed hunter-gatherers is even lower. Nancy Howell (1979, p. 123) found that 62 Dobe !Kung women aged 45 years and older had borne only 4.69 offspring on average. Even this, she says, may have been an overstatement, due to a tendency of childless women to migrate out of the territory and hence fall out of the sample. An analysis of registration data for Australian aborigines of the Northern Territory in 1958–60 showed a TFR of 4.23 (Jones, 1965, p. 242). In a survey of population control among hunter-gatherers in general, Brian Hayden (1972) found that these societies use only a fraction of the reproductive potential available to them. "Out of a maximum possible fertility of 20–30 living offspring per female," he says (p. 209), "this is reduced to 5–6 or fewer primarily by prolonged lactation, physiological controls, abstinence and abortion." Progeny are further curtailed by infanticide, especially female infanticide, which is surprisingly widespread in hunter-gatherer societies (Hausfater and Hrdy, 1984).

Clearly, the idea that our remote ancestors had a high, biologically determined "natural" fertility, because they did not use modern contraception, is false. The highest birth rates are found, not under primitive, but under modern circumstances. Among 94 married Hutterite women aged 45–49 in 1950, Joseph Eaton and Albert Mayer (1954, p. 20) found that the mean number of births per woman was 9.9; T. E. Smith (1960, p. 95) found that the average number per woman in the Cocos-Keeling Islands was 8.4; and as mentioned already, the UN *Demographic Yearbook* reports the TFR for Jordan in 1979 as 8.34. Compared with such examples, the fertility of hunter-gatherers or of ancient man seems quite moderate. If we imagine a TFR scale with ten births per woman at the top and one birth per woman at the bottom, our preagricultural hominid ancestors would probably fall somewhere near the middle, with four to six births per woman. That is not low compared with TFRs in today's industrial countries, which would fall near the bottom of the scale, but it shares with them a common outcome—namely, zero or negative natural increase.

In other words, the circumstantial evidence suggests that throughout hominid evolution the long-run birth rate was kept as low as possible consistent with survival—as low, that is, as the death rate. Why? The answer seems to be that the hominids were exploiting a unique evolutionary niche by relying on culture, learning, and social organization as their mode of adaptation. To do this, they had to invest heavily in prolonged care and training of offspring. They succeeded best in this task when the offspring were widely spaced.

Helpless infants were particularly burdensome in hunting and gathering societies because of the nomadism generally characterizing those groups (Lee, 1979, ch. 11; Carr-Saunders, 1922). Present-day hunter-gatherers frequently give as reasons for wide spacing of offspring the burden of trying to carry two nursing infants at one time and the danger to an older child if the mother has a new birth too soon. A similar motivation often underlies infanticide following the birth of twins, most often of one infant only (Lee and DeVore, 1968, pp. 11, 236ff., Hausfater and Hrdy, 1984, pp. xiii–xiv, xxvi–xxxii; Scrimshaw, 1984, p. 446; Daly and Wilson, 1980, pp. 492–493; Lee, 1979, ch. 11).

There was a limit, however, on how low the birth rate of ancient man could be. It could not be regularly lower than the death rate. Of the two processes—mortality and fertility—hominids found it far easier to control fertility. As a result, the prehistoric birth rate was determined by the death rate. This meant that to attain the advantages of moderate fertility, our remote ancestors had to achieve a moderate mortality as well, something they found difficult to attain.

The struggle against death

The hominids' best approach to combating mortality was to maximize production, which they did by strengthening the very possession (culture) that comprised their evolutionary advantage. They gradually created and improved a cultural system that could satisfy basic needs for food, shelter, clothing, and security. This achievement, peculiar to humans, evolved with extreme slowness at first (during at least 2 million years; Washburn and Lancaster, 1968b), but it was cumulative and increasingly had the potential for keeping the death rate low compared with rates among other animals. This approach, however, had its own limitation. Beyond a certain point, improvement of the means for exploiting the environment meant a degradation of the environment. In some cases this may have meant outright extinction of prey fauna (Martin, 1973; Martin and Klein, 1984; Nitecki, 1984), but more often it meant a local or seasonal scarcity.

Another strictly human method of combating mortality was care of the sick and wounded (Washburn and Lancaster, 1968a; Jolly, 1972, pp. 289–290). This behavior, which may have arisen as part of the food-sharing complex early in human evolution, must have saved lives because rest and food were often all that an incapacitated individual needed to get well. It did require, however, a home base or at least a temporary shelter or campsite. If the sufferer was permanently injured or sick, and therefore a complete drain on the group, he or she was probably left to die. In present-day hunting and gathering societies, the care of the sick and wounded is generally the responsibility of close kin.

A third development that saved lives was the use of fire for cooking and warmth, for protection from predators, and for stampeding prey (Fagan, 1979, pp. 87–89). But a fourth method—also unique to man—proved singularly unsuccessful. This was the development of medicine, a deliberate effort to prevent and cure illness. The emergence of medical practitioners—the shaman, a combined priest, showman, and doctor; the midwife; the diviner—doubtless was among the earliest examples of a division of labor based on presumed skill rather than gender, age, or kinship (Corlett, 1935; Maddox, 1923; Landy, 1977, chs. 14, 15, 17, 22). Unfortunately, these specialists, by and large, never developed much ability to benefit the patient.

Significantly, all four of early man's strategies for combating mortality were cultural and therefore unique to humans. Taken together, these efforts must have given the hominids a death rate that was high by today's standards but nevertheless low in comparison with that of other animals of equal size (see Johansson and Horowitz, 1985; Cohen and Armelagos, 1984). These strategies did, however, run up against severe limitations. One of these (environmental degradation) has already been mentioned. Another, much more long-run in character, was deterioration of the hominid genetic constitution. During hundreds of millennia our distant ancestors tended to lose through relaxed selection what they gained in cultural adaptation.

Another barrier to lowering the death rate was the inability to control infectious and parasitic diseases. Since these, under primitive conditions, usually comprise the main causes of death, this failure guaranteed a rather high mortality compared with present-day societies (Acsádi and Nemeskéri, 1970, ch. 4; Schaller, 1965, p. 334).

In sum, the barriers to mortality control acted as feedback mechanisms. If under favorable conditions a hunting and gathering population expanded, it would become more dense, the environment would become depleted, contagious diseases would spread, or warfare would set in. The result would be a rise in the death rate and a return to the status quo ante. In some instances, where local resources were great, Late Pleistocene man could become sedentary, but in general, through millions of years, the evolving hominid species remained scarce creatures. They were equipped by their cultural apparatus to spread to new environments, but as hunter-gatherers they were not equipped to multiply within the same area. Overwhelmingly, their population expansion depended on geographical expansion. Spreading out first, apparently, in Africa, they moved into Europe and Asia, and eventually invaded Australia and the Americas. Population numbers must have grown, but since this worldwide dispersion took millions of years, the rate of human population increase was virtually zero. There was apparently some acceleration of population growth after the appearance of modern man around 40,000 years ago as the hunting and foraging technology became more efficient, but a significant departure from zero growth did not occur until the agricultural revolution.

Agriculture and population imbalance

If this description is correct, our low fertility in contemporary society is not an aberration. It is rather an approximation of a sine qua non for human evolution. The genius of the species has not been to rely on a birth rate so high that it can overcome almost any death rate, no matter how high. The genius of the species is rather to have few offspring and to invest heavily in their care and training, so that the advantages of a cultural adaptation can be realized. Throughout 99 percent of hominid history, then, fertility was kept as low as it could be, given the current mortality. Zero population growth was the rule, not the exception. The abnormal situation is that of present-day less developed countries—Bangladesh, the African states, many countries of the Middle East—where death rates have been rapidly reduced but total fertility rates have stayed at, or risen to high levels such as six to nine births per woman. These are societies demoralized by a drastic reduction in mortality without compensating changes in economic and social institutions. They illustrate the principle that an excess of reproduction militates against trained skills in a population.

What happened to the long-term balance of births and deaths that characterized the hunting and gathering way of life?

The answer in a word is "agriculture." But that response is inadequate. What were the mechanisms by which agriculture destroyed the demographic balance?

According to my estimates, the growth of the human population for some 12,000 years preceding the industrial revolution—the period of the rise and spread of agriculture—was 4.4 percent per century. This was a snail's pace by present-day standards, but it was nine times faster than the estimated growth during the 40,000 years preceding the agricultural epoch.

As a technological change, the agricultural revolution was remarkable for its speed and impact. Although some Upper Paleolithic peoples had reached an impressive level of technological sophistication, no antecedent technological advance was so great or so rapid as the domestication of plants and animals. Among other things, it destroyed some of the feedback mechanisms of the hunting and gathering economy. There, if fertility exceeded mortality for a period, the balance tended to be restored by contagious disease, warfare, and/ or deterioration of the environment. But under agriculture the improvement of the productive apparatus was so fast (in terms of human evolution) that it temporarily suspended some of the important feedback mechanisms. With respect to fertility, for instance, women no longer needed long birth intervals, because they did not need to carry their infants for long distances. They could wean their offspring earlier, because cultivation provided more reliable alternative food sources. Also, insofar as cultivation increased per capita food consumption, it may have hastened menarche and improved the likelihood of conception. In any case, children were more useful in an agrarian than in a hunting and gathering economy, because the variety of tasks suitable to the young was greater. The traditional brakes on fertility were therefore lifted.

On the mortality side, there is considerable evidence that initially the switch to agriculture may have raised mortality, owing to increased reliance on starchy staples and increased density of settlement, but later, as agriculture provided more reliable food sources, better shelter, and greater resistance to disease, the death rate was probably no higher than it had been in hunting and gathering societies and may have been lower. The symposium volume edited by Mark Cohen and George Armelagos (1984) adduces evidence for most parts of the world that the transition to agriculture at first meant a worsening rather than an improvement in mortality. The somewhat stepped up rate of population growth must therefore have been due to a rise in fertility.

Eventually, the demographic imbalance created by the speedy adoption of agriculture would have righted itself, and it probably did in many worn-out farming areas. But once the genie was out of the bottle, further technological progress and the spread of agriculture to new areas compensated for feedback mechanisms that otherwise would have driven up mortality or depressed fertility and thus have halted population growth. At last the reliance on a cultural mode of adaptation was beginning to pay off in an evolutionary sense—in the sense of permitting, for the world as a whole and for a much longer period than ever before, a birth rate higher than the death rate.

The industrial revolution

If left alone, the agricultural revolution would doubtless have spun itself out and eventually would have ceased to sustain population growth. As it was, the main stimulus to growth came from expanding agriculture into new areas, not from piling up ever more people in the same area. But the industrial age came along while the expansion of agriculture around the world was still going on. It thus did not permit a return to the zero population growth rate that would eventually have characterized a world limited to agriculture; instead, it sharpened the imbalance between birth rates and death rates that agriculture had already fostered.

Despite temporary exceptions in particular cases, industrialism generally produced a lower death rate in several ways. First, it facilitated the improvement of agricultural output per man and per worker through irrigation, plant breeding, machinery, and fossil fuel. Second, it improved the efficiency of transportation, permitting more varied diets and more secure supplies around the world. In other words, the agricultural age did not disappear when faced with industrialization, the way hunting and gathering societies disappeared in the face of agricultural encroachment; instead, agriculture was enormously improved by the advent of industrialism. Third, man's age-old effort to develop a specialized medical technology finally began to bear fruit after about 1850 (Starr, 1982, ch. 3). With continued improvement of economic production, and with medical technology rapidly diffused to all nations, man could control mortality as he had never done before. The speed of this control was unique, and the later it occurred in a country the faster mortality fell.

In all modern societies there were, and are, offsetting factors tending to nullify the mortality improvements (warfare, self-destruction through drugs and alcohol, new diseases), but these are weak in the face of the continued drive to save lives. Consequently, in the advanced nations most of the burden of restoring a balance between births and deaths has fallen, as it did in hunting and gathering societies, on the fertility side. After a century or more of rapid population growth and the resulting congestion, the advanced nations have finally adjusted their fertility to their mortality. Since their mortality is now extremely low, the adjustment has given rise to birth rates so low as to be unprecedented for entire nations. The advanced countries have reached these low rates by pushing the principle underlying human social organization—reliance on a division of labor based on acquired skills—to its limit. The destiny of the child (and hence of the parent) has come to depend on the child's training and education. The social structure that generates this kind of adaptation is characterized by social mobility, planned innovation, formal schooling, urbanization, separation of home and workplace, and bureaucracy. Unless these traits are somehow reversed or overcome, the industrial countries will continue to have fertility rates near or below replacement, and as other countries become developed, they too will record low fertility.

Causes of below-replacement fertility

When we ask why industrial societies eventually exhibit below-replacement fertility, the answer can be given in more than one universe of discourse. For instance, from a global point of view it would be impossible for these societies to do otherwise. A hunting and gathering technology enabled people to live modestly by harvesting the wild bounty of nature, but, except as it expanded into new areas, the population could not grow. By contrast, the agricultural and especially the modern industrial societies have learned how to alter and manipulate nature in order to increase its bounty. The result is a miraculous gain in the level of consumption and, initially at least, an equally miraculous increase in the human population. It needs little perspicacity, however, to see that in a finite world the twin forces of population and per capita consumption cannot both long continue to increase. Neither one can grow indefinitely, but the two together can grow for only a brief moment in history. To see this, one can take any basic resource and calculate the drain on it under certain assumptions regarding growth. For example, if the entire world were to consume energy at the rate the United States did in 1980, total world consumption would be 5.6 times what it actually was. If one assumes that the world not only reaches the US 1980 level but surpasses it by a rate of increase corresponding to that for the United States between 1950 and 1980, one finds that by 2010 the world consumption would be more than 12 times the actual 1980 level. Even if quantities of coal, oil, and uranium, or new substitutes, could be found sufficient to meet this enormous demand, it is doubtful whether the environment could withstand the assault of the resulting contaminants.

In industrial societies, then, the combination of ever more goods and services per person and ever more persons is creating an impossible situation in terms of congestion and environmental damage. It is this situation to which below-replacement fertility is an adjustment. People cannot, or will not, limit the goods and services supplied by their ever more complex technology, but they can forgo children, who, if produced in abundance, would greatly add to the congestion.

Ordinarily, however, people do not curb their fertility out of concern for society at large. They may invoke environmental problems as a rationalization, but their main motivation is more personal. To understand today's extremely low fertility, then, one must turn to the special features of industrial societies that dampen the individual's enthusiasm for childbearing. Since these features are interrelated, it makes little difference where we start. Let us begin with marriage.

Postponement of marriage

In the past, marriage was the approved institutional arrangement for bearing and rearing offspring. With remarkable persistence, from hunting and gathering societies to modern times, it was a focus of public interest and ritual. But in today's advanced nations it is in trouble (Davis, 1986). One sign of this is that it is increasingly being postponed. In the United States in 1960, for example, only 19.2 percent of women aged 20–39 had never married; the corresponding figure in 1984 was 37.1 percent (US Bureau of the Census, 1970, p. 11; *Statistical Abstract of the United States 1986*, p. 36). The latter figure may seem high, but in Sweden (in 1981) 49.6 percent of women aged 20–39 had never married.

It is difficult to predict how far marital postponement will eventually go. In the past some countries, such as Ireland and the Scandinavian nations, approached female marital ages as high as 30 on average, and a high proportion of women (26 percent in Ireland and 22 percent in Sweden in 1940) reached menopause without ever marrying (Sklar, 1977, p. 360). Today, marriage is again being postponed, this time with a rising percent of births that are illegitimate. Postponement is not being used as a respectable mode of birth control, as it long was in Western Europe, but rather as a means to reduce uncertainty with respect to marriage and parenthood.

If one asks why marriages are being postponed, the answer lies largely in the other traits of modernity that we shall consider. High rates of divorce make marriage a risky business; widespread cohabitation and numerous births out of wedlock provide alternatives to marriage; wives' employment disturbs the division of labor between husband and wife. These changes decrease the need for marriage, especially for the young, at the same time that they increase the penalties.

The rise of nonmarital reproduction

Of course, postponement of marriage does not necessarily bring a commensurate decline in births, because illegitimate births may wholly or partially offset the decline. In most advanced countries, the percentage of all births that are illegitimate has been rising. In the United States in 1960, the fraction was

5.3 percent; by 1984 the percent had reached 21.0 (US National Center for Health Statistics, 1985, p. 31). With such a speedy rise, illegitimate reproduction can compensate for a considerable portion of the loss of legitimate births. In the United States there were 1.1 million fewer legitimate births in 1983 than in 1960, but there were 0.5 million more illegitimate births. Illegitimacy thus offset 45 percent of the decline in legitimate births, the rest being accounted for by marital postponement and reduced marital fertility.

In general, a similar pattern seems to characterize other developed nations. Married women still have higher fertility than unmarried women (nearly six times higher in the United States), but the difference is narrowing. Further, because of marital postponement, the proportion of young women who are unmarried has risen greatly. These two trends—rising illegitimate fertility compared with legitimate fertility, and swelling proportions of young women who are unmarried—have given rise to a spectacular increase in the proportion of births out of wedlock. Table 1 shows the trend for the United States between 1940 and 1983. Until 1960 much of the rise was due to increasing fertility among unmarried as compared with married women, but since then it has been due more to marital postponement.

The figures furnish stark evidence that marriage is not only failing in procreation but is losing its monopoly of births. Traditionally the institution in which reproduction was expected and rewarded, lawful wedlock now competes in producing children with other kinds of sexual relationships (Carlson, Espenshade, and Spanier, 1986). It should not be inferred, however, that these other relationships are highly prolific. If people are unwilling to commit themselves to a durable legal relationship (marriage), they are usually reluctant to commit themselves to parenthood in any other situation. In other words, a switch from marital to unorganized and unregulated mating will not result in

TABLE 1 Percent of births that are illegitimate, and fertility rate of unmarried women, United States, 1940–83

	Percent of all births illegitimate	Total fertility rate per unmarried woman
1940	3.8	.17
1950	4.0	.38
1955	4.5	.59
1960	5.3	.75
1965	7.7	.82
1970	10.7	.71
1975	14.3	.57
1980	18.4	.68
1983	20.3	.71

SOURCES: US National Center for Health Statistics, 1981, pp. 54–55; and "Advance report of natality statistics," 1980 and 1983.

high fertility, as people occasionally assume, but in low fertility. According to the second column of Table 1, unmarried women in the United States in 1965 (their peak year for fertility) were bearing children at a rate that would have resulted in less than one child per unmarried woman at the end of their childbearing years. If the nation had to depend exclusively on nonmarital reproduction, it would quickly become depopulated. This explains why Sweden, with the world's lowest proportion married and one of the world's highest divorce rates, also has one of the world's lowest birth rates. In this regard the following Swedish and American "antimarriage" indicators for 1981 are of interest:[2]

	Sweden	United States
Percent of women aged 20–39 not married	49.6	38.1
Divorces per thousand wives under age 50	24.7	42.2
Total fertility rate, per woman	1.63	1.82

High divorce rates

Marriage formerly served as a reproductive institution in part because it was durable and therefore, with close kin, provided a stable milieu for rearing children. Today, as high divorce rates testify, that stability has been substantially lost. Although the rise in the divorce rate in the United States has ceased since 1977, the rate has stabilized at a very high level. In nearly all other advanced countries, it has continued to increase. Among 24 industrial countries selected because they had the necessary data, not one showed a decline in divorce during the 13 years between 1970 and 1983. The average number of divorces per thousand population for the 24 countries was 1.32 in 1970 and 2.29 in 1983. The unweighted average increase in the rate was therefore 4.3 percent per year. At that pace of increase, the divorce rate would double every 16.5 years. It was back in 1956 that the United States had a divorce rate equal to the 1983 average divorce rate of the 24 countries (2.3 per thousand population); so the industrial countries as a whole are approximately 27 years behind the United States in divorce. It thus seems probable that in the industrialized countries the divorce rate will continue to climb, at least for the next quarter of a century. Already in the United States, over half of all marriages end in divorce (Weed, 1980, p. 19).[3]

Divorce tends to reduce fertility in various ways. First, it lessens the time that men and women spend in marriage. Using 1975 data, James Weed (1980, p. 13) finds that without divorce the average first marriage in the United States would last 41.4 years. Actually it lasts only 25.8 years. Thus 38 percent of the potential first-marriage duration is lost to divorce. Second, a high divorce rate implies a high degree of marital instability. Hence decisions about childbearing, which necessarily involve long-run planning, must often be made in an atmosphere of apprehensive uncertainty. As a result, couples often postpone having a child, in which case divorce may intervene. Third, a high divorce rate diminishes the financial security that a wife gets through marriage (Weitzman, 1985; 1986, ch. 12). Young women consequently tend to work outside the home and to seek more education as a means of upgrading their marketable working skills.

Wives and work

Less direct than marital postponement, divorce, and illegitimacy, but nevertheless influential is the high and rising participation of married women in the labor force. This phenomenon is well documented (Davis, 1984c; Pepitone-Rockwell, 1980; US Bureau of the Census, 1986), and it characterizes virtually all of the industrial nations. For a long time, single women normally entered employment, and when marriage was postponed, increasing the number of single women, the female labor supply grew. The expanding activity of married women, however, is relatively new. As late as 1910 in the United States, only 9 percent of married women were gainfully employed; by 1985 the figure had climbed to 54.2 percent. If we take only married women in the prime working ages (20–59), we find that the proportions are higher:

	Percent of married women aged 20–59 in labor force
United States, 1985	64.4
Norway, 1980	65.6
England and Wales, 1981	56.0
New Zealand, 1981	42.1

Wives' participation in the labor force outside the home has a chilling effect on fertility in several ways. To begin with, it motivates single women to seek more education in order to get better jobs. To avoid entrapment in household duties, they postpone marriage, perhaps opting for cohabitation in the interim. Once married, having already been in the labor market, they appreciate having an income of their own. Men, in turn, experiencing increased competition from women for jobs, are motivated to get more education and to conserve their assets. They, too, are likely to postpone marriage, and if they do get married they are in no position to demand that their wives quit work. They may assume some household duties, but not enough to eliminate the "double burden" confronting their working wives.

In addition to contributing to marital postponement, the employment of married women contributes to marital instability. By giving the wife an income of her own, it lessens her need for a husband; by providing social contacts at the workplace, it enables her to meet other men; and by focusing her attention on an occupation, it gives her a role—a personal identity—apart from that of childcare and household responsibility. For these reasons, a high divorce rate goes hand in hand with a high rate of married women's employment.

In addition, regardless of marital stability or instability, work outside the home takes time and energy that would otherwise go into domestic activities. Just as in a hunting and gathering regime, so in a present-day industrial society the wife's role in economic production makes low fertility necessary. Indeed, the conflict is even greater now, because a mother cannot carry her offspring to work with her and because training the young in a complex society is more burdensome. If a young woman today has only two children, she can work out daycare arrangements, can minimize the time lost from work due to pregnancy and infant care, and can expect to spend less than a fifth of her postmarital life with children under age seven. Unlike the mother in a hunting and gathering regime, she experiences less difficulty if she bears her children close together rather than far apart. On the other hand, she has far more reason to limit the total number of offspring she bears. Also, while the work of husband and wife in a hunting and gathering regime was complementary, in modern industrial societies it is, normally at least, unrelated. For husband and wife, then, there is nothing in the modern workplace that encourages either marriage or reproduction.

Underlying causes of below-replacement fertility

I have chosen to discuss what is happening to marriage in industrial societies, because it is through the institution of marriage that most factors affect fertility. Certainly, the four major trends considered—marital postponement, nonmarital reproduction, divorce, and wives' employment—go far toward explaining the below-replacement fertility of industrial nations.

Explanation in terms of such causes, however, does not satisfy everybody. Some investigators seek the underlying causes. They want to know why the trends described have occurred. Why is it that advanced industrial societies penalize marriage and marital reproduction?

The best answer I can hazard is that there is an incompatibility, or tension, between the family on the one hand and the industrial economy on the other. The fundamental principle of the family is ascription of status. Members of the family are connected with one another and with extended kin through reproduction. Husband and wife, for example, are connected to each other through common offspring. Kinship has been a major basis of social organization throughout human history, but the family's role in status ascription goes beyond kinship. Insofar as societies are divided into groups, membership has tended to be based on who one's parents were. One is a Muslim, Jew, or Christian because one's parents were. In fact, the major cleavages in human societies today—tribal, caste, racial, religious, ethnic, linguistic—are between groups whose membership is overwhelmingly determined by birth. This is why radical social reformers, seeking to achieve equality and freedom, often want to abolish the family.

The principle of industrial society is the opposite. By rewarding people for achievement, for what they do rather than who they are, industrialism generates competition and mobility. The result is a system so powerful that it dominates the world and inspires the dreams of backward countries.

Replacement of the population, however—at least insofar as it depends on biological motives—has not been "industrialized." It has been left to the family, which remains much as it has always been, a center of close personal contact, primal emotions, and (as we have seen) status ascription. In a sense, then, industrial societies have left the important function of population replacement to a unit that is not only alien in principle to industrialism but which is vestigial, a social fossil. Until recently, this arrangement worked well enough—too well in fact, for the population in the industrializing nations grew rapidly. But of late the encroachments of modernity have so demoralized the family that it is failing to fulfill its reproductive function.

Since the family includes people of different age and sex in close and durable contact, and since it involves appetitive and emotional behavior, its existence requires strong normative controls. These tend to break down when people live in large cities, strive for social mobility, work in an impersonal environment, receive income as individuals rather than as family members, and acquire formal education in schools beyond parental control. Under these conditions family norms increasingly are violated with impunity, and an ideology arises that justifies the violations as being "up to date" or "modern," while conformity is labeled as "old-fashioned" or "conservative." Any catalog of "liberal" or "enlightened" views will include numerous antifamily attitudes. Homosexuality is only a matter of "sexual orientation" and must be accepted; no-fault divorce is a good thing because it reduces recrimination; women bearing children out of wedlock should not be blamed for their situation but given financial help and special attention; abortion is a matter for the woman and her doctor to decide (the husband is ignored); teenagers should have access to contraceptives and abortions without their parents' knowledge; cohabitation without marriage is acceptable.

Unavoidable consequences

If industrial societies thus inherently discourage procreation, they are not likely to experience automatically a new baby boom. Despite some minor cyclical fluctuation, their very low fertility will probably persist unless it is changed by deliberate policy. Presumably, the purpose of pronatalist policy is to avoid the undesired consequences of below-replacement fertility. What are these?

One consequence, the much-discussed aging of the population, has perhaps been exaggerated (the problem depends more on policies with respect to the aged than on the number of the elderly), but almost any conceivable pronatalist policy, even if successful, would make the population younger by only a small degree. In a stable population with present-day mortality, raising the total fertility rate from 1.6 to 2.0 (a 25 percent increase) lowers the proportion aged 65 and over from 26 to 20 percent (Coale and Demeny, 1983, p. 104). At any reproduction rate below replacement, the age structure will be top-heavy.

Further consequences arise from the confinement of very low fertility to the industrial nations. With fertility still high in the less developed countries, this creates in the advanced countries a new and powerful demographic vacuum. Between 1980 and 1985, for example, the population of the less developed countries grew at roughly three times the rate of industrial countries (United Nations, *Demographic Yearbook*, 1984, p. 143):

Rate of population increase per year, 1980–85 (in percent)			
Developed		Less developed	
Europe	0.3	Africa	3.0
Japan	0.6	Western Asia	2.9
Northern America	0.9	Central America	2.7
Australia-New Zealand	1.2	Pacific Islands	2.5

Nobody knows how long the high fertility in the less developed countries will continue. In recent years much optimism has been generated by sharp declines in birth rates in some of these countries, but at least for the time being the decline appears to have lost much of its momentum. For example, in eight poor countries[4] for which reasonably reliable information is available, the average crude birth rate fell impressively during the 1960s and early 1970s but more slowly thereafter:

	Average crude birth rate (per 1000)	Annual percent decline in prior period
1960–64	41.3	
1965–69	37.2	−2.1
1970–74	33.2	−2.3
1975–79	32.2	−0.6
1980–84	30.0	−1.4

It seems that women in these countries are determined not to have big families of six or more children. Whereas in the past they would have had that many births but fewer living children, the reduction of mortality has now, with the same number of births, given them large living families.

Regardless of any foreseeable changes in fertility per woman, however, the less developed countries are facing a period of heavy reproduction because, owing to past high fertility, the generation now entering the reproductive ages is extremely large. In fact, some 90 percent of the world's next generation will be born in the three-fourths of the world that is less developed; even the United Nations projections (medium variant), which assume drastic declines in fertility, expect a population growth rate of almost 1 percent per year as late as 2020–25.[5]

This spectacular demographic imbalance between rich and poor nations is aggravating international tensions in numerous ways. It is increasing the size of the debt owed by the Third World to the developed nations. It is putting enormous pressure on the developed nations to absorb migrants from the Third World—migrants who compete with native labor and whose contribution to the economy, many would argue, is outweighed by their driving up government welfare, educational, and medical expenditures and by the ethnic conflict that their presence often generates. The difference in population growth between the advanced and less advanced countries is also adding to dissension over the use of resources, the developing countries frequently favoring schedules and rates of exploitation different from those favored by developed nations.

Clearly the fate of the industrial nations does not depend solely on their own low fertility, but on the course of fertility in the rest of the world. If the entire world were experiencing zero population growth, or at least moving rapidly toward it, a major source of international friction and environmental contamination would be alleviated; but as things stand, the advanced nations are suffering certain disadvantages from their low fertility that they would not suffer if the less developed countries achieved a similar level. With some notable exceptions such as China, however, the movement in that direction seems to be more a function of general development and modernization than of deliberate population policy (Hernandez, 1984).

The impulse of the advanced nations is to adopt pronatalist policies. Such policies, however, can be expected to boost the birth rate only moderately (Frejka, 1980; McIntosh, 1981). If they should do more than that, the resulting population growth would add to the existing congestion and pollution. A more effective and humane policy would be to encourage very low fertility in the less developed world as well as at home. This, if successful, would bring the Earth back to the virtually zero population growth it had before humans ventured into agriculture and industrialism.

Conclusion

From an evolutionary point of view, humans have been extremely successful. They now number about 5 billion and are increasing by some 80 million each year. For an insect, this would not be many, but for a large resource-consuming and environmentally destructive mammal, it is a big number. In the human case, however, success in an evolutionary sense is not viewed with equanimity by everyone. A sizable proportion of humans view the explosive multiplication of their species as a global catastrophe that has helped to expand poverty, to extinguish thousands of other species, to pollute the air, to waste resources, to create congestion. No wonder, then, that a substantial and increasing number of people are in favor of either fewer or at least no more people than there are now.

For many observers, then, the current below-replacement fertility in the industrial countries is a blessing, not a calamity. It is a solution to a major problem, not a problem in itself. Since these countries are in a minority, however, their self-restraint with respect to fertility reduces global population growth only slightly. Instead it gives the industrial countries aging populations and international complications. Like everything else, then, below-replacement fertility has its costs. While these costs are leading some governments to pursue or consider pronatalist programs, they are hardly great enough to justify programs that will do much more than achieve zero growth (Vining, 1984; Tomlinson, 1984).

To evaluate the present below-replacement fertility of the industrial nations, one must recall the millions of years when humans, like other animals, hunted and foraged. Under those conditions, a rapid expansion of human numbers was suicidal, because it would lead to feedback mechanisms such as environmental exhaustion, tribal warfare, and disease. In some animals, population stabilization is achieved by very high mortality, but in others, including humans, it is achieved by moderate fertility, which fits the evolutionary niche that humans have carved for themselves—namely a reliance on culture and technology. This reliance has succeeded best when emphasis was placed on the training of offspring rather than the number of offspring.

With agriculture, however, man began to live by controlling rather than simply skimming his environment. The switch was so profound and sudden that normal feedback mechanisms restraining population growth became partially inoperable. As agriculture improved and spread, population increased many times faster than it had grown before.

By greatly expanding production in agriculture and in other sectors of the economy, and by finally inventing scientific medicine, industrialism lowered death rates dramatically, with consequent unbridled population growth. Since, however, an industrial system must invest ever more heavily in the training of the young, it soon exerts a downward pressure on fertility. With full industrialism, the family, which has survived up to this point, becomes a weak institution and the output of babies becomes inadequate to replace the population. When and if the whole world becomes industrialized, the growth of the human population may, mercifully, reverse itself.

Notes

1 The term "hominids" designates the human family after it separated from the ape family. The time of the separation is variously estimated as between 7 and 30 million years ago. The hominids include several fossil species in addition to modern man. See Fagan, 1979, ch. 5, and Campbell, 1974, pp. 372–397.

2 Calculated from data in United Nations, *Demographic Yearbook*, 1982-84 editions.

3 Weed's finding is that 47.4 percent of first marriages in the United States and 48.9 percent of remarriages will end in divorce, but his calculation uses 1975 data. The divorce rate rose by 12 percent between 1975 and 1979, after which it stabilized. It is therefore safe to say that the probability of divorce now exceeds 50 percent.

4 The countries are Egypt, El Salvador, Fiji, Malaysia, Mauritius, Panama, Sri Lanka, and Tunisia. Calculated from United Nations, *Demographic Yearbook*, various editions, and *Population and Vital Statistics Report*. See also Davis, 1984a.

5 Calculated from United Nations, 1985, p. 33.

References

Acsádi, Gy., and J. Nemeskéri. 1970. *History of Human Life Span and Mortality*. Budapest: Akadémiai Kiadó.

Campbell, Bernard G. 1974. *Human Evolution: An Introduction to Man's Adaptations*, 2nd edition. Chicago, Illinois: Aldine Publishing Company.

Carlson, Elwood. 1986. "Couples without children: Premarital cohabitation in France," in Davis, 1986, pp. 113–130.

Carr-Saunders, A. M. 1922. *The Population Problem: A Study in Human Evolution*. Oxford: Clarendon Press.

Coale, Ansley J., and Paul Demeny. 1983. *Regional Model Life Tables and Stable Populations*, 2nd edition. New York: Academic Press.

———, and Melvin Zelnik. 1963. *New Estimates of Fertility and Population in the United States*. Princeton, New Jersey: Princeton University Press.

Chiglieri, Michael Patrick. 1984. *The Chimpanzees of Kibale Forest: A Field Study of Ecology and Social Structure*. New York: Columbia University Press.

Cohen, Mark Nathan, and George J. Armelagos (eds.). 1984. *Paleopathology at the Origins of Agriculture*. New York: Academic Press.

Corlett, William Thomas. 1935. *The Medicine-Man of the American Indians*. Baltimore, Maryland: Charles C. Thomas.

Daly, Martin, and Margo Wilson. 1980. "Sociobiological analysis of human infanticide," in Hausfater and Hrdy, 1984, pp. 487–502.

Davis, Kingsley. 1984a. "Declining birth rates and growing populations," *Population Research and Policy Review* 36 (January).

———. 1984b. "Demographic dilemmas in the mid-1980s," in *To Promote Prosperity: U.S. Domestic Policy in the Mid-1980s*, ed. John H. Moore. Stanford, California: Hoover Institution Press, ch. 21.

———. 1984c. "Wives and work: The sex role revolution and its consequences," *Population and Development Review* 10, no. 3 (September): 397–417.

——— (ed.). 1986. *Contemporary Marriage: Comparative Perspectives on a Changing Institution*. New York: Russell Sage Foundation.

Eaton, Joseph W., and Albert J. Mayer. 1954. *Man's Capacity to Reproduce: The Demography of a Unique Population*. Glencoe, Illinois: The Free Press.

Espenshade, Thomas J. 1986. "The recent decline of American marriage: Blacks and whites in comparative perspective," in Davis, 1986, pp. 53–90.

Fagan, Brian M. 1979. *World Prehistory: A Brief Introduction*. Boston, Massachusetts: Little, Brown and Company.

Frejka, Thomas. 1980. "Fertility trends and policies: Czechoslovakia in the 1970s," *Population and Development Review* 6, no. 1 (March): 65–93.

Goodall, Jane van Lawick. 1971. *In the Shadow of Man*. Boston, Massachusetts: Houghton Mifflin Company.

Hausfater, Glenn, and Sarah Blaffer Hrdy (eds.). 1984. *Infanticide: Comparative and Evolutionary Perspectives*. New York: Aldine Publishing Company.

Hayden, Brian. 1972. "Population control among hunter/gatherers," *World Archaeology* 4, no. 2 (October).

Hernandez, Donald J. 1984. *Success or Failure? Family Planning Programs in the Third World*. Westport, Connecticut: Greenwood Press.

Howell, Nancy. 1979. *The Demography of the Dobe !Kung*. New York: Academic Press.

Johansson, S. Ryan, and S. Horowitz. 1985. "Life expectancy and age at death in skeletal populations," mimeo.

Jolly, Alison. 1972. *The Evolution of Primate Behavior*. New York: Macmillan.

Jones, F. Lancaster. 1965. "The demography of the Australian aborigines," *International Social Science Journal* 17, no. 2: 232–245.

Klein, Richard G. 1984. "Mammalian extinctions and Stone Age people in Africa," in Martin and Klein, 1984, pp. 553–573.

Landy, David (ed.). 1977. *Culture, Disease, and Healing: Studies in Medical Anthropology.* New York: Macmillan.

Lee, Richard B. 1979. *The !Kung San: Men, Women, and Work in a Foraging Society.* Cambridge: Cambridge University Press.

———, and Irven DeVore (eds.). 1968. *Man the Hunter.* Chicago, Illinois: Aldine Publishing Company.

McIntosh, C. Alison. 1981. "Low fertility and liberal democracy in Western Europe," *Population and Development Review* 7, no. 2 (June): 181–207.

Maddox, John Lee. 1923. *The Medicine Man.* New York: Macmillan.

Martin, Paul S. 1973. "The discovery of America," *Science* 179 (March): 969–974.

———, and Richard G. Klein (eds.). 1984. *Quaternary Extinctions: A Prehistoric Revolution.* Tucson, Arizona: The University of Arizona Press.

Nitecki, Matthew H. 1984. *Extinctions.* Chicago, Illinois: University of Chicago Press.

Pepitone-Rockwell, Fran (ed.). 1980. *Dual-Career Couples.* Beverly Hills, California: Sage Publications.

Schaller, George B. 1965. "The behavior of the mountain gorilla," in *Primate Behavior: Field Studies of Monkeys and Apes,* ed. Irven DeVore. New York: Holt, Rinehart and Winston, pp. 324–367.

Scrimshaw, Susan C. M. 1984. "Infanticide in human populations: Societal and individual concerns," in Hausfater and Hrdy, 1984, pp. 439–462.

Sklar, June. 1977. "Marriage and nonmarital fertility: A comparison of Ireland and Sweden," *Population and Development Review* 3, no. 4 (December): 359–375.

Smith, T. E. 1960. "The Cocos-Keeling Islands: A demographic laboratory," *Population Studies* 14 (November): 94–130.

Spanier, Graham B. 1986. "Cohabitation in the 1980s: Recent changes in the United States," in Davis, 1986, pp. 91–111.

Starr, Paul. 1982. *The Social Transformation of American Medicine.* New York: Basic Books.

Tomlinson, Richard. 1984. "The French population debate," *The Public Interest,* No. 76 (Summer): 111–120.

United Nations. 1984 and earlier. *Demographic Yearbook.* New York.

———. 1985. *World Population Trends, Population and Development Interrelations and Population Policies,* 1983 Monitoring Report, Vol. 1. New York.

———. 1986 and earlier. *Population and Vital Statistics Report,* Series A, 1 January.

United States Bureau of the Census. 1970. "Marital status and family status: March 1969," Series P-20, No. 198 (25 March).

——— Bureau of the Census. 1986 and earlier. *Statistical Abstract of the United States.* Washington, D.C.

——— National Center for Health Statistics. 1981. *Vital Statistics of the United States, 1980, Volume 1, Natality (1981).*

——— National Center for Health Statistics. 1985. "Advance report of final natality statistics, 1984," *Monthly Vital Statistics Report* 34, no. 4 (18 July).

Vining, Daniel R., Jr. 1984. "Family salaries and the East German birth rate: A comment," *Population and Development Review* 10, no. 4 (December): 693–696.

Washburn, Sherwood L., and C. S. Lancaster. 1968a. "The evolution of hunting," in Lee and DeVore, 1968, pp. 293–303.

———, and Jane B. Lancaster. 1968b. "Human evolution," in *International Encyclopedia of the Social Sciences,* Vol. 5. New York: Macmillan, pp. 215–221.

Weed, James A. 1980. "National estimates of marriage dissolution and survivorship: United States," National Center for Health Analytical Studies, Series 3, Number 19 (November).

Weitzman, Lenore J. 1985. *The Divorce Revolution: The Unexpected Social and Economic Consequences for Women and Children in America.* New York: The Free Press.

———. 1986. "The divorce law revolution and the transformation of legal marriage," in Davis, 1986, ch. 12.

MODELS

Altruism and the Economic Theory of Fertility

Gary S. Becker
Robert J. Barro

The economic approach to fertility emphasizes the effects of parents' income and the cost of rearing children. With the exception of work by Richard Easterlin (1973) and a few others (e.g., Becker, 1981, Chapter 7), this approach has neglected the analytical links between decisions by different generations of the same family. Moreover, despite Malthus's famous precedent, fertility has not been integrated with the determination of wage rates, interest rates, capital accumulation, and other macro variables (exceptions include Razin and Ben-Zion, 1975; Willis, 1985).

Economic analyses of fertility have assumed that the utility of parents depends on the number and "quality" of children, usually without any specification of how or why children affect utility. Although agnosticism about preferences is common among economists, a more powerful analysis of fertility and population change is available by building on recent discussions of altruism toward children.

The importance of altruism within families began to be recognized systematically by economists during the 1970s (two early studies are Barro, 1974, and Becker, 1974). Obviously many parents are altruistic toward children in the sense that the utility of parents depends positively on the utility of their children. This article relies heavily on the assumption of altruism toward children to generate a dynamic analysis of population change.

We assume that each person lives for two generations, childhood and adulthood. We pretend that each adult has children without "marriage." We believe the production of children through marriage of men and women would complicate, but not affect the essence of, the analysis (although, see Bagwell and Bernheim, 1985). We also bypass issues related to the spacing of children by assuming that parents have all of their children at the beginning of adulthood.

If the utility of a parent is an additively separable function of own consumption, denoted c_0, and the utility of each child, and with the important assumption that parents' utility depends linearly on children's utility, parents' utility U_0 would be given by

$$U_0 = v(c_0) + a(n_0)n_0 U_1 \quad, \tag{1}$$

where v is a standard utility function (with $v' > 0$, $v'' < 0$), n_0 is the number of children, and U_1 the utility per child. The term $a(n_0)$ measures the degree of altruism toward each child, and converts the utility of children into that of parents. We assume that, for given utility per child U_1, parental utility is increasing and concave in the number of children n_0. This property requires the altruism function to satisfy the conditions,

$$a(n_0) + n_0 a'(n_0) > 0 \text{ and } 2a'(n_0) + n_0 a''(n_0) < 0 \quad, \tag{2}$$

where we neglect integer restrictions on the number of children.

The utility of grandchildren U_2 would appear in the utility function if U_1 of equation (1) is replaced by terms that depend on c_1, n_1, and U_2. By continuing to substitute later consumption and fertility, we arrive at a *dynastic* utility function that depends on the consumption and number of children of all descendants of the same family line. This dynastic utility function can be expressed as

$$U_0 = \sum_{i=0}^{\infty} A_i N_i v(c_i) \quad, \tag{3}$$

where A_i is the implied degree of altruism of the dynastic head toward each descendant in the ith generation, as given by

$$A_0 = 1, A_i = \prod_{j=0}^{i-1} a(n_j), \quad i = 1, 2, \ldots \quad, \tag{4}$$

n_j is the number of children per adult in generation j, N_i is the number of descendants in the ith generation, as given by

$$N_0 = 1, N_i = \prod_{j=0}^{i-1} n_j, \quad i = 1, 2, \ldots \quad, \tag{5}$$

and c_i is the consumption per adult in generation i.

Each adult supplies one unit of labor to the market and earns the wage w_i. Adults leave a bequest of (nondepreciable) capital, k_{i+1} (possibly human capital), to each child. We assume as a convention that bequests occur at the beginning of period i. Since the capital k_i earns rentals at the rate r_i, an adult in generation i spends his total resources, $w_i + (1 + r_i)k_i$, on own consumption, c_i, on bequests to children, $n_i k_{i+1}$, and on costs of raising children. We assume that each child costs β_i, so that $n_i \beta_i$ is the total cost of raising children to adulthood. Therefore, the overall budget condition for an adult in generation i is

$$w_i + (1 + r_i)k_i = c_i + n_i (\beta_i + k_{i+1}) \ . \tag{6}$$

The parameter β_i represents a cost of raising children that is independent of the "quality" of children (as measured by their consumption, c_{i+1}, wage rate, w_{i+1}, or inheritance, k_{i+1}). We assume also that debt can be left to children—that is, bequests k_i can be negative as well as positive, although parents cannot leave negative levels of human capital.

The optimization problem as seen by the dynastic head is to maximize utility U_0 in equation (3), subject to the budget constraints in equation (6), and to initial assets k_0. In carrying out this maximization, each head takes as given the path of wage rates, w_i, interest rates, r_i, and childrearing costs, β_i. The chosen path of consumption per adult, $c_0, c_1, c_2, \ldots$; capital stock per adult, $k_1, k_2, \ldots$; and number of descendants, $N_1, N_2, \ldots$, must be consistent with this maximization problem.[1]

The first-order conditions are obtained in the usual manner, with allowance for a Lagrange multiplier for each period that corresponds to each of the budget constraints in equation (6). One set of first-order conditions is

$$\frac{v'(c_i)}{v'(c_{i+1})} = (1 + r_{i+1}) a(n_i), \quad i = 0, 1, \ldots \ . \tag{7}$$

The analysis of the other conditions simplifies if the degree of altruism toward children has a constant elasticity with respect to the number of children—that is,

$$a(n_i) = \alpha (n_i)^{-\epsilon} \ . \tag{8}$$

In this case the degree of altruism toward descendants, A_i in equation (4), depends only on the number of descendants in generation i, $N_i = \prod_{j=0}^{i-1} n_j$—specifically, $A_i = \alpha^i (N_i)^{-\epsilon}$. Then the condition $0 < a(1) < 1$ requires $0 < \alpha < 1$, and the condition that parental utility is increasing and concave in the number of children for given utility per child (as ensured by the inequalities in expression (2)) corresponds to $0 < \epsilon < 1$. By substituting the altruism function from equation (8) into the expression for dynastic utility in equation (3), we get

$$U_0 = \sum_{i=0}^{\infty} \alpha^i (N_i)^{1-\epsilon} v(c_i) \ . \tag{9}$$

Dynastic utility in equation (9) is a time-separable function of the number of descendants and consumption in each generation, and does not depend explicitly on the fertility of any generation. Demand functions derived from time-separable utility functions depend only on the marginal utility of wealth and the prices of variables with the same date. Consequently, if we hold constant the marginal utility of wealth, the number of descendants and consumption in any generation would not be affected by price changes in other generations.

With the utility function in equation (9), the other set of first-order conditions[2] is

$$v(c_i)[1 - \epsilon - \sigma(c_i)] = v'(c_i)[\beta_{i-1}(1 + r_i) - w_i], \quad i = 1, 2, \ldots \quad (10)$$

where $\sigma(c_i)$ is the elasticity of $v(c_i)$ with respect to c_i. There is also the dynastic budget constraint, which equates the present value of all resources to the present value of all expenditures,

$$k_0 + \sum_{i=0}^{\infty} d_i N_i w_i = \sum_{i=0}^{\infty} d_i (N_i c_i + N_{i+1} \beta_i) , \quad (11)$$

where $d_i = \prod_{j=0}^{i}(1 + r_j)^{-1}$.

Equation (7) is an arbitrage condition for shifting consumption from one generation to the next. Aside from the term that depends on fertility, n_i, this equation expresses the familiar result that the utility rate of substitution between consumption in periods $i+1$ and i, $v'(c_i)/v'(c_{i+1})$, depends directly on the time-preference factor ($a(1) = \alpha$), and the interest-rate factor, $1 + r_{i+1}$. The standard conclusion is that a rise in time preference, α, or in the interest rate, r_{i+1}, increases c_{i+1} relative to c_i. In our modified arbitrage condition, an increase in fertility, n_i, lowers altruism per child, given by $a(n_i)$, and thereby increases the discount on future consumption. Therefore, higher fertility is associated with a reduction in c_{i+1} relative to c_i, for given values of r_{i+1} and α.

Changes in the level of interest rates or in the degree of altruism mainly affect fertility, n_i. We can rewrite equation (7) with $a(n) = \alpha n^{-\epsilon}$ to solve for the fertility rate:

$$n_i = [\alpha(1 + r_{i+1})v'(c_{i+1})/v'(c_i)]^{1/\epsilon}, \quad i = 0, 1, \ldots \quad (12)$$

Equation (10) pegs the intertemporal-substitution term, $v'(c_{i+1})/v'(c_i)$, for $i = 1, 2, \ldots$, because c_i in each future generation depends only on the net cost of producing descendants. For example, if the cost were the same for all generations, the intertemporal-substitution term would be unity. Since substitution in consumption is pegged, the fertility rate, n_i for $i = 1, 2, \ldots$, rises with increases in the interest rate, r_{i+1}, or the rate of altruism, α.

Easterlin, a pioneer in analyzing the effects of intergenerational relations on fertility, has argued (1973) that fertility depends negatively on the wealth of parents compared with own wealth because growing up in a wealthy family shifts preferences toward own consumption at the expense of children. Put differently, fertility is said to be positively related to the growth in wealth from the previous to the present generation. Fertility in our model also depends on the rate of growth between generations, but it depends *negatively* on the growth between own consumption and consumption per capita of the *next* generation. Moreover, in our model, preferences are invariant with wealth and have the same form for each generation.

Our model has surprising implications about the effects of changes in the cost of producing children on the demand for children. For consider a tax on raising children in generation j that raises β_j but does not change β_i for $i \neq j$. Furthermore, to abstract from wealth effects, assume a compensating increase in initial assets, k_0, that leaves the marginal utility of wealth, $v'(c_0)$, unchanged. Equation (10) indicates that c_{j+1} rises, but all other c_i do not change. Equation (12) implies that fertility in generation j falls—after all, children are now more costly to produce in that generation. What is surprising, however, is that fertility in generation $j + 1$ rises, and by an amount that exactly offsets the fall in generation j. Therefore, the tax in generation j would not change the number of descendants after the $(j + 1)$st generation.

As it were, the fertility rates of adjacent generations are perfect substitutes in the production of descendants. Any change in the net cost of producing descendants in one generation causes enough substitution from the fertility in the succeeding generation to leave unchanged the number of descendants in subsequent generations.

Consider now a compensated permanent increase in the cost of children that raises the net cost of children, $\beta_i(1 + r_{i+1}) < w_{i+1}$, by the same proportion for each generation $i \geq j$. Equation (10) implies that consumption per person rises in generation $j + 1$ and in each subsequent generation. Further, if we now assume as an approximation that the elasticity of utility is the constant σ, then the increases in c_{j+1}, c_{j+2}, ... are equiproportional. The arbitrage condition for consumption over time in equation (10) simplifies in this case to

$$(c_{i+1}/c_i)^{1-\sigma} = \alpha(1 + r_{i+1})/(n_i)^\epsilon, \quad i = 0, 1, \ldots . \tag{13}$$

Equiproportional increases in c_i for $i = j + 1, \ldots,$ imply that fertility in generation j falls (because c_j/c_{j+1} declines), while fertility in all other generations is unchanged. Consequently, given interest rates, even a permanent (compensated) tax on children reduces fertility only in the generation where the tax is first enacted. However, the decline in fertility in one generation alone has lasting effects because the number of descendants in all later generations also declines.

Economic growth, child mortality, and social security

We have assumed for simplicity that the cost per child β_i is independent of the number n_i. We have shown that a temporary change in the cost of children in one generation induces an oscillation in fertility over that generation and the subsequent one, whereas a permanent change in cost starting in a particular generation alters fertility only in that generation. A permanent fall in fertility would require a continuous rise in the cost of children. Assume, for example, that the interest rate is the constant r, while wages, the cost of rearing children, and hence the net cost of descendants are each rising at a constant rate—due say to steady economic growth. Then, if the elasticity of utility is the constant σ, the consumption of descendants, c_i, would rise at the same rate as the net cost of descendants. A higher rate of growth in consumption per person would reduce fertility permanently, given the values of α and r (see equation (13)).

The decline in fertility observed since the mid-nineteenth century in most Western countries has sometimes been explained by rapid economic growth that continues to raise the cost of children through raising the value of parents' time (see, for example, Becker, 1981, Chapter 11). This explanation has not been based on a formal model that links fertility to economic growth, and our model does not have this implication. If interest rates do not change, a steady rate of economic growth that induced a steady growth in the net cost of descendants, and hence also in consumption per capita, would permanently lower fertility, but would not generate a persistent fall in fertility. A persistent fall requires either that interest rates fall steadily, economic growth continues to accelerate, or that the net cost of descendants accelerates for other reasons.

The secular decline in fertility has also been explained by the secular decline in child mortality that continued to reduce the number of births required to produce a target number of surviving children. Our analysis has novel implications for the effects of declines in child mortality on birth rates and the demand for surviving children.

We assume that wage rates and interest rates are constant over time, and that parents ignore the uncertainty about child deaths and respond only to changes in the fraction, p, of offspring who survive childhood. Let β_s be the constant marginal cost of rearing a child to adulthood, and β_m be the cost of a child who dies prior to becoming an adult. Since the latter cost includes any psychic losses from child mortality, β_m could exceed β_s. The expected cost of n_b births is $[p\beta_s + (1-p)\beta_m]n_b$. The ratio of this expected cost to the expected number of survivors n—which corresponds to our previous cost per (surviving) child—is

$$\beta = \beta_s + \beta_m(1-p)/p \ . \tag{14}$$

As before, parents choose own consumption, the expected number of surviving children, and bequests to surviving children, but now subject to a budget constraint that depends on the expected cost β.

A permanent decline in the level of child mortality lowers the cost of raising surviving children in all generations. Our prior analysis implies that the demand for surviving children per adult, n_i, rises in the initial generation, but is unchanged in later generations. Since the demand for surviving children increases in the initial generation, birth rates may also rise then, although the higher probability of survival, p, reduces the number of births, n_b, needed to produce a given number of survivors. Birth rates definitely fall in later generations because the demand for surviving children in these generations would not be affected by the increase in p.

The cost of rearing surviving children would continue to fall over time, and hence the demand for surviving children per adult would increase for more than one generation, if child mortality continues to fall over time. However, the rate of decline in child mortality slows down once the latter approaches zero, as it has in the West during the past 40 years. As the rate of decline slows, the rate of decline in the cost of producing survivors also slows and eventually more or less ceases. Thereafter, the *cumulative* increase in the child survival probability does not affect the demand for surviving children. Birth rates, however, are reduced by the same percentage level as the increase in survival probability.

Our analysis explains why the transition to regimes of low child mortality has only temporary positive effects on rates of population growth. It can also explain why birth rates often rise before they decline (see the evidence in Dyson and Murphy, 1985), and why declines in birth rates lag behind declines in child mortality. Eventually, the decline in birth rates must accelerate until the percentage decline from prior levels equals the percentage increase in the probability of surviving to adulthood.

Summary and conclusions

This article develops the implications of altruism toward children, where utility of parents depends on their own consumption, their fertility, and the utility of each of their children. Altruism toward children implies that the welfare of all generations of a family is linked through a dynastic utility function that depends on the consumption, fertility, and number of descendants in all generations. The head of a dynastic family acts as if he maximizes dynastic utility subject to a dynastic budget constraint, which involves the wealth inherited by the head, interest rates, the cost of rearing children in all generations, and the earnings of all descendants.

We neglect uncertainty, marriage, the spacing of births, and capital-market restraints over life cycles and across generations. Nevertheless, even a highly simplified model of altruism toward children and the behavior of dynastic families appears to us to capture important aspects of the dynamic behavior of fertility and consumption. If so, a new approach would be warranted to the analysis of trends and long-term fluctuations in fertility, population growth, and consumption.

Notes

A longer version of this article to be published elsewhere develops an economic analysis of linkages in fertility across generations. It also considers the interaction between fertility and various macro variables for a dynastic family and in open economies when wage rates and interest rates are parameters. A sequel will consider the determination of interest rates, wage rates, population growth, and capital accumulation in closed economies (see Barro and Becker, 1985, for an earlier version of our approach).

1 We pretend that the dynastic head can pick the entire time path. However, descendants face a problem of the same form, and have no incentive to deviate from the choices made initially. In other words, decisions are time-consistent across generations. Note also that, as long as all the capital stocks k_i are positive, bequests from parents to children are also positive.

2 The second-order condition is $\epsilon + (1 - \epsilon)vv''/(v')^2 < 0$. If $\sigma(c_i)$ is the constant σ, then this condition reduces to $\sigma + \epsilon < 1$.

References

Bagwell, Kyle, and B. Douglas Bernheim. 1985. "Is everything neutral?," working paper, Stanford University.

Barro, Robert J. 1974. "Are government bonds net wealth?," *Journal of Political Economy* 82, no. 6: 1095–1117.

———, and Gary S. Becker. 1985. "Population growth and economic growth," paper presented at the Workshop in Applications of Economics, University of Chicago.

Becker, Gary S. 1974. "A theory of social interactions," *Journal of Political Economy* 82, no. 6: 1063–1093.

———. 1981. *A Treatise on the Family*. Cambridge, Mass.: Harvard University Press.

Dyson, Tim and Mike Murphy. 1985. "The onset of fertility transition," *Population and Development Review* 11, no. 3: 399–440.

Easterlin, Richard A. 1973. "Relative economic status and the American fertility swing," in *Family Economic Behavior: Problems and Prospects,* ed. E. B. Sheldon. Philadelphia: Lippincott.

Razin, Assaf, and Uri Ben-Zion. 1975. "An intergenerational model of population growth," *American Economic Review* 65, no. 5: 923–933.

Willis, Robert J. 1985. "A theory of the equilibrium interest rate in an overlapping generations model: Life cycles, institutions, and population growth," discussion paper no. 85-8, Economics Research Center/NORC, University of Chicago.

Comment: Paul A. David

The contributions so concisely summarized in the article by Gary Becker and Robert Barro can best be appreciated, in my view, if one first puts aside what has been learned empirically about the socioeconomic determinants of fertility behavior in modern societies. Their article, which explores the economic implications of altruism toward children along lines initially indicated by the authors' previous theoretical writings (see Barro, 1974; Becker, 1974), well might have been subtitled: "What Every Loving, Utility-Maximizing Mother Knows About the Ricardian Equivalence Theorem." We should accept it as making a significant extension to that rambling analytical structure erected by economists on the assumption that the actions of individuals may be connected not only through participation in markets that determine the constraints on individual choice, but more directly, through the interdependence of individuals' utility functions.

Economists, it has been said, are people who, on seeing anything working in practice, will soon be determined to find out whether it could work also in theory. The authors in this instance, no doubt having first-hand experience of the practice of altruism toward children, now wonder whether, and how, such a thing might work in the economic theory of fertility, and how that in turn would fit into a more general theory of intertemporal accumulation—involving inanimate as well as human forms of "wealth." Thus Barro and Becker elsewhere (1985) have pursued the ambitious goal of formulating a complete dynamic model of fertility determination and capital accumulation, for a population whose members' current welfare is linked with that of future generations by virtue of their altruism toward their own offspring. On this occasion, however, they have concentrated largely upon presenting the model's microeconomic underpinnings and showing us what these imply about the behavior of fertility in successive generations of a representative family lineage.

Such lineages are described in their article as "dynastic families," presumably because the members must attend to the succession of economic welfare down through the generations of their descendants, as hereditary rulers formerly had to concern themselves with arranging for the transmission of sovereignty so as to guarantee the retention of power throughout their own lifetimes. Economic theory works in many wondrous ways to illuminate the world around us. So, whatever one thinks about the realism of the constrained intertemporal optimization problem addressed by Becker and Barro, something useful may be learned about the causes of below-replacement fertility in contemporary societies—merely from the observation that readers seem to find the authors' reference to "dynasties" a heuristic aid in this context. Consider, for the moment, how profound has been the historical transformation in Western culture that makes it a plausible literary device nowadays to equate the obligations incumbent upon responsible, caring parents with the considerations that formerly occupied potentates. For modern parents, children appear not only as love-objects, but as masters whose future needs must be gratified; whereas for the dynasts of old it was the children who served as instrumentalities of political power. John Caldwell (1982), among others, suggests we should consider the implications for fertility behavior of such shifts in the balance of responsibilities between children and parents, a theme on which I shall later essay some further variations.

But to do justice to Becker and Barro's article as a contribution to the economic theory of fertility—rather than subject its text to close examination as an informative cultural exhibit—I should first set out some of my reservations about three aspects of their analysis. These are, first, its extremely atomistic conception of society; second, the dependence of many of its theoretical conclusions upon assumptions whose empirical content is not examined; third, its implied view of uncertainty as a peripheral rather than central aspect of the phenomenon of voluntary below-replacement fertility. My concerns under each heading can be stated briefly.

First, the radically atomistic conception of society that infuses this article is a paradoxical feature in a piece devoted to examining the economic implications of altruism. Altruism is a tricky substance to use in economic modeling, as it resembles crazy-glue in its propensity to bond everything in the model-kit together with everything else. Becker and Barro are not like the amateur hobbyists who labor in my garage, fortunately. They have used their great expertise in carefully applying just enough altruism where it is needed to cement individuals into "dynastic" families, while preventing any of the families thereby constructed from becoming socially interactive with one another. This in itself is a remarkable achievement. But, when one adds to it the authors' retention of partial equilibrium analysis as their expositional mode, the result is a representation of the economy as a large sea surrounding many family-islands; and of society as the aggregation of individuals who, being stuck on these islands, remain forever isolated from the effects of actions taken by anyone other than the forebears of their lineage. One must question the ultimate usefulness of a framework such as this, within which it will be difficult, if not impossible, to seriously examine any of the social policy issues that arise from the "externalities" produced by microdemographic behavior.

My second set of reservations concerns some of the specific assumptions made in setting up the fertility-choice problem that supposedly faces the progenitors of dynastic families. The novel feature of Becker and Barro's theory is that it treats the demand for children, and changes therein, as essentially epiphenomenal in nature. At the core of the analysis one does not find the old calculus of the pleasures and pains of having children, *qua* children—although the range of considerations made familiar by Becker's previous contributions can also be fitted into the new model. But even if people had no direct use

Comment: Paul A. David

for children, we now are told, they would put up with them for the sake of having descendants. The unique attribute for which children are sought is, in other words, their ability to confer upon their parents a form of consumer-immortality. Through the miracle of altruism toward one's progeny, the utility functions of people in successive generations can become firmly bonded in just the right way, permitting anyone capable of producing a child to go on vicariously deriving pleasure—unto eternity—from the consumption of mundane market goods.

With this comforting prospect in view, Becker and Barro quite logically proceed to ask how fertility would be managed by a person who sought her own happiness by optimizing the time path of consumption activities carried on not only in her household but by all her descendants. There is probably little of value to be gained by debating whether this intriguing conceptualization is deeply insightful or preposterous. I would rather have us recognize that many of Becker and Barro's specific propositions about fertility behavior derive not so much from the foregoing, general conceptualization, as from some very restrictive assumptions—about the detailed form of the utility function, and the constraints upon maximizing parents—that the authors have made in translating it into a concrete and mathematically tractable dynamic model. It seems to me that among all the species of social scientists, economists, especially economists who believe in the efficacy of markets, should be made to pay for their assumptions—rather than have them as free goods. Only then will there be an end to the recurring threadbare jokes, such as the one about the economist who, being shipwrecked on a desert island with a crate of canned beans, figured out how to save himself from starving: "It will be assumed," he wrote in the sand, "that I also have found a can-opener."

The third thing about Becker and Barro's article that gives me pause is that it closes by suggesting that their model of intertemporal allocation in a single lineage, with perfect foresight extending to the infinitely distant horizon, can "explain why" various demographic phenomena—such as the lag in birth rates behind declines in child mortality—are observed in the world around us. Modest though their concluding statements may be, I find such claims of direct empirical relevance still too strong. In particular, I question whether the implications of Becker and Barro's analysis are robust enough to survive the introduction into the model of uncertainty, for it strikes me that the relative degree of uncertainty attending the business of producing and caring for human offspring needs to be considered in order to understand the main empirical phenomenon that has prompted this volume—an increasing tendency of people in the high-income nations of the world to avoid reproducing themselves biologically. I suspect that a root cause, if not *the* root cause of the emerging pattern of below-replacement fertility may be found in the combination of increasing relative risk aversion associated with wealth, and the special, irreducible hazards to which altruistic parents must submit themselves.

Since it may be difficult to extract much of my meaning from the foregoing, compressed remarks, I owe it to Becker and Barro and their readers to expand somewhat on each of these points. The balance of my comments therefore is organized as responses to three questions, corresponding to the three sources of reservations I have just indicated: Can a family be an island? Why assume we have a can-opener? Is altruism toward children perhaps a cultural trait with low survival value?

Can a family be an island?

In maintaining their focus primarily upon the determinants of the relative sizes of successive generations in a closed population, Becker and Barro shut down the parts of their apparatus that generate macroeconomic, general equilibrium phenomena. They present their analysis, therefore, as pertinent to the situation of individual families; and, equally, to the representative family in an economy that is completely "open" to trade in goods and to capital movements, and so faces a parametrically determined wage rate and interest rate. This expositional strategy has an effect that is probably unintended, but nevertheless unfortunate. It closes off discussion of policy issues arising from divergences between private optimality and social optimality in regard to fertility decisions; a "social optimum" will not have any efficiency consequences distinguishable from the collectivity of private optima when individual agents, in this case families, do not interact. Becker and Barro here have assumed away the possibility of interaction through markets, and with it the possibility that families pursuing their private welfare may cause the population to grow (or shrink) in ways detrimental to the welfare of all.

This suppression of market-mediated interactions further reinforces the two structural features of their model that serve to rid it of all taint of "non-market externalities." First, altruism, in the form recognized by the authors, suffices to internalize all interactions between members of different generations belonging to the same family lineage. The effects of one's actions on members of the lineage are completely taken into account by the decisionmakers for these "happy families." Future generations cannot affect their forebears in any unforeseen ways in this perfect certainty model, and the latter gain satisfactions (directly and indirectly) from the utility of their descendants. Moreover, since the article assumes that all generations have (conveniently) identical utility functions—identical degrees of parental altruism, rates of time-preference, and preferences regarding own consumption—no Becker–Barro child can ever reproach its mother for not having done enough on its behalf. One who did so would receive the instant retort: "So, tell me, what would you have done differently, were you in my place?"

The second socially "isolating" assumption is that the population in question is unisexed, so that when their members reach adulthood they can beget children "without 'marriage,'" as Becker and Barro have phrased it (p. 69). Recourse here to the assumption of a unisexed population is not just a simple gesture intended to make the formal demographers among us feel at home; nor are the authors being quaintly discreet in substituting "marriage" when they mean "heterosexual copulation." They do say exactly what they mean: it is the institution that is awkward to accommodate within their analytical framework, and from which, accordingly, they seek to abstract. The formation of unions joining members of different family lineages, that is to say, the institution of nonincestuous marriage, is a source of nonmarket externalities which—whatever their socially redeeming features in other respects—have a quite devastating potential for this particular theoretical enterprise.

Once one admits marriage into the picture, what stops two distinct lineages from winding up with an interest in, and an effect upon, the welfare of the partners in a marital union? Worse yet, if Becker and Barro would permit it, two sets of grandparents, involving four distinct lineages, could have an interest in each of that couple's offspring. Will lineages recognize their eventual mutuality of interests and so act in universal concert, or will they behave noncooperatively and attempt to free-ride on the altruistically motivated actions of other lineages that affect the welfare of their own descendants? Rather than have to work through such tangles, Becker and Barro simply cut the Matrimonial Knot. One must qualify John Donne to describe properly the resulting analytical conception of human society on which this analysis is founded: "No man is an island . . . though, conveniently, every family is."

Why assume we have a can-opener?

A host of mathematically convenient but otherwise unsupported assumptions about people's tastes, and the range of actions open to them in matters affecting their children, have gone into the construction of the Becker–Barro model. They make little effort to justify these assumptions, or even to state them in less abstract terms that might invite discussion of their empirical relevance. This is a matter more of style than anything else, and it does not necessarily signify an absence of empirical correspondence between the model and the world we inhabit. Indeed, there is a sense in which one may read in Becker and Barro's mathematical specifications the emergent tastes and mores of a society that is coming to terms with below-replacement fertility. Consider the following psychosocial profile drawn from the utility function of a typical native, by an economic ethnographer recently returned from Becker–Barroland:

    1 These people are not their brothers' and sisters' keepers; they have not developed any taste for altruistic involvement with siblings, either as children or as adults. Presumably, it has been found there is little point to inculcating in them a virtue that will find scant occasion for expression.

    2 As parents, the Becker–Barrolanders are aware that they possess only a fixed emotional capability for deriving satisfaction from the well-being of their offspring, so the average degree of altruistic involvement they can have with any one child must decline as the number of their progeny rises. The quality of altruism toward children that has been cultivated in them is quite unlike "mercy," in that it definitely does become "strained." Perhaps this is due to their having so few children with whom to practice.

3 The grandparental role is much attenuated among these folk: they seem incapable of deriving any direct satisfactions from the existence of grandchildren, or from the happiness thereof. Indeed, they appear to have been thoroughly socialized never to complain of any deprivation regarding grandchildren, and insist that they care about having grandchildren only to the extent that their own children are made happier by having children of their own. (The Becker–Barrolanders' secret rites for ridding parents of all cravings for grandchildren are assigned great importance and are closely guarded from discovery by strangers.)

4 A taste for joint consumption activities, such as family meals and family vacations—in which the pleasure that loved ones are seen to be having serves to enhance one's own satisfactions from additional consumption—apparently is alien to the Becker–Barrolanders. On the other hand, the extra pleasure they take from the incremental consumption-satisfactions enjoyed by their grown-up children seems to be equally intense whether they themselves are starving or sated. (When asked to describe in the local dialect this absence of feelings of interdependence of kinfolk's consumption activities, our informant says that her utility function is additively separable into her own consumption and the utility she derives from the utility experienced by all her grown-up children.)

The fact that the people of Becker–Barroland have these particular taste patterns has a lot to do with the detailed dynamic properties of the fertility behavior the article describes. It is through these assumptions that the authors derive an objective function for the dynastic family head that turns out to be a *time-separable* function of the number of descendants and the rate of consumption maintained in every generation—and also one that *does not depend explicitly upon the fertility of any generation*. With a time-separable utility function, each generation's derived demands for consumption and for descendants will be determined with regard only to the prevailing shadow prices of those "goods" for the generation in question (and, of course, the marginal utility of wealth). This means that if any change were to reduce the number of descendants demanded, say, by the second generation, fertility would have to rise subsequently to restore the number of descendants to the level desired by the third, fourth, and later generations. Such is the implication, unless the cause of the original change persisted and so also altered the number of descendants demanded by later generations.

Because the desired consumption rate for any generation will not be affected directly by the fertility of that generation, or of any other, the dynamics of adjustment in the model are further simplified. Fertility becomes merely the mechanism through which utility-conveying descendants are accumulated. Thus the fertility rate needs to be adjusted only when the stock of descendants *desired* by a generation is out of alignment with the *actual* stock of descendants that otherwise would result—from the fertility-adjustments made by preceding generations.

One reason everything turns upon the adjustment of fertility levels in this analysis is that parents in Becker–Barroland lack any direct means of inducing a change in the consumption behavior of their offspring. Should they wish to increase their own vicarious satisfaction by having their children consume at a higher rate (as would be the case were the real interest rate to rise), they cannot give them income (inefficiently) in the form of goods that the youngsters might enjoy but otherwise would not buy for themselves, like the old car, or the season subscription to the opera. Nor can they dictate a pattern of consumption as a condition of a bequest. Since they have to treat all their identical children identically, they cannot even threaten to give the family fortune to the most spendthrift among their brood unless the rest agree to do their fair share of extra consuming. It's a tough thing to be an altruistic parent under such conditions. Their only open course is to have more kids, and spread the available bequest-wealth more thinly among them. In that way they each will have less fungible wealth to pass on to future generations, but the aggregate consumption rate among them will be higher—which is what the parents are trying to achieve.

The analytical results that derive from these special features of the model's objective function and constraints are not likely to survive a respecification, especially not a respecification of "tastes" that would recognize the direct interests of grandparents in their grandchildren, of children in the happiness of siblings, or the effects of one's close relatives' happiness upon the marginal utility derived from one's own consumption pursuits. But if we wait long enough at low fertility levels, the world increasingly may come to resemble Becker–Barroland. Then the tastes just mentioned, having ceased to command any social reinforcement, will be remembered only as obsolete cultural vestiges of a defunct demographic regime.

Is altruism toward children a cultural trait with low survival value?

Economic models are not supposed to replicate reality, but rather to assist us to think clearly about the greater complexities of reality. While ruthlessly stripping things down to bare essentials is the name of the game, not everything essential is simple. Such were the thoughts that formed in my mind when I found Becker and Barro (p. 74) saying, "We assume . . . parents ignore the uncertainty about child deaths. . . ." Were they to retain uncertainty in this analysis, would it still be the case that altruism supports the level of fertility— that the stronger is the degree of satisfaction parents take from their children's enjoyment of consumption, the more they would seek to enlarge their brood? Or will the dependence of one's happiness upon that of one's offspring be revealed as the real enemy of the procreative drive?

My simple thought was this: whether one regards children as commodities or as assets, they appear to be peculiarly characterized by risk. An irreducibly high proportionate variance surrounds both the costs they entail and the benefits they provide. To be sure, much of the variance associated with the illness and death of children has been reduced through medical progress. Contraceptive technology has been developed to the point of permitting people to pretty well control when the birth of a child will *not* occur. The costs of selecting against fetuses' carrying undesired genetic traits are likewise being reduced. But there remain obtrusive sources of risk emanating from imperfect control, and these risks appear to be hard for parents to insure against.

A brief catalogue will surely suffice to clarify my meaning. The stochastic nature of conception, and the risks of miscarriage, make production scheduling an uncertain affair. Genetic processes are not controlled sufficiently to allow people to mate selectively and produce offspring with specified attributes, although they may try. The rearing of youngsters has yet to be elevated to a dependable management science: "What did we do wrong?" is an expression of the fundamental uncertainty that overcomes parents, making it difficult for one generation to learn anything really useful from the evident mistakes of its predecessor. Moreover, success offers no haven from worry. Bringing into the world an independent, well-integrated child, with whom one develops strong bonds of affection, ultimately exposes the parent to an enormous range of positive and negative "externalities." One does go on worrying about the kids even when things are going well.

One would scarcely stop to remark upon these facts of life, were it not for the ever more obtrusive contrast between the uncertainties adhering to the range of child-related activities and the increasingly predictable, insurable, and controllable alternative ways of employing resources that are becoming available to people in the high-income societies of the West. The infinite chain of descendants, linked together by altruism in the model of Becker and Barro, has a distinctly unappealing cast when viewed from this vantage point. If the fortunes of successive generations within a lineage are significantly correlated, being indirectly "plugged in" to the utility states of all those descendants, extending far into the unknowable future, is positively scary.

Now, living with real scariness—measured by high variance relative to expected outcomes that one cares about, and not by the whiteness of one's knuckles during horror movies—is a condition I believe most people strive harder and harder to avoid as their real income rises. Relative certainty, the inverse of proportionate-variance, is a superior good in my model of our world. Indeed, because the demand for greater control over life's vicissitudes tends to grow more rapidly than the rise in real incomes, market incentives in the rich countries are channeling more and more resources into developing better control-technologies, information-technologies, and insurance devices—both private and governmental. Courts are now asked to provide recourse not only when the negligence of others leads to wrongful death, but equally when it results in unplanned, and thus "wrongful" birth—as in cases when vasectomies and tubal ligations fail to work. Social institutions also are adapting to the pressures for control over the terms of one's existence. Divorce has been made easier, for example, permitting exit from the quintessential condition in which individuals otherwise have to reconcile themselves to never being fully sure what is going to happen next. This has had the unfortunate side effect of increasing the uncertainties of parenthood, if only in the form of never being quite sure of the last names of one's daughter's children, or the first name of one's son's wife.

In his article in this volume, "The family that does not reproduce itself," Nathan Keyfitz has drawn attention to the unattractive aspects of childrearing as an occupation compared with other jobs. Parents continually are on call to cope with a wide range of problems that they find difficult to schedule, just like the old-fashioned general practitioner who made house calls, except without the signs of prestige and authority (not to mention the fees) that marked even the family doctor's dealings with patients. Keyfitz, extending the analogy by noticing the improvement in hours and working conditions that has accompanied the development of specialties within the practice of medicine, ends his article with a call for greater professionalization of childrearing.

I find Keyfitz's remarks responsive to the same problem on which I have focused; his proposal aims precisely at limiting some of the risks and uncertainties of the parenting role, rendering it a more "controllable" activity—at least on the input side. To deal with the output side, proceeding along the Keyfitz route, one would need also to provide cheap insurance against suits for *parental* malpractice. Yet, such palliatives at best can be of only limited help in dealing with the ineluctible difficulty: just as the persistence of parental altruism makes it impossible to "divorce" the kids (in the sense of throwing them out of one's utility function), so it must thwart efforts to transform parenthood into a state of professionalized, clinical detachment.

Thus, simply allowing uncertainty into the Becker–Barro model may yield a further reformulation, in which altruism toward children is suddenly revealed to be the root cause of the inexorable progress of populations toward below-replacement fertility. Altruism will prevent the risks connected with the business of accumulating descendants from being reduced *pari passus* with the risks surrounding other competing activities and assets. In the end, rational potential parents afflicted with this taste must try to confine their exposure to the narrowest possible span within the life cycle, unless they opt out of the perilous business entirely, to seek more certain satisfactions elsewhere.

And so, to close on the most pessimistic of notes, the main grounds for hope that the human species will escape voluntary, utility-maximizing extinction would not seem to reside in faster technological progress, but may rest with the possibility that altruism is a heritable trait. In that case, it would be purged from the gene pool through natural selection.

Note

While retaining full responsibility for the opinions expressed and for any mistakes made herein, the author acknowledges the perceptive comments and suggestions offered by Timothy Bresnahan, Tom MaCurdy, and John Pencavel. Clarifications supplied by Robert Barro and Gary Becker were helpful in revising an earlier version of these comments.

References

Barro, Robert J. 1974. "Are government bonds new wealth?," *Journal of Political Economy* 82, no. 6: 1095–1117.

———, and Gary S. Becker. 1985. "Population growth and economic growth," paper presented at the Workshop in Applications of Economics, University of Chicago.

Becker, Gary S. 1974. "A theory of social interactions," *Journal of Political Economy* 82, no. 6: 1063–1093.

Caldwell, John C. 1982. *Theory of Fertility Decline*. New York: Academic Press.

The Value and Allocation of Time in High-Income Countries: Implications for Fertility

T. Paul Schultz

Several sets of economic hypotheses have been proposed to account for the long-run decline in fertility in modern industrial societies. This article restates one of these theories, reviews some evidence bearing on its predictions, and considers the conditions that would, according to the theory, help forecast future levels of fertility in high-income countries such as the United States. The theory links the decline in fertility to the increase in real wages and to the increase in wages of women relative to those of men.

Let me indicate at the outset those issues I will consider here and those I will set aside. The issues selected for emphasis embody, I think, important constraints that affect long-run trends in aggregate fertility levels in high-income countries. Showing how these constraints may affect fertility levels is my first task; the second is to suggest the developments that have modified these constraints in the past and are likely to continue to influence them in the future.

This article will not attempt to separate the exogenous biological supply and endogenous behavioral demand factors in fertility determination; rather, my working assumption is that changes in the determinants of desired fertility dominate the overall level of fertility today, and, moreover, that this dominance of demand factors will become progressively greater in the future as birth control technology improves and becomes more widely available (Westoff, 1981; Pratt and Horn, 1985; Rosenzweig and T.P. Schultz, 1985a, b). Thus the neglect here of supply factors.

Another aspect of fertility neglected here is the timing of births and implicitly the timing of marriage and remarriage. Although this dynamic dimension of fertility is beginning to be studied by economists (Wolpin, 1984; Newman, 1985; Heckman, Hotz, and Walker, 1985), it is not central to this article. More research is needed to discover whether the onset of childbearing and resumption of childbearing upon remarriage are responsive to life cycle liquidity constraints or other economic conditions.

The juxtaposition of parental choices of the quantity of children and the human capital resource intensity (or quality) of children focuses attention on two central, and undoubtedly related, human behaviors that change with modern economic growth (Becker, 1960; T. W. Schultz, 1974). But despite our fascination with this empirical regularity across households between fertility and the resources parents provide each of their children (proxied generally by schooling), such parallel changes in family choices may arise for many reasons. Quantity and quality may interact in the budget constraint in the sense that the marginal cost of increasing quality depends on quantity and vice versa, as formulated by Gary Becker and Gregg Lewis (1974). But this specification is generally indistinguishable from conventional explanations that interpret the correlation between quantity and quality as evidence that the goods are substitutes in the usual sense (Rosenzweig and Wolpin, 1980). Economists (e.g., T. P. Schultz, 1983) and demographers (e.g., Caldwell, 1982) have yet to demonstrate a satisfactory causal explanation that arises from outside the household economy and is responsible for these two aspects of parents' investment strategy in children.

Two developments are assumed here to increase the relative price of children and hence decrease the number of children parents desire or demand. Under the first hypothesis, (1) if children are more time-intensive than the average consumption commodity, and (2) the real value of human time increases, then the price of children will increase relative to other goods, and some of these other cheaper goods will partially substitute for children in the parents' budget constraint, which is defined to include both time and goods.[1] The second hypothesis is also founded on a feature of production technology and a trend in prices: (1) if child care is more intensive in the mother's time than in the father's time, and (2) the value of women's time increases relative to the value of men's time, then children will be more expensive and fewer children will be sought. These secular trends in the relative prices of child inputs should also induce households to conserve on the increasingly costly inputs and rely more heavily on the progressively cheaper inputs (Mincer, 1963; Becker, 1965).

The first section to follow develops the household demand model, to define more precisely how the opportunity cost of time of men and women may affect fertility. US data are then used to estimate the relationship between fertility in the cross-section and the wage opportunities of husband and wife. A subsequent section reviews recent trends in education, wages, and labor force participation of men and women in several high-income countries. Finally, a framework is proposed to account for the changing relative educational attainment of women and men. As these fragmentary relationships are assembled into a consistent story, a clearer understanding should emerge of the causal dynamics underlying modern economic and demographic development.

The household demand framework

To structure the empirical analysis and make the assumptions underlying my two hypotheses explicit, it is convenient to start with the standard household demand framework. A couple is assumed to decide how many children to have over their lifetime based on their physical assets at marriage (A)—a vector of prices (P), wages (W), and asset returns (R). The utility of parents (U) depends on the enjoyment of two commodities: number of children (C) and other goods (G), the latter including investments in child "quality." Parents produce both commodities with known household technologies using their own time (T_w, T_h) and market goods (X), where the subscript w refers to the wife and h to the husband:

$$U = U(C,G)$$
$$C = C(T_{wc}, T_{hc}, X_c)$$
$$G = G(T_{wg}, T_{hg}, X_g)$$

The economic opportunities available to the parents are summarized in a full income (F) budget constraint:

$$F = W_w T + W_h T + V = Y + W_w(T - T_{wm}) + W_h(T - T_{hm})$$

where $V = RA$ is the return on the physical assets, Y is market income, and T is the total time available to each parent, which is the sum of time producing C and G and that supplied to the market labor force T_{jm}. Thus,

$$T = T_{jc} + T_{jg} + T_{jm} \quad \text{for } j = w \text{ and } h$$

The full income constraint can also be stated as the sum of the commodities produced and consumed by the parents valued in terms of the opportunity cost of the time and market good inputs used in their production (shadow prices π), if the household technology is assumed to be subject to constant returns to scale and there is no jointness between the production of C and G:

$$F = \pi_c C + \pi_g G$$

These last two technological assumptions of Becker's (1965) framework are needed if the shadow prices are to be treated as exogenous and consequently invariant across households in which parents vary in their output/consumption decision (Pollak and Wachter, 1975).

For numbers of children to be parent time-intensive means that the share of the opportunity cost of children due to parents' time inputs (s_{jc}) exceeds the parents' time input value share in other goods (s_{jg}), namely:

$$(T_{wc}W_w + T_{hc}W_h)/(\pi_c C) = (s_{wc} + s_{hc}) > (s_{wg} + s_{hg}) = (T_{wg}W_w + T_{hg}W_h)/(\pi_g G)$$

Analogously, for children to be more female time-intensive than male time-intensive means that the female time-intensity of children relative to that of the other consumption commodity exceeds the male time-intensity of children relative to the other commodity:

$$(s_{wc} - s_{wg}) > (s_{hc} - s_{hg})$$

The utility-maximizing demand of parents for numbers of children depends on the underlying exogenous variables in the model: wages, prices, endowments, and preferences. Preferences are generally set aside by economists because they are not objectively observed and are conventionally assumed to be uncorrelated with other exogenous variables:

$$C = D_c(W_w, W_h, V, P_g, P_c) \tag{1}$$

where P_g and P_c are the exogenous prices of the market inputs to the two basic commodities. While it is common to assume that market prices do not vary substantially in the cross-section, it is important to distinguish between variation in market-determined prices of children, which is exogenous, and variation in the resource intensity of parental investments or consumption expenditures on children, which reflects parents' choice and is therefore another endogenous variable.

The derivative of numbers of children demanded by parents with respect to wage rates and nonearned income can be expressed as a weighted combination of compensated price and income effects:

$$dC/dW_w = (C/W_w)(\eta^*_{c\pi_c}(s_{wc} - s_{wg}) + \eta_{cy}(W_w T_{wm}/Y)) \tag{2}$$

$$dC/dW_h = (C/W_h)(\eta^*_{c\pi_c}(s_{hc} - s_{hg}) + \eta_{cy}(W_h T_{hm}/Y)) \tag{3}$$

$$dC/dV = \eta_{cy}(C/Y) \tag{4}$$

where $\eta^*_{c\pi_c}$ is the income-compensated demand elasticity with respect to the full opportunity price of children, and η_{cy} is the market income elasticity of demand for children. Demand theory implies that the compensated own-price elasticity is negative. Some economists suspect that the income elasticity of demand for children is positive if appropriately defined (Becker and Lewis, 1974), but economic theory does not preclude wealthier parents' demanding to have fewer children and to invest more resources per child.

The empirical demand estimation equation for fertility is initially assumed to be linear, or, more specifically, semi-logarithmic in the wage parameters:

$$C_i = \beta_0 + \beta_1 \ln W_{wi} + \beta_2 \ln W_{hi} + \beta_3 V_i + e_i \tag{5}$$

where i indexes individual couples in the sample of observations on fertility, their permanent wages, and nonearned income, and e is a residual error due to many minor omitted factors and misspecifications of functional form, which is assumed independently distributed with respect to the other explanatory variables and symmetrically distributed.

The income elasticity of children is readily obtained from a regression of the form (5), $\eta_{cy} = \beta_3(Y/C)$. If the effects of price of time on the price of children are suitably captured by the husband's and wife's wage variables, then nonearned income will reflect merely an expansion of the parents' opportunities and may exert a small positive effect on fertility. The compensated price components of the wife's wage (w^*) and the husband's wage (h^*) can be constructed from the estimates of (5) and the sample mean values of fertility and market labor supply:

$$w^* = \eta^*_{c\pi_c}(s_{wc} - s_{wg}) = \beta_1/C - \beta_3 T_{wm}$$
$$h^* = \eta^*_{c\pi_c}(s_{hc} - s_{hg}) = \beta_2/C - \beta_3 T_{hm}$$

Our two hypotheses regarding time-intensity of children may now be empirically evaluated. For the time-intensity of children to exceed that of other goods, $w^* + h^* < 0$. This condition would hold if the sum of the uncompensated wage effects per child $((\beta_1 + \beta_2)/C)$ is negative and the income elasticity is either positive or, if negative, smaller than the sum of the previous wage effects. Empirical studies of fertility that have sought to estimate the distinctive effects of the wage opportunities for men and women generally find β_1 to be negative while β_2 tends to be negative in high-income urban populations and frequently positive in low-income agricultural populations (T. P. Schultz, 1981). Regardless of the sign of β_2, the absolute magnitude of β_1 generally exceeds that of β_2, and the fertility effect of nonearned income, β_3, is positive.

The second hypothesis—that children are female relative to male time-intensive—implies that $w^* - h^* < 0$. This is a more difficult condition to satisfy if the income elasticity is positive. The difference in the uncompensated wage/price effects per child (i.e., $(\beta_1 - \beta_2)/C$) must in this case be larger (negative) than the time-weighted difference in income effects (i.e., $\beta_3(T_{hm} - T_{wm})$). Thus, confirmation of the female relative to male time-intensity hypothesis requires more than the standard finding that the wife's uncompensated wage coefficient is more negative than the husband's. In other words, wages of men and women may increase by the same percentage, contributing to a reduction in fertility if $\beta_1 < \beta_2$, but this empirical regularity need not imply that children are more female than male time-intensive.

It would be useful, in addition, to have measures of market prices of basic child inputs, P_c, holding constant in some sense the quality or resource intensity of children (Lindert, 1980). But I know of no satisfactory proxies for such prices over time or across regions. Studies have attempted to calculate the cost of a child, but these investigations do not recognize that expenditures on children and the number of children parents have are to some degree jointly and simultaneously determined. Thus, when these studies hold constant for fertility and the wife's work behavior to calculate the expenditures on children (Espenshade, 1984), it is not clear how the estimates are to be interpreted. Existing measures of market expenditures on childrearing are determined not only by market prices, but also by parents' choosing their expenditure level to satisfy their own preferences. Exercises using demand systems to estimate compensating variations in income that appear to offset precisely the consumption "requirements" of an added child are merely more sophisticated ways of treating fertility and family composition as if they were exogenous (Deaton, 1982; Lazear and Michael, 1980). These studies do not permit us to infer expenditure "effects" of an added child, since they yield inconsistent estimates if parents influence their own fertility, and the distribution of children thereby becomes correlated with the tastes of the consumer.[2]

Fertility estimates: United States, 1967

To describe how fertility varies with wage opportunities of women and men in the United States, the reduced-form fertility equation (5) is estimated as suggested by the household demand framework. The data are from the 1967 Survey of Economic Opportunity (SEO), an augmented version of the Current Population Survey (CPS). Fertility regressions are reported in Table 1 for the 14,631 husband–wife families, stratified by age and race groups. Age is introduced as a linear control for differences in both the experiences of specific birth cohorts and variation in stage of their life cycle. Nonemployment income is the realized income flow from wealth and excludes work-conditioned public and private transfers such as unemployment, social security, pension, and welfare payments. These work-conditioned payments may be endogenous, since they may be administratively linked to family size or fertility, as well as to past and current labor force behavior.

A woman's realized wage is clearly a function of her past accumulation of labor market experience, and consequently it tends to be inversely related to her fertility and directly related to her life cycle investments in labor market skills. The realized hourly wage rate is, therefore, endogenous to the couple's reproductive choice or plans, or, in other words, the unexplained error in the fertility equation (5) is likely to be correlated with the wife's past, current, and anticipated labor market and human capital investment behavior. Exogenous instrumental variables are therefore used to predict a wage for each wife (and husband) based on an estimated semi-logarithmic hourly wage function that does not include as explanatory variables endogenous fertility, family composition, or labor market experience. It does include schooling, a quadratic in postschooling age, functional health disabilities, and local labor market characteristics in the residential region. (See T. P. Schultz, 1975 for more detail.) The predicted wage variables may be subject to selection bias, but experimentation with standard probit corrections (Heckman, 1979) for this

TABLE 1 Fertility regressions for US married women in 1967, by race and wife's age

Wife's age group	Log of predicted wage (dollars per hour) Wife	Log of predicted wage (dollars per hour) Husband	Nonearned income ($1000 per year)	Wife's age (years)	Intercept	F-statistic (sample size)	Dependent variable: children ever born (standard deviation)
Whites							
18–24	−1.80	.417	−.0814	.313	−5.42	87.8	1.13
	(13.4)	(3.06)	(−1.23)	(17.7)	(14.2)	(1209)	(1.06)
25–34	−2.10	.402	.0232	.144	−1.05	85.8	2.58
	(11.4)	(2.46)	(.51)	(13.7)	(3.07)	(2199)	(1.58)
35–44	−.888	−.371	−.0108	−.0243	4.92	20.4	3.04
	(3.42)	(2.30)	(.32)	(1.99)	(9.78)	(2980)	(1.92)
45–54	−1.37	−.270	−.00318	−.0373	5.45	28.5	2.62
	(5.66)	(2.40)	(.19)	(2.71)	(7.84)	(2651)	(2.05)
55–64	−1.50	−.623	−.0227	.0047	3.46	56.8	2.54
	(7.58)	(4.52)	(.83)	(.25)	(3.05)	(1689)	(2.28)
Blacks							
18–24	−2.34	1.13	1.89	.277	−4.57	26.7	1.91
	(6.47)	(3.31)	(.59)	(8.62)	(6.29)	(433)	(1.37)
25–34	−1.33	−.370	−4.60	.171	−.842	31.8	3.55
	(4.33)	(.99)	(1.59)	(4.33)	(1.02)	(807)	(2.39)
35–44	−1.76	−.631	−2.64	−.101	8.74	48.7	3.92
	(5.40)	(1.77)	(1.04)	(3.44)	(7.43)	(1161)	(3.05)
45–54	−1.10	−.942	1.72	−.121	9.78	25.7	3.09
	(2.95)	(2.53)	(1.03)	(3.55)	(5.83)	(937)	(3.12)
55–64	−1.85	−.273	1.47	−.0042	5.37	14.2	2.67
	(3.69)	(.61)	(.71)	(1.03)	(2.14)	(565)	(2.92)

NOTE: The absolute values of the t-statistics are shown in parentheses beneath the regression coefficients.
SOURCE: Calculated from the 1967 Survey of Economic Opportunity.

source of bias in the wage and fertility equations did not indicate that the bias was statistically significant.[3]

In every age and race regression the wife's predicted wage is negatively associated with fertility. The coefficient on the husband's predicted wage changes sign over the life cycle (or across birth cohorts), adding to the number of children ever born for younger wives—aged 18–34 for whites and 18–24 for blacks—but contributing to lower fertility among older wives. If this pattern in the age cross-section were to persist for a cohort over time, higher wages for husbands would encourage earlier childbearing, but the earlier onset of childbearing is counterbalanced by a much lower rate of childbearing at later ages. For white wives over age 35 and for black wives aged 35–54, a higher predicted husband's wage is significantly associated with lower completed fertility. The elasticities of fertility with respect to the wage rates of wives and husbands are of similar magnitude for blacks and whites, although for blacks the level of fertility is higher and wage levels are lower.

In no regression is the estimated effect of nonearned income on fertility statistically significantly different from zero at the 5 percent confidence level. Alternative net worth (stock) measures of potential nonearned income were substituted for the flow of nonearned income, but the explanatory power of the relationship was not improved. These estimates do not confirm that the timing of cumulative fertility or the completed number of children among currently married couples is affected substantially by nonearned or wealth income. This evidence supports the view that η_{cy} is essentially zero.

These estimates give credence to the hypothesis that children are time-intensive. In all age and race regressions the sum of the coefficients on the wife's and husband's wage rates is negative and increases generally for the older age groups. The hypothesis is most appropriately tested for these later age groups, since the model describes completed fertility and not the timing of childbearing. The adjustment for the income elasticity is small and, more often than not, negative. The hypothesis that children are more female than male time-intensive is also consistent with these estimates. The value of $w^* - h^*$ is always negative, but is smaller for older white cohorts and not particularly stable for older black cohorts.

In sum, cross-sectional linearized reduced-form fertility regressions from the late 1960s suggest that in the United States the standard technology assumptions advanced by the household demand model are reasonable. Although women's wages did not increase relative to men's from the 1950s to the early 1970s (O'Neill, 1985), equiproportional growth in real wages for both men and women could have been responsible for substantial declines in fertility at all ages. An increase in both spouses' real wage rates by 50 percent, as occurred from 1960 to 1980, is associated in these regressions with an average reduction in fertility of .6 to 1.2 children ever born. This large reduction in fertility would have been anticipated on the basis of the reported regression estimates and the actual US trends in male and female real wage levels. But if, as some economists forecast (Smith and Ward, 1985), female wages relative to male wages are likely to increase in the United States for the rest of this century, will US fertility continue to fall?

Wages and labor force behavior of women and men

The fertility consequences of change in real wages of women and men depend on a couple's allocation of their time among child care, housework (proxied by G), and market labor force participation, as summarized in equations (2) and (3). Data for high-income countries are currently insufficient to measure directly the difference in male and female time-intensities of children and other household commodities—or, in our notation, $s_{wc} - s_{wg}$ and $s_{hc} - s_{hg}$. But impressionistic evidence suggests that a gradual convergence in the time allocation patterns of men and women may be occurring. If this continues, one would anticipate that the fertility effects of male and female wages will also become more similar. The increasing value of women's time relative to men's should contribute to changing the relative household production roles of husbands and wives, and to a substitution of child care activities from the family to the marketplace. These adjustments in factor proportions within household production and the locus of production contain the seeds of change that should dampen the responsiveness of fertility to future increases in women's relative wage.

The record is much clearer when it comes to documenting the increasing share of women's time allocated to labor market activities (Mincer, 1962; Cain, 1966; Evenson, 1983). This change is particularly notable among married women and, most recently, among married women with preschool-age children. Since male participation rates have tended to drift downward slowly with secular increases in real wage levels, the ratio of female to male participation has often risen markedly, averaging an increase of about 60 percent from 1960 to 1980. Table 2 shows these tendencies in labor force participation rates for men and women after age 25, when schooling is generally completed, and before age 55, when retirement becomes evident for both men and women. Needless to say, there are still differences across countries and time periods that have influenced the level and rate of increase in women's labor force participation (Stafford, 1980; Davis and van den Oever, 1982; Evenson, 1983). In some countries, such as Japan, this reallocation of women's time to the market is entirely concealed in overall labor force statistics, because married women were frequently enumerated in previous periods as economically active in family businesses, such as small farms, and were therefore counted as unpaid family workers or self-employed. Thus, in countries such as Japan, the traditional family segment of the female labor force has contracted while wage and salary employment for women has expanded, leaving total participation rates temporarily unchanged (Hill, 1983).[4]

Women over the first half of the twentieth century have tended to get married earlier in high-income countries. And since married women have

TABLE 2 Market labor force participation rates for males and females aged 25–54: Selected high-income countries, 1960 and 1980

Country	Labor force participation rate (percent)				Ratio of female-to-male participation rates	
	Males		Females			
	1960	1980	1960	1980	1960	1980
Australia	97.9[a]	93.7[b]	26.7[a]	54.9[b]	.273[a]	.586[b]
Belgium	94.1[c]	n.a.	25.1[a]	n.a.	.266[a]	n.a.
Canada	96.3	94.8	30.6	60.1	.318	.634
Finland	95.7	88.5	56.8	77.6	.593	.877
France	96.3	96.4	45.1	63.0	.468	.654
West Germany	96.7	93.5	45.1	53.9	.466	.576
Greece	92.9[a,d]	89.6[d]	35.6[a,d]	36.7[d]	.384[a,d]	.410[d]
Ireland	97.3[a]	95.1	23.4[a]	28.4	.240[a]	.300
Italy	95.2	93.1	32.4	39.9	.340	.429
Japan	96.0	97.0	57.6	56.7	.600	.585
Netherlands	98.0	94.5[c]	17.2	42.5[c]	.175	.454[c]
New Zealand	98.2[a]	95.7[b]	24.9[a]	45.3[b]	.254[a]	.473[b]
Norway	96.9	95.0[c]	22.2	72.0[c]	.230	.758[c]
Portugal	96.5	94.6[b]	15.9	56.2[b]	.165	.594[b]
Spain	97.1	94.4[b]	16.2	32.7[c]	.167	.346[c]
Sweden	96.1	95.4	56.0	82.9	.583	.879
Switzerland	98.4	97.7	32.9	51.8	.334	.530
United Kingdom	98.1	96.9	40.4	63.6	.412	.656
United States	95.7	94.0	42.8	63.8	.447	.678

[a]1961. [b]1981. [c]1982. [d]ages 25 to 64.
n.a. = not available.
SOURCES: US Bureau of the Census, *Statistical Abstract of the United States 1982–83* (103rd ed.). Washington, D.C., 1983, Table 1534, p. 872; International Labour Office, *Yearbook of Labour Statistics 1982*, Geneva, 1983, Table 1; United Nations, *Demographic Yearbook 1964*, New York, 1965, Table 8; *Labour Force Statistics 1963–1983*, OECD, Paris, 1985.

historically participated less in the market labor force than single women, this secular change in marital status composition helps to explain why participation rates for married women can increase, while overall female participation rates remain more stable (Layard and Mincer, 1985). The shift of married women into market employment has occurred in some countries through acceptance of part-time jobs, the United Kingdom being an example. In the United States, on the other hand, the share of the female labor force in part-time jobs has been relatively stable for two decades.[5] The increase in hours that women have supplied to the labor market is not frequently reported, and it need not, thus, follow precisely the path of participation rates.

The overall trend toward increasing female participation in market labor force activity does not necessarily imply that female workers are accumulating labor market experience more rapidly than male workers. On the contrary, James Smith and Michael Ward (1985) and June O'Neill (1985) document that one reason for the stability of female relative to male wages in the United States since World War II was the tendency during the early postwar years for the accumulated work experience of women to decline relative to that of working men. The market wage opportunities available to the average woman in the population may have been increasing, as more women worked in the labor force for part of their lives. But a change in the experience composition of the women who worked concealed this fact. In the next decade this short-term compositional shift in experience of working women will have run its course, and the average experience of working women should begin to increase relative to that of working men, with implications for women's wages relative to men's.

The educational attainment of women in most societies is lower than that of men. The United States is an exception in this regard. White women born between 1856 and 1921 attained more schooling than white men in their birth cohort (Smith, 1984). This pattern reversed for men and women born between 1925 and 1954, with men attaining slightly more schooling than women. Although the differences in schooling of US men and women were small, changes in the average schooling of those women who decided to enter the labor force were more substantial. Here too, the educational level of women who worked during the 1950s and 1960s declined relative to that of all women, contributing to a compositional decline in the schooling of female workers relative to male workers (O'Neill, 1985; Smith and Ward, 1985). As the participation rate of women increases, changes in the educational composition of female workers relative to that of the female population are likely to diminish in importance.

Across a national labor market, wages of both men and women are strongly associated with their educational attainment, particularly when age or postschooling experience is held constant. Therefore, the tendency for women's educational attainment to increase relative to men's is a crucial factor in raising the market wage opportunities of women relative to men. Moreover, the process is self-reinforcing through its impact on female labor supply behavior, as illustrated in the estimates of Table 3 for US married women based on the same SEO sample used for the previous fertility estimates. An increase in market wage opportunities for women contributes to more women entering the labor force and working more hours (Smith, 1980). This outcome permits women to accumulate greater labor market experience and thereby to further increase their market wage opportunities (Mincer and Polachek, 1973). This tendency for male and female wages to converge relatively in the long run is likely to continue, but the speed of convergence remains uncertain, not only because of the cross-currents in compositional change noted earlier, but also because technologically determined derived demand for male and female labor may differ from country to country and over time as the composition of output changes during modern economic growth (T. P. Schultz, 1985b).

Increases in educational levels, particularly in female relative to male levels of schooling, have an important long-run bearing on female relative to male labor force participation ratios, and directly and indirectly influence female-to-male opportunity wage ratios. The educational levels that were taken as given in the preceding section's analysis of fertility, labor force participation, and wages in a US cross-section must, therefore, now be reexamined. To

TABLE 3 Linear probability estimates of wife's labor force participation: US married women in 1967, by race and age

Explanatory variable	Whites		Blacks	
	35–44	45–54	35–44	45–54
Wife's market wage[a]	.111	.168	1.07	.100
	(4.01)	(6.31)	(3.14)	(2.33)
Husband's market wage[a]	−.0787	−.0894	−.0390	−.0872
	(5.65)	(6.44)	(1.16)	(2.04)
Nonemployment income	−.00226	−.00142	.00851	−.00305
	(2.69)	(3.70)	(1.95)	(1.10)
Farm residence	−.149	−.165	−.181	−.319
	(4.28)	(4.94)	(2.77)	(4.50)
Wife's health disability	−.149	−.196	−.264	−.249
	(5.32)	(7.86)	(6.60)	(6.40)
Constant	.406	.383	.435	.585
	(9.49)	(8.68)	(7.93)	(9.47)
R^2	.0295	.0624	.0726	.0780
F (degrees of freedom)	17.97	34.23	17.77	14.32
	(5,2959)	(5,2570)	(5,1135)	(5,847)
Standard error of estimate	.465	.467	.481	.480
Sample size	2965	2576	1141	853
Sample mean of participation	.332	.366	.462	.451

NOTE: t-ratios are reported in parentheses beneath regression coefficients for comparative purposes but they are not unbiased. See T.P. Schultz, 1975 for comparably specified logistic estimates.
[a]Wage variables are endogenous and estimated by means of instrumental variables for participating persons: schooling, region of residence, experience, experience squared, farm residence, city size, and health disability (T. P. Schultz, 1975).
SOURCE: Calculated from the 1967 Survey of Economic Opportunity.

complete my story I need an initial cause, or the forcing developmental variables that might have set into motion in industrially advanced countries the secular decline in fertility along with the increase in women's market labor force participation. These forcing variables must be shown to determine investments in schooling and ultimately differential investments in the schooling of men and women.

Determinants of schooling of women and men

Simple specifications of the technical production function relating the inputs of the educational system to the output of school services can be combined with consumer demand relationships to explain the quantity of schooling that a population seeks. An explicit expression is thereby obtained for the factors that determine the equilibrium level of public educational services produced in terms of (1) the income of consumers, (2) the relative prices of school inputs to the public sector, and (3) various technological and demographic constraints that might influence the unit costs or consumer benefits of these services. This production demand framework, which has been employed to explain the level and distribution of national public expenditures on education, is used here to analyze female and male enrollment rates by schooling level (T. P. Schultz, 1985a). Public expenditures on all educational levels are expressed in constant 1970 local currency prices, and converted to US dollars according to prevailing average exchange rates in 1969–71, as reported by the International Monetary Fund.[6] To summarize the output of schooling services, gross enrollment ratios at all three school levels are aggregated.[7] Between these two measures of the financial input into the educational system per child and the quantitative output of years of schooling per child there lie several intervening links that may represent qualitative dimensions of public school expenditures per child. More specifically, the quality of schooling produced and the mix of factors used in the schools may adjust to the relative price of inputs entering the educational system and the productive values of more resource-intense years of schooling, as well as more years of schooling of a given quality.

The principal input to education is teacher salaries, which represent between 75 and 95 percent of the current expenses of national educational systems. The price of teachers will, therefore, be closely correlated with educational expenditures and, like any price, will be responsive to unexplained variations in the current demand for school services. Thus, the relative price of teachers is treated as an endogenous variable for the purpose of understanding the long-run determinants of the demand for educational services. The price of teachers is estimated by instrumental variables, where the instruments are ten-year lagged values of gross national product per adult, urbanization, and the secondary school enrollment rate. The previous production of secondary school graduates within the country provides the pool of trained personnel who could work as teachers, and, as anticipated, the size of this pool should be inversely related to current teacher salaries (T. P. Schultz, 1985a). The expenditures and enrollments of the educational system are thus regressed against real incomes per working-age adult (aged 15–65); the endogenous relative price of teachers; urbanization as a measure of population density, which is expected to reduce unit costs; and the proportion of the population of school age (ages 6–17), an indirect measure of population growth that could raise unit costs or erode benefits to providing schooling for an exceptionally large cohort of children.

Table 4 reports the estimates of the sex-specific enrollment rates and the public school expenditures per school-age child. The sample includes all countries with over one million population in 1984 for which all of the relevant variables could be obtained after 1960. The sample contained 67 countries, mostly observed in the 1970s, while several countries provided repeated observations at five- and ten-year intervals.

Income, not surprisingly, explains much of the international cross-sectional variation in schooling expenditures; the R^2 is .95. The income elasticity of public school expenditures is 1.35; a doubling of real incomes per adult is associated with an increase of 135 percent in real expenditures on schooling per child. An increase in the relative price of teachers lowers school

TABLE 4 School enrollments of women and men and expenditures on education: Cross-country regressions, 1960–80

Explanatory variable	Log of expected years enrolled[a]			Log of public expenditures on education per child aged 6–17 (1970 US$)
	Female	Male	Total	
GNP per adult (log of 1970 US$)	.510 (5.24)	.256 (3.98)	.351 (4.79)	1.35 (21.6)
Relative price of teachers to workers (log)[b]	−.916 (5.14)	−.690 (5.85)	−.793 (5.92)	−.156 (1.36)
Proportion of population urban	−.835 (2.01)	−.481 (1.75)	−.624 (1.99)	−.510 (1.91)
Proportion of population aged 6–17	1.46 (1.17)	.413 (.50)	.782 (.84)	−5.38 (6.75)
Intercept	−.543 (.63)	1.29 (2.26)	.631 (.97)	−3.38 (6.10)
R^2	.572	.548	.587	.942
Mean of dependent variable	1.71	2.02	1.89	3.89
(standard deviation)	(.726)	(.461)	(.550)	(1.44)

NOTE: Instrumental variable estimates with the absolute value of the asymptotic t-ratio are reported in parentheses below each regression coefficient. See T. P. Schultz (1985a) for description of data, derivation of model, comparison with alternative specifications, and estimation methods. Sample size is 133.
[a]The expected years enrolled is defined as six times the primary and secondary school enrollment ratios and five times the higher education enrollment ratio as reported by UNESCO. These ratios are based on six-, six-, and five-year population denominators.
[b]The relative price is endogenous and probably measured with error. It is estimated by instrumental variable methods where the instruments are gross national product per adult, urban proportion of the population, and the secondary school enrollment ratio, all measured ten years earlier.
SOURCES: Calculations based on a variety of data sources, including the World Bank data file and various issues of the *UNESCO Statistical Yearbook*.

expenditures slightly, but not by a statistically significant amount, whereas enrollments decline markedly and primary school teachers are used more intensively as average classroom size increases (T. P. Schultz, 1985a). With urbanization there is a small reduction in public school expenditures and enrollments, other things being equal. Rapid population growth that increases the share of the population of school age is not associated with a decline in enrollment rates, but public outlays per student in large birth cohorts do decline as classroom size increases and teacher salaries fall.

For the purpose of understanding the factors accounting for the increasing levels of schooling obtained by women, the estimates in Table 4 document the differential effect of income and teacher prices on female and male enrollment rates. The income elasticity of female enrollment is twice as large as that for males, .51 versus .26, and female enrollments are also more responsive to prices than are male enrollments, −.92 versus −.69. Evidence in this contemporary cross-section of countries suggests that rising real incomes and decreasing relative prices for schoolteachers have paralleled the advance of women's educational status relative to men's

Although the enrollment rates analyzed above are collected and published in relatively standardized form, comparable figures on educational attainment for adult populations by sex and age are not available. Years of schooling completed by age and sex can be estimated from certain national census tabulations, but these approximations depend on attributing an estimate of years of education to many special school categories, and hence may embody considerable errors. Nevertheless, these crude calculations for a few industrially advanced countries are presented for illustrative purposes in Table 5. The near parity in educational attainment of US men and women was already noted. This may be contrasted with the lower female-to-male ratio of educational attainment in more recently industrialized countries, such as Yugoslavia and Italy. The higher female-to-male educational attainment ratios for Finland, France, and Ireland remain a puzzle that is not explained by the general cross-sectional pattern illustrated in Table 4. But most estimates of educational attainment confirm the expected increase in female relative to male schooling

TABLE 5 Estimated educational levels for men and women in selected high-income countries

Country (year of census)	Female-to-male aggregated years of enrollment, 1970[a]	Female-to-male, years of education, by age			Years of education, males aged 35–44
		25–34	35–44	45–54	
Australia (1966)	.97	.98	.96	.96	8.90
Belgium (1970)	.96	.95	.96	.95	8.77
Canada (1976)	.96	.95	.95	.97	10.28
Finland (1970)	1.07	1.04	1.05	1.02	7.32
France (1975)	1.02	1.05	1.02	.99	7.63
Greece (1961)	.87	.86	.82	.78	6.14
Ireland (1966)	.99	1.03	1.03	1.03	6.62
Italy (1971)	.90	.84	.81	.76	6.00
Japan (1970)	.94	.92	.93	.93	10.55
Netherlands (1960)	.88	.97	.95	.96	8.22
New Zealand (1981)[b]	.95	1.01	.98	1.00	11.46
Norway (1970)	.99	.95	.92	.92	9.71
Portugal (1970)	.90	1.01	.99	.96	6.31
Spain (1970)	.90	1.00	1.02	1.01	6.28
Sweden (1970)	.98	1.01	.95	.93	7.83
Switzerland (1960)	.96	.94	.92	.92	7.20
United States (1970)	.96	.98	.98	.99	11.62
Yugoslavia (1971)	.90	.66	.60	.60	6.35

[a]Expected years of enrollment defined as six times the sum of gross enrollment rates at the primary and secondary levels plus five times the enrollment rates at the third level of schooling.
[b]Only the age group 25–44 is reported in the New Zealand census.
SOURCES: Enrollment data are from various issues of the UNESCO Statistical Yearbook; educational attainment data are taken from census tabulations reported in various issues of the United Nations Demographic Yearbook.

levels over the last three decades. A continuation of these trends should narrow any disadvantage women have in terms of education and will translate, over time, into a rise in the ratio of female-to-male wages, as more women enter and remain more permanently attached to the labor market.

Conclusions

The household demand framework assigns importance to the parent-specific time requirements of having (and enjoying) children and the distinct price effects of the opportunity value of women's and men's time in market and nonmarket production. The framework implies that if child care duties can be transferred to the market without loss of parental satisfaction, then the link between the opportunity value of the parents' time and the shadow price of children would be partially broken. Increasingly the family may use the market for specialized preschool child care and extended adolescent schooling. But this development is unlikely to prevent the opportunity cost of children from continuing to rise, though it may dampen the rate of increase. Fertility may not, therefore, rebound substantially and permanently from its current trough, though it may become less sensitive to women's wages for reasons indicated below. Intermittent periods of fertility increase can be expected, however, as the timing of fertility becomes subject to perfected methods of birth control. Moreover, below-replacement fertility could be a viable long-run national strategy, so long as there is excess demand for immigration into high-income countries and assimilation of immigrants can be accomplished without unacceptable social strains.

The household demand framework predicts that in traditional nuclear families, in which the wife specializes in nonmarket production activities, increases in the market wage opportunities for women relative to men will lead to downward pressure on desired fertility. But households will also attempt to substitute the male's time for the female's in some child care activities, and will transfer some of these child care duties and schooling functions to lower cost providers in the market. Thus, there are two forms of household adjustment that should diminish over time the sensitivity of fertility to the upward trend in women's wages. The reallocation of women's time from nonmarket to market work is clearly proceeding apace in virtually all high-income countries. Although more difficult to document, it is probably also true that men have assumed a moderately increased share of child care activities, if for no other reason than that much domestic child care is being transferred to the marketplace. Women's gains in education relative to men, also evident in many countries, must be a factor in the growth of women's wages relative to men's. With their increased participation in the market labor force, women have accumulated the market experience necessary to narrow their occupational separation from men, and this development should continue to narrow relative wage differences over the remainder of this century.

Cross-sectional differences in US fertility and labor force participation confirm some of these patterns in industrially advanced high-income countries. Many questions remain unanswered, however, and most data on economic and demographic characteristics of these populations remain unanalyzed for what answers they would yield. A linear reduced-form fertility equation was fit to 1967 data from the US Survey of Economic Opportunity for white and black married couples. Estimated coefficients on the wife's predicted wage are consistently more negative than the coefficient on the husband's predicted wage. These estimates were shown to be consistent with the hypothesis that children are both generally time-intensive and in particular female time-intensive.[8] The wife's labor force participation equation was also estimated from these data, to illustrate the strength of market opportunity-wage effects on labor force behavior. There was no evidence that nonemployment income or physical wealth increased fertility among US couples circa 1967. Nonhuman wealth may influence the timing of fertility, but it does not appear to be an important factor in the final size of US families. A single set of cross-sectional estimates of the fertility relationship such as these is only the start of the research required to confirm the usefulness of the household demand framework for interpreting fertility trends. The difference between the estimated coefficients on female and male predicted wages must now be shown to diminish in a predictable fashion as households substitute for mother's time in child care. This finding would lend support to the household demand framework. The next challenge would then be to account for time-series changes in fertility, and on this score the record of economic research is even more sparse.[9]

Finally, there remains the question of what has caused the secular convergence in educational investments in women and men. One straightforward explanation given above for this fundamental development stressed the growth in real incomes and the decline in the relative cost of teachers as affecting the level and composition of public and private expenditures on schooling. There is undoubtedly more to this trend than increasing income and lowering relative prices of schooling. Aversion to inequality within the family may increase with personal wealth, leading parents and society to demand schooling for girls and boys on a more equal basis. Certainly the increased expectation of life, the decreased share of that life needed to bear and rear children, and the capacity of household durables to reduce the time requirements of housework have all provided women with stronger economic incentives to invest in their market-specific training. Another source of this trend might be the change in the character of skills demanded by the modern industrial and service economy. For example, greater male than female physical stature may have commanded a larger wage premium in the labor market in the past than it does today, while skills in which females may have a comparative advantage are of increasing value today. But I would be cautious in assigning much weight to predisposing biological factors. Particular changes in the composition of US aggregate output in this century have been implicated in the increased derived demand for educated women workers, but these connections from the composition of output to women's schooling and market labor force participation need to be placed on a firmer analytical foundation and tested against data from a variety of countries (Fuchs, 1968; Goldin, 1983; T. P. Schultz, 1985b; Smith and Ward, 1985).

Tracking down the economic origin of the advance in women's schooling and market productivity relative to that of men should help in forecasting fertility trends. Nonetheless, it should come as no surprise that the family is an adaptable unit. The increasing value of women's time relative to men's, a relatively new development, is certain to motivate many individual and institutional accommodations; undoubtedly parental roles and household technology will adapt, and new opportunities for specialization in child care between the family and the market will be found. If the secular downturn in fertility in high-income countries halts, or even reverses, it will probably be due to these largely uncharted possibilities of factor and sectoral substitutions within the family and not to a reversal in the trend toward greater similarity in men's and women's labor market participation and wage rates.

Notes

The author appreciates the research assistance of Andrew Yuengert and the comments of J. Hotz, R. Lee, D. Meltzer, J. Newman, M. Rosenzweig, and K. Wolpin.

1 An aggregate counterpart to the increasing real value of time is the increasing share of national income received by labor. Kuznets (1959), the architect and analyst of national income statistics, assembled the evidence from many countries to show the tendency for labor's share of national income to increase with industrialization and modern economic growth. This pattern can be "explained" by functional specification of the aggregate production function (Solow, 1958), or in terms of the changing composition of output that favors with development the expansion of labor-intensive sectors, such as services, at the expense of capital-intensive sectors (Johnson, 1954), or in terms of increases in the relative share of human capital in the national stock of capital (T. W. Schultz, 1961).

2 What descriptive evidence one gleans from these studies of expenditures on children suggests that outlays per child in the United States have risen rapidly in recent years as fertility has declined. But they do not clarify the extent to which parents have managed to substitute childrearing from the family to the market. Reed and McIntosh (1972) report that the direct expenditures per child in 1969 dollars are estimated at $29,000 to $39,000 for urban families with low and moderate income levels. Reed and McIntosh estimate the opportunity cost of the mother's reduced time in the labor force as $20,000 for the first child and between $4,000 and $7,500 for subsequent children, depending on whether the children are born at two- or four-year intervals. The most recent calculation of direct expenditures to age 18, by Espenshade (1984) in 1981 dollars, ranges between $75,000 and $98,000 for low and high socioeconomic status husbands. Espenshade reports the additional cost of college education for the child at a public four-year college as $15,000 and at a private four-year college as $27,500 (1984, Table 5). The lack of parallel figures for the opportunity costs of the wife's time makes it difficult to even roughly compare these cost estimates over time. Has there been a substitution of market services for the wife's in the period that would have reduced the amount of time she withdrew from the labor force during her childrearing years? Has the share of income spent by parents per child on education increased or decreased? Even simple descriptive statistics are

not available on expenditures for and opportunity costs of children.

3 Almost a majority of the survey respondents report no nonearned income. Therefore, the logarithmic specification of this variable seemed inadvisable, because it would require one to fix some arbitrary minimum value below which the variable could not fall. The logarithmic specification with the minimum set at 1, 10, and 100 dollars per year did not yield in any race or age group a statistically significant regression coefficient for nonearned income at the 5 percent level. Hence, the arithmetic treatment of nonearned income is adopted here. The wage variables were predicted in a logarithmic earnings function and are thus reasonably predicted in logarithmic form here as a function of years of schooling, completed years of postschooling experience and experience squared, functional health disability, and whether the individual resided in an SMSA of two size classes, outside an SMSA, on a farm, or in the Southern Census region. The variables used in the wage prediction equations are described in T. P. Schultz (1975: Appendix A).

4 A similar pattern is noted by Durand (1975), who observes that female agricultural labor force participation rates vary widely across countries for no obvious reason. Much of this variation appears to be due to relatively arbitrary statistical conventions or cultural practices that lead to the enumeration or not of women as labor force participants when they work in family farming activity.

5 In the United Kingdom the proportion of women in the labor force who worked less than 30 hours per week increased from 5.2 percent in 1951 to 22.4 percent in 1981. See Layard and Mincer (1985: S-154).

6 Gross national product and public expenditures on education reported in constant local prices must be converted into common units. The conventional procedure adopted here is to use foreign exchange rates and express all monetary units in US dollars as of 1970. Alternatively, purchasing-power-parity price deflators constructed by Summers and Heston (1984) can be employed, in which case the estimated real income elasticity of enrollments is increased by about 15 percent.

7 See footnote a to Table 4 for the definition of expected number of years enrolled in school. It is a period-specific estimate of the number of years an average child could expect to be enrolled in school if enrollment ratios remained constant at today's levels. The data do not include years repeated and thus may not yield an approximation for the completed years of schooling reported in censuses.

8 Willis's (1974) fertility regression was estimated from the US 1960 census public-use sample of urban white once- and currently married women aged 35–64. The estimated specification omitted the squared terms implied by his model, but retained the interaction between the husband's predicted income at age 40 and the wife's years of education. At sample means, the elasticity of fertility with respect to husband's income is $-.067$, and the elasticity of fertility with respect to wife's education is $-.412$ (Table 3, p. 63). Converting the wife's education to a wage elasticity requires the proportionate wage effect of the wife's education. From analogous wage equations estimated for white, currently married women in the 1967 SEO, this effect is about .074. Consequently, we can approximate the elasticity of fertility with respect to the wife's wage in Willis's regression as $-.53 = -.0889/(.074 \times 2.265) = \beta/(dW/dE)\,(W)\,(C)$. The negative male income elasticity is about one-eighth the magnitude of the female wage elasticity, and both $w^* + h^* < 0$ and $w^* - h^* < 0$, confirming the general time-intensity of children and the female time-intensity of children, as hypothesized. Clearly, the ratio of female-to-male uncompensated wage effects is larger in the 1960 estimates than in the 1967 estimates, but many other features of these estimates also differ. Repeated estimates of fertility regressions are needed to confirm trends based on a common empirical specification and using both the linear and interactive approximations.

9 Butz and Ward (1979) are virtually alone in venturing to estimate a demand equation for fertility based on aggregate US time series. They regressed period fertility rates on a series for male median income and a special series representing female hourly earnings derived from an occupation-specific wage series for personal services from the US Bureau of Labor

Statistics. These quasi sex-specific wage series are interacted with the wives' labor force participation rate, which is viewed as simultaneously determined with fertility. Instrumental variable estimates of the fertility equation are identified on the basis of current and one-period-lagged values of the wage series. A distinct rise in the occupational wage series for women relative to men's incomes after 1962 parallels the decline in fertility and the rise in the proportion of wives working. The concurrent rise in female wages and the participation of wives could be consistent with the predominance of household responses to exogenous wage developments or, for that matter, with a change in tastes toward having a smaller family and more women working. To discount this latter possibility, women's wages must also be treated as an endogenous variable (T. P. Schultz, 1985b), which is determined in part by the past accumulation by women of market-relevant experience and education, and identified by an exogenous demand factor.

In sum, any interpretation of time series must explain what factors were responsible for male wages rising more rapidly than female wages in the 1950s, if they did, and for the reverse trend developing in later years, if it did. Only then is it possible to discriminate among competing hypotheses regarding the underlying causes of fertility trends and swings about these trends. The lack of an education/experience standardized wage series for women is a serious current limitation to time-series research on US fertility determinants.

References

Becker, G. S. 1960. "An economic analysis of fertility," in *Demographic and Economic Change in Developed Countries,* Universities-National Bureau Committee for Economic Research. Princeton: Princeton University Press, pp. 209–230.

———. 1965. "A theory of the allocation of time," *Economic Journal* 75, no. 3 (September): 493–517.

———, and G. Lewis. 1974. "Interaction between quantity and quality of labor," in *Economics of the Family: Marriage, Children and Human Capital,* ed. T. W. Schultz. Chicago: University of Chicago Press, pp. 81–90.

Butz, W. P., and M. P. Ward. 1979. "The emergence of countercyclical U.S. fertility," *American Economic Review* 69 no. 3 (June): 318–328.

Cain, G. 1966. *Married Women in the Labor Force.* Chicago: University of Chicago Press.

Caldwell, J. C. 1982. *Theory of Fertility Decline.* New York: Academic Press.

Davis, K., and P. van den Oever. 1982. "Demographic foundations of new sex roles," *Population and Development Review* 8 no. 3 (September): 495–512.

Deaton, A. 1982. "Inequality and needs: Some experimental results for Sri Lanka," in *Income Distribution and the Family,* ed. Y. Ben-Porath. Supplement to *Population and Development Review* 8: 35–49.

Durand, J. D. 1975. *The Labor Force in Economic Development.* Princeton: Princeton University Press.

Easterlin, R. A., R. A. Pollak, and M. L. Wachter. 1980. "Toward a more general economic model of fertility determination: Endogenous preferences and natural fertility," in *Population and Economic Change in Developing Countries,* ed. Richard A. Easterlin. Chicago: University of Chicago Press, pp. 81–149.

Espenshade, T. J. 1984. *Investing in Children: New Estimates of Parental Expenditures.* Washington, D. C.: Urban Institute Press.

Evenson, R. E. 1983. "The allocation of women's time: An international comparison," *Behavioral Science Research* 17, no. 3-4 (Spring-Summer): 193–215.

Fuchs, V. R. 1968. *The Service Economy.* New York: National Bureau of Economic Research (distributed by Columbia University Press).

Goldin, C. 1983. "The changing economic role of women," *Journal of Interdisciplinary History* 13, no. 4 (Spring): 707–733.

Heckman, J. J. 1979. "Sample bias as a specification error," *Econometrica* 47, no. 1 (January): 153–162.

———, V. J. Hotz, and J. R. Walker. 1985. "New evidence on the timing and spacing of birth," *American Economic Review* 75, no. 2 (May): 179–184.

Hill, M. A. 1983. "Female labor force participation in developing and developed countries: Consideration of the informal sector," *Review of Economics and Statistics* 65, no. 3 (August): 459–468.

Johnson, D. G. 1954. "The functional distribution of income in the United States, 1850–1952," *Review of Economics and Statistics* 34 (May): 173–182.

Kuznets, S. 1959. "Quantitative aspects of the economic growth of nations IV. Distribution of national income by factor shares," *Economic Development and Cultural Change* 7, Part II (April): 1–100.

Layard, R., and J. Mincer (eds.). 1985. "Trends in women's work, education and family building," *Journal of Labor Economics* 3, no. 1, Part 2 (January).

Lindert, P. H. 1980. "Child costs and economic development," in *Population and Economic Change in Developing Countries*, ed. R. A. Easterlin. Chicago: University of Chicago Press, pp. 5–69.

Lazear, E. P., and R. T. Michael. 1980. "Family size and the distribution of real per capita income," *American Economic Review* 70, no. 1 (March): 91–107.

Mincer, J. 1962. "Labor force participation of married women," in *Aspects of Labor Economics*, ed. H. G. Lewis, Universities-National Bureau Conference Series No. 14. Princeton: Princeton University Press.

———. 1963. "Opportunity costs and income effects," in *Measurement in Economics*, ed. C. Christ et al. Stanford: Stanford University Press.

———, and S. Polachek. 1973. "Family investment in human capital: Earnings of women," *Journal of Political Economy* 82, no. 2, Part 2: S76–S108.

Newman, J. 1985. "The use of dynamic fertility models," mimeo. Tulane University, New Orleans.

O'Neill, J. 1985. "The trend in male-female wage gap in the United States," *Journal of Labor Economics* 3, no. 1, Part 2 (January): S91–S116.

Pollak, R. A., and M. L. Wachter. 1975. "The relevance of the household production function and its implications for the allocation of time," *Journal of Political Economy* 83, no. 2: 255–278.

Pratt, W. F. and M. C. Horn. 1985. "Wanted and unwanted childbearing: United States, 1973–82," *NCHS Advance Data*, No. 108. Washington, D. C.: National Center for Health Statistics (May 9).

Reed, R. N., and S. McIntosh. 1972. "Costs of children," in *Economic Aspects of Population Change*, ed. Elliott R. Morss and Ritchie H. Reed, Commission on Population Growth and the American Future. Washington, D. C.: US Government Printing Office, pp. 333–350.

Rosenzweig, M. R., and T. P. Schultz. 1982. "The behavior of mothers as inputs to child health," in *Economic Aspects of Health*, ed. V. Fuchs. Chicago: University of Chicago Press.

———, and T. P. Schultz. 1985a. "The demand and supply of births: Fertility and its life cycle consequences," *American Economic Review* 75, no. 5 (December): 992–1015.

———, and T. P. Schultz. 1985b. "Schooling, information and nonmarket productivity: Contraception use and its effectiveness," Center Discussion Paper No. 490, Yale University Economic Growth Center (September).

———, and K. I. Wolpin. 1980. "Testing the quantity-quality fertility model: The use of twins as a natural experiment," *Econometrica* 48, no. 1: 227–240.

Schultz, T. P. 1975. *Estimating Labor Supply Functions for Married Women*. Santa Monica: The Rand Corporation. Reprinted in Smith (1980).

———. 1981. *Economics of Population*. Reading: Addison Wesley Publishing Company.

———. 1983. Review of John C. Caldwell, *Theory of Fertility Decline, Population and Development Review* 9, no. 1 (March): 161–168.
———. 1985a. "School expenditures and enrollments, 1960–1980: The effects of income, prices, and population growth," Center Discussion Paper No. 487, Yale University Economic Growth Center (July).
———. 1985b. "Changing world prices, women's wages, and the fertility transition: Sweden 1860–1910," *Journal of Political Economy* 93, no. 6 (December): 1126–1154.
Schultz, T. W. 1961. "Investment in human capital," *American Economic Review* 51, no. 1 (March): 1–17.
———. 1974. "Fertility and economic values," in *Economics of the Family*, ed. T. W. Schultz. Chicago: University of Chicago Press.
Smith, J. P. (ed.). 1980. *Female Labor Supply*. Princeton: Princeton University Press.
———. 1984. "Race and human capital," *American Economic Review* 74, no. 4 (September): 685–698.
———, and M. P. Ward. 1985. "Time series growth in the female labor force," *Journal of Labor Economics* 3, no. 1, Part 2 (January): 559–590.
Solow, R. M. 1958. "A skeptical note on the constancy of relative shares," *American Economic Review* 48, no. 4 (September): 618–632.
Stafford, F. P. 1980. "Women's use of time converging with men's," *Monthly Labor Review* 103: 57–59.
Summers, R., and A. Heston. 1984. "Improved international comparisons of real product and its composition, 1950–1980," *Review of Income and Wealth* 30, no. 2 (June): 207–262.
Westoff, C. F. 1981. "Planned and unplanned births in the US," *Family Planning Perspectives* 13, no. 2 (March/April): 70–73.
Wolpin, K. I. 1984. "An estimable dynamic stochastic model of fertility and child mortality," *Journal of Political Economy* 92, no. 3 (August): 852–874.
Willis, R. J. 1974. "Economic theory of fertility behavior," in *Economics of the Family*, ed. T. W. Schultz. Chicago: University of Chicago Press, pp. 25–75.

Comment: Ronald D. Lee

We have here the chance to contrast and discuss two theories—Richard Easterlin's relative income theory and that of the New Home Economics—and attempt to get at the fundamental similarities and differences between them. T. Paul Schultz's article has four parts: first, a presentation of a version of an economic approach to fertility and derivation of the demand equation for children; second, empirical estimates of the demand equation for children; third, theoretical and empirical analysis of female labor supply; and fourth, a consideration of the determinants of the driving force behind changing fertility and labor supply, namely rising educational attainment. I have comments on each of these sections, in order.

There are two points I want to make about the theoretical section. First, consider the role of education in these models. Although the value of time, typically measured by the wage rate, is the driving variable in the theory, in practice it is education that carries the weight, for wages cannot be used directly as observed, but must be imputed, and education is the principal instrument of imputation. My question is this: is education really an exogenous or predetermined variable here? The problem is not just that unplanned births may truncate the planned education of young women, although this effect may be quantitatively important. But more basically, it seems likely to me that young women formulate decisions about education jointly with decisions about their future work or career goals, their marriages, and their fertility. A girl who in high school chooses to take academic courses so as to be able to go on to college may well do so because she is envisaging a future life in which she has a job, marries late, and has few children. If this is so, then much of the association of fertility and education observed in the cross-section may be a mere collinearity of two endogenous variables.

My second point on the theory section is that I can make no sense of a production function for numbers of children, when characteristics of the children are not specified. Schultz has argued convincingly for excluding quality as a separate argument in the utility function, but leaving it out of the analysis causes very serious problems. Constraints on the production of simple numbers of children at the subsistence level hardly seem relevant, and I do not believe this is what is intended. But what does production of numbers of children entail, and how is it constrained? Surely at this point we would have to introduce a sociological concept of what constitutes an acceptable standard for resources devoted to childrearing—shades of Leibenstein and Duesenberry, not to mention Easterlin's hypothesis.

Now let me move on to the empirical estimation of the fertility demand equation. Let me repeat my caution about education in this context; the problem should be particularly severe in the cross-section. My other difficulty is with the independent variables used. The economic variables (wages and nonlabor income) all refer to the sample date, 1967. But the oldest age group considered is 55–64 in 1967 and was at mean reproductive ages in 1932. What is the relevance of 1967 data? Of course the problem is less severe for the younger cohorts, but nonetheless it remains for all of them to some degree.

On the positive side, I particularly liked the exercise of using the cross-sectional estimates of wage effects to predict the time series decline in fertility to be associated with the actual 50 percent increase in both male and female real wages between 1960 and 1980.

I will skip over the section on female labor supply, except to make two comments about the role of market provision of child care, which the article downplays on the grounds that child care provided by the market is also time intensive and so subject to the same consequences of trends in the value of time. First, this might be so for trends, but it won't be so in the cross-section, since the cost of child care is not very different for high-wage and low-wage women. Second, the economies of scale are so great in market child care, where one woman can care for four to six children, that the time costs are minimized. Therefore, more extensive use of child care may indeed alter the economics of fertility.

I turn now to the last section, dealing with changes in educational attainment, which are the "initial cause," in Schultz's words, "setting into motion" the changes in fertility and labor supply. This section reports on pathbreaking work on the demand for and supply of education. However, I was surprised at the treatment of secular changes in education here; it appears that education is treated as a sort of consumer good with a high income-elasticity whose demand is therefore driven by rising per capita income. I expected to see it treated here, as it has often been elsewhere, by others and by Schultz himself, as an investment decision in response to rising returns to education. The returns to education rise and stay high because of continuing technical progress, itself perhaps resulting from increased education. Thus the incentive to provide education for oneself or for one's children is that it increases the value of time, which is the same reason that it leads to subsequent reductions in fertility. Viewed in these terms, the ultimate cause of the secular rise in education and the value of time, on the one hand, and secular decline in fertility, on the other, remains unclear.

Competitive Human Markets, Interfamily Transfers, and Below-Replacement Fertility

Mikhail S. Bernstam

Fertility below replacement has been experienced in the last 15 years or so throughout the developed world. It exists in high-income countries of North America and Western Europe as well as in socialist countries with much lower income levels, including Cuba, Romania, and European populations of the Soviet Union. This article seeks possible common causes of low fertility in the area of interfamily transfers. Involuntary transfers of incomes and future opportunities of children occur between families and over age groups through the mechanisms of social security for the elderly, public education, and seniority of earnings and promotions on the labor market. It is argued here that such transfers in highly competitive modern societies may cause additional fertility reduction on the margin sufficient to reduce fertility below replacement.

The first section presents a microeconomic approach to fertility that combines the Chicago school analysis of the demand for children (Becker, 1981) with the relative income literature (Oppenheimer, 1982). A novel feature of this approach is that it focuses on relative opportunities of children from different families. A formal model of the race between children is presented in the appendix.

The second section presents cross-sectional and time series evidence from the United States and the Soviet Union of the age-specific fertility effects of various interfamily transfers. The United States and the Soviet Union have the two largest populations in the developed world. They differ vastly from each other in many socioeconomic respects but not in those respects described in this article. Other countries with fertility below replacement have similar systems of interfamily transfer arrangements (Soderstrom, 1983; Inkeles, 1986).

A competitive market approach to below-replacement fertility

In the economic literature on the family, marriage is treated as a process in the competitive market (Becker, 1981). A similar approach is applied here to reproduction. This approach follows from simple considerations that parents are concerned about the future of their children and that this future depends, among other things, on the expected conditions of labor markets. This means that the future of one's own children may depend on the levels of skill, training, education, and other human capital of the future labor force, and on the family backgrounds, biological endowments, and inherited nonhuman capital of other participants in the labor market. Thus, opportunities of one's own children, given their inherited and acquired income-earning capacities, may depend on opportunities of other children. In this sense, own children and other children may be called competitors. These competitors of own children may come from the preceding generations of children who are ready to enter the labor market and remain there over a significant part of the life cycle of own children. Competitors may also come from the concurrent generations. For the reasons just given, incomes both of the parents' generational peers and of older parents from the preceding generations may be relevant in planning the family strategy.

Parents' information about absolute and relative future opportunities of their children is grossly imperfect. One has to assume that their rational expectations are based on their current comparisons and some past income and opportunities dynamics. As parents anticipate relative opportunities for their children, they can decide whether to have children at all, when to have them sequentially, and how much to spend on each one in order to increase their relative opportunities. The eventual number of children will thus depend on the parents' expected lifetime income and their chosen anticipated expenditures per child. The latter, as already noted, depend also on the parents' assessment of the intensity of competition with other children on the competitive human market.

Correspondingly, various fertility levels can be treated as outcomes of a given level of competition for the future of own children between families with different incomes and backgrounds, and facing different prices of children's upbringing. This allows us to follow George Stigler and Gary Becker (1977) in dealing with the production function with stable preferences. Here it is the production of children who will succeed in life, given opportunities and backgrounds of other children on the market and incomes of other children's parents. To secure own children's success in relation to opportunities of other children, parents may be willing to bear greater than originally planned expenditures per child. This, in turn, may induce an additional substitution of the quality of children for their quantity within the family. Intensification of this process by some additional socioeconomic forces may lead to further fertility reductions.

The above-sketched approach is presented in the appendix as a formal model that sheds light on demographic transitions.[1]

Intensity of competition between children and fertility levels

One can briefly consider noncompetitive, moderately competitive, and highly competitive socioeconomic environments. The more closed and the more rudimentary are markets, the less economically mobile is the society, the lower are the average opportunities, and the lower is the competition between families. If there are virtually no labor markets outside the family household, as in an autarkic agrarian environment, competition between children may be confined within the family. The more open and diverse are markets, the higher is potential individual economic mobility, the more fluid is the society, the higher are individual opportunities, and the more likely competition between families for their children's future is intensive. In an open society, there is room for everyone as determined by level of biological endowments, luck, inherited wealth, and acquired human capital. Most parents, however, want their children to end up closer to the top than to the bottom and strive to increase the probability of such an outcome.

One can surmise that fertility levels are inversely related to the intensity of competition. Historically the development of private farming plus economically mobile and competitive environments led to demographic transition in France, the United States, Hungary, and some other areas before incomes increased and before industrialization and modernization took their course (Demeny, 1972; Cook and Repetto, 1982). The emergence of competitive markets for individual economic opportunities and the relaxation of the implicit price constraint of rigid socioeconomic barriers, rather than rising incomes and industrial development, seem to me to stand behind the early demographic transition. An elimination of competitive markets for human and nonhuman capital may lead to the reversal of that transition. One major example is the reverse movement from controlled fertility in rural Russia to fertility without parity-specific control that occurred in the 1920s when the rural commune with its land entitlements was restored and private land property and transactions were prohibited (Ptukha, 1960; Bernstam, 1986). I would submit that demographic transition need not be linear and thus need not imply an unlimited fertility decline. Otherwise, current fertility decline below replacement would not need further explanation beyond the transition's inherent linearity.

Moderately competitive environments mean that children's future is more or less predetermined over their life cycle, although some individual mobility outside the parental household may exist. The system of life cycle agricultural service and life cycle inheritance of tenancy rights, which prevailed in Northern and Western Europe until some time during the second half of the nineteenth century, is such an environment (Hajnal, 1982). This may partly explain why parity-specific control started later in more industrial England than in less industrial France.

One can safely claim that in the modern developed world parents and children operate in a highly competitive environment. Children's future depends heavily and often primarily on parental expenditure per child. In such an environment, fertility can be expected to be generally low. The crucial question for the present article concerns how low fertility declines in this setting. Put differently, the question is whether income elasticities of expenditures per child must always be so high that they render the effective income elasticity of the number of children negative. The model of the race between children suggests that parents increase fertility in response to a rise in *own* incomes, but they have to increase expenditures per child in response to rises in incomes of *other* parents and opportunities of other children in the competitive setting.

This approach has common implications with some of the findings of Becker (1981, p. 130) as well as with the fertility response to the cyclic course of relative income in the works of Richard Easterlin (1973, 1980) and Yoram Ben-Porath (1973, 1975). In the cyclic case I would reemphasize high relative opportunities of cohorts who entered the labor market after the cohorts that did so during the Great Depression in the United States. The same can be said about the children born to parents who benefited from the boom that followed the devastations of World War II in Western Europe. This would imply a one-time boom rather than a continuous self-generating demographic cycle.

When a highly competitive setting is well established and equal opportunities are provided for all in the economically highly mobile society, fertility levels should depend primarily on changes in incomes of different families. Suppose that incomes increase over time and over the life cycle of parents in the same way for different generations. In the long run, steady-state low fertility with increasing child qualities could emerge, subject to short-term fluctuations. Prolonged below-replacement fertility does not necessarily follow from a pure competitive setting, that is, if no additional forces intensify competition and induce incremental expenditures per child to increase faster than incomes.

Intensified competition and below-replacement fertility

So far, I have sketched the relationship of family incomes, child prices, and fertility under market conditions where the life cycle distribution of wealth follows some natural pattern of earnings and accumulation of human and nonhuman capital. But many societies have various transfers of incomes and opportunities of children between families over the life cycle of both parents and children. The traditional life cycle service system of Northern and Western Europe assured opportunities for children by securing their employment as farmhands before they inherited tenancy rights and then by helping them start their farming and reproduction (Hajnal, 1982). This contributed to lower child prices to the family and hence to higher fertility. This system, by implication, helped to secure safe early retirement of parents, who bequeathed their farm and tenancy to their children knowing that cheap agricultural servants from the next cohort would lower the cost of farming. Among families, the system can be considered as a form of social security. Another form of social security, the communal provision for the elderly from insolvent households, existed in the Russian rural commune. These forms of social security might have produced a positive fertility effect by reducing own savings and expenditures on children. However, the fertility effect of other forms of interfamily transfers over the life cycle may be negative.

Increasing the levels of mandatory education up to certain levels is one simplified example. Unless the difference between the costs of mandatory and nonmandatory education is financed by taxing only nonfecund individuals, more will be spent by all parents on the quality of the average child at a given average income level. The net demographic effect will be fewer, more expensive children, unless families reduce other components of their and their children's consumption. (I am not assessing this arrangement for financing education as an economic or social policy but only pointing out its fertility outcome.)

One can also look briefly at several other arrangements that are common to all countries with below-replacement fertility. I will focus here on social security for old age, public education, and earnings seniority in labor markets. All three are widely recognized as interfamily transfers between different generations. Their effects are many and often offsetting; several important works have studied their life cycle effects on incomes, opportunities, family welfare, and fertility behavior.[2] In the following, one has to distinguish between the life cycle effects and the fertility effects of these transfers. Over the life cycle, total individual wealth may be unchanged, but fertility decisions may be influenced at particular stages of the life cycle of parents.

A major aspect of social security, public education, and the earnings seniority system (hereafter, SS-PE-ES) is the transfer from young adults of prime childbearing ages to older adults whose children are school-aged. On the public education side, the benefit of this transfer increases with age while its financing does so to a lesser extent. Thus public education can be a net transfer from younger parents to older parents, hence subsidizing quality of older children. Public education also makes higher education more attractive, increasing enrollment and obtainment of higher degrees—but typically with a class bias favoring the better-off.[3] In addition to reducing prices of education—that is, child-quality unit prices—for parents of older children at the expense of younger families, public education induces more intense competition. When the average quality of children on the market increases, some younger parents have to hire tutors for the next cohort of children, opt for more expensive private schools, strive to enroll them into the top universities, and so on. Even when reimbursement is received at a later stage through public financing of higher education of own children, intensified competition might already have resulted in increased expenditures per child and reduced numbers. Public education may be socially beneficial by increasing the average level of human capital and thus contributing to economic growth and rising average incomes. Its negative fertility effect at a particular stage of the life cycle is postulated here, subject to empirical verification later in this article.

On the social security side, workers of all ages, including young parents, support the elderly. Without mandatory social security, most individual savings for own retirement and allocations for own parents are concentrated at the middle and later ages of workers. The mean age of the supporting population, in the absence of social security, is the mean age of retirees minus their mean age of childbearing, both adjusted for mortality. Under social security, the mean age of the supporting population is the mean age of the labor force. In the latter case, the mean age of the supporting population is roughly ten years lower than in the former. Part of the social security burden for middle-aged workers is alleviated by contributions of younger workers. Middle-aged parents can thus enhance the quality and income-earning capacities of their children. This may intensify competition for children's opportunities on the part of younger parents. Whether the later reimbursement from the next cohorts of workers will raise the net effect of these transfers on fertility to replacement level is, again, an empirical question. This will be tested in the next section.

In the case of a partially funded social security system, such as in Japan, only a portion of the transfers occurs between families (US Department of Health and Human Services, 1984). Nonetheless, individuals' mandatory transfers over their own life cycle can produce the same effect on fertility of parents of consecutive age groups as in the pay-as-you-go case. Middle-aged workers are relieved of the burden of supporting their parents' old age, while young adults are forced to save long in advance. This produces steep real after-tax income seniority, in addition to earnings seniority. Also, the employers' and the government's portions of the benefits are derived in the same manner as in the pay-as-you-go system.

The transfer effect of the labor market seniority of earnings and promotions is in the same direction as public education and social security. Although seniority often forces earlier retirement, firings, and the like, these usually occur after major expenditures on children are completed.

An additional reimbursement of younger parents can come from their own retired or middle-aged parents. Robert Barro (1974) made such a life cycle case for the United States. Additionally, much evidence from the Soviet Union and European countries suggests that young parents are to an extent compensated by their own middle-aged and elderly parents in terms of cash allowances, apartment purchases, and payments in kind (Blekher, 1979). Again, whether relative incomes of different cohorts are affected over the life cycle of children is an empirical question.

Generally, under the SS-PE-ES system, the possibility arises that incomes of parents increase over age and effective prices of their children decline, in both cases relative to the schedule of incomes and prices without such arrangements. This can enhance older children's opportunities, education, and various investments in their human and nonhuman capital beyond what would have been the case without the SS-PE-ES transfers. If so, the level of quality augmentation increases on the average over consecutive generations and at each given amount widens the opportunity gap between children of older and younger parents. Although reimbursements occur later in life for each generation at the expense of the next one, it is likely that a new intensive margin of child quality is produced each time. As a result, competition between parents for future opportunities for their children intensifies over consecutive generations. This additional quality augmentation may be beneficial for the society at large, for economic growth, and for individual children who are born in such a society, although some marginal children may not be born because of the child price caused by increases in these transfers.

Demographic responses to these developments may include postponement of first birth, with or without postponement of marriage, postponement of the entire age-specific fertility schedule, lower completed fertility, substitution of expenditures away from children, and, in extreme cases, childlessness. In terms of such aggregate demographic measures as total fertility and gross and net reproduction rates, this may mean additional declines. In a moderately competitive setting, such as in Soviet Central Asia, fertility may shift from very high to moderately high levels. In many less developed countries with tribal or caste systems, and thus with narrowly confined opportunities, existing interfamily transfer arrangements over age groups may produce a negligible effect. In highly developed market societies with diverse opportunities and high individual mobility, a marginally negative fertility effect of the SS-PE-ES interfamily transfers can reduce fertility to very low levels. If the race between families intensifies faster than can be compensated for by increases in income over time, a demographic depression may result even in the absence of economic depression.

It is an empirical question to what extent the SS-PE-ES system may intensify interfamily competition and reduce fertility, especially at prime childbearing ages, in a highly developed society. Elasticities of the demand for children with respect to the above interfamily transfers that are both negative and sufficiently high at prime fertile ages may explain the current below-replacement levels of fertility. This hypothesis is examined in the following section.

Tests and evidence

Several propositions must be tested and illustrated here. The first is whether the overall fertility effect of social security, public education, and earnings seniority is negative, holding other important socioeconomic influences constant. Second, one must check whether such an effect has a consistent age-specific pattern. The asserted pattern is that the negative effect must be increasing from older to earlier fertile ages or, conversely, be declining over the age-specific fertility schedule. One implication is, for example, that areas with lower interfamily transfers should have higher fertility at younger ages (e.g., 20–24) and relatively lower fertility at older ages (e.g., 30–34) than areas with higher transfers. If fertility declines rapidly from high levels in the newly emerged SS-PE-ES settings, the age pattern of the Coale–Trussell index of fertility control should be opposite to the conventional transitional pattern. In other words, the level of fertility control should decline, not increase, over age. Third, one has to look at whether the negative effect of the SS-PE-ES system is strong at prime fertile ages and whether the demand is sufficiently elastic in response to transfers to produce an overall depressing effect.[4]

Cross-sectional tests from US state-level data

Tables 1 and 2 present the results of regressing age-specific fertility rates for whites and blacks in the 50 US states against social security benefits relative to men's mean real incomes at ages 25–34, public education expenditures per pupil relative to the same incomes, various measures of men's relative incomes, and a host of other variables. The data, unless otherwise specified, were derived from the US decennial censuses of 1970 and 1980 (US Bureau of the Census, 1970, 1980).[5] Due to their collinearity, the public education and social security variables were used in separate but otherwise identical equations.

Dependent variables are specially derived white and black fertility rates at ages 15–19, 20–24, 25–29, and 30–34 that are taken as approximations of individual demand for children at those ages. Bernstam and Peter Swan (1986) argued that in the United States, the Soviet Union, and some other countries marital and illegitimate fertility have different demand functions and are complements rather than substitutes. In accordance with this proposition, illegitimate births and mothers of illegitimate children were excluded in calculating the demand variable for the present text. Thus marital births over the total number of women less out-of-wedlock mothers in a given state in a given year constitute the dependent variables.[6] This choice of the dependent variable implies that decisions to marry, to produce a child while being married, and to delay or forgo childbearing are treated as simultaneous at each given age. Although marital fertility may not be below replacement, the demand for marriage and marital childbearing are below certain levels that would secure overall replacement.

The *public education* variable is the ratio of the per pupil expenditure on public education in a given state to men's average income at ages 25–34.[7] Higher education was not included in educational expenditure because students at that level often enroll in other states. The *soc. sec. income* variable is the ratio of the average old-age social security benefits in a given state to the above denominator.[8] This variable is a proxy for the transfer from young workers to middle-aged workers as the former may be relieving the latter of part of the burden of supporting social security, hence its expected negative fertility effect. The *soc. sec. particip.* variable is the social security participation rate at ages 65 and over.[9] It allows for the alternative hypothesis of the old-age security motive in producing children; it is often argued that social security arrangements negatively affect fertility because parents do not need as many children when old-age support is provided from nonfamily sources. The *rel. income by education* variable is the ratio of incomes of male college graduates to male high

TABLE 1 Elasticities of age-specific fertility rates with respect to various measures of interfamily transfers and labor market variables: US whites and blacks, 1970 and 1980

Dependent variables	Age-specific fertility rates (excluding illegitimate births)							
	Age 15–19	Age 15–19	Age 20–24	Age 20–24	Age 25–29	Age 25–29	Age 30–34	Age 30–34
Independent variables								
Constant	4.085	2.980	4.613	3.927	6.209*	3.749	−0.516	−2.380
	(1.285)	(1.049)	(1.801)	(1.814)	(2.853)	(1.582)	(−0.123)	(−0.513)
Public education	−0.836*		−0.357*		−0.284*		−0.271	
	(−6.320)		(−2.707)		(−3.581)		(−1.883)	
Soc. sec. income		−1.929*		−0.860*		−0.664*		−0.576**
		(−6.535)		(−3.601)		(−4.568)		(−2.272)
Soc. sec. particip.	−1.508**	−0.891	−0.145	0.244	0.686	0.783**	0.771	0.790
	(−2.273)	(−1.432)	(−0.297)	(0.532)	(1.635)	(1.968)	(1.345)	(1.443)
Rel. income by education	0.469	0.793*	−0.155	0.076	−0.234	−0.148		
	(1.327)	(2.635)	(−0.565)	(0.289)	(−1.064)	(−0.714)		
Rel. income 18–24	1.861*	2.630*	0.254	0.737**				
	(5.590)	(7.108)	(0.806)	(2.077)				
Rel. income 25–34					−0.792*	−0.109	0.212	0.866
					(−3.110)	(−0.339)	(0.418)	(1.198)
Rel. cohort size 15–24	−0.483**	0.384						
	(−2.073)	(1.359)						
Rel. cohort size 20–29			0.013	0.164	0.022	0.145		
			(0.060)	(0.699)	(0.152)	(1.017)		
Rel. cohort size 30–39							0.019	0.084
							(0.062)	(0.303)
Female emp. 20–24	0.400	0.081	0.250	−0.073				
	(1.694)	(0.302)	(1.234)	(−0.343)				
Female emp. 25–29					−0.034	0.033		
					(−0.261)	(0.251)		
Female emp. 30–34							0.251	0.243
							(1.576)	(1.765)
Year dummy 1980	−0.735*	−0.095	−0.424*	0.216**	−0.336*	−0.139	−0.207	−0.033
	(−8.643)	(−0.648)	(−6.279)	(−2.287)	(−5.794)	(−1.859)	(−1.560)	(−0.181)
$\bar{R}^2$	0.701	0.714	0.483	0.515	0.520	0.560	0.113	0.146
N	154	154	154	154	154	154	165	165

NOTE: Eight age-specific fertility equations represent different model specifications.
t-statistics are in parentheses and computed on the basis of heteroskedastic-consistent standard errors.
* significant at .01 level.
** significant at .05 level.

TABLE 2 Elasticities of age-specific fertility rates with respect to various measures of dynamic relative income, interfamily transfers and labor market variables, US whites and blacks, 1980

Dependent variables	Age-specific fertility rates (excluding illegitimate births)											
Independent variables	Age 15–19	Age 15–19	Age 20–24	Age 20–24	Age 20–24	Age 20–24	Age 25–29	Age 25–29	Age 25–29	Age 25–29	Age 30–34	Age 30–34
Constant	8.541** (2.156)	13.688** (2.577)	−3.403 (−1.142)	−4.837 (−1.655)	−1.571 (−0.442)	−3.850 (−1.011)	−5.744 (−1.980)	−2.792 (−0.908)	−4.051 (−1.577)	−1.461 (−0.539)	4.565 (1.359)	3.835 (1.007)
Public education	−1.004* (−8.391)		−0.300** (−2.584)	−0.244** (−2.102)			−0.194* (−3.271)	−0.231* (−3.359)			0.007 (0.083)	
Soc. sec. income		−1.791* (−5.362)			−0.917** (−4.745)	−0.580** (−2.018)			−0.607* (−2.966)	−0.788** (−3.846)		−0.163 (−0.626)
Soc. sec. particip.	−0.286 (−0.313)	0.635 (−0.607)	2.098* (3.087)	2.292* (3.387)	2.259* (2.442)	2.453* (2.710)	2.217* (3.528)	1.259 (1.965)	2.165** (3.701)	1.153** (2.368)	0.079 (0.123)	0.332 (0.401)
Dynamic rel. inc. 1	1.556* (4.216)	1.322* (3.599)	0.988* (2.952)	0.766** (2.373)								
Dynamic rel. inc. 2				1.400* (4.925)		1.305* (3.474)	1.171* (7.846)		0.878* (3.833)			
Dynamic rel. inc. 3								1.052* (5.998)		0.628** (2.632)	0.673** (3.679)	0.577** (2.296)
Rel. income by education	1.030* (3.042)	0.829** (2.288)	0.293 (0.801)	0.263 (0.865)	0.279 (0.966)	0.283 (1.081)	0.173 (0.816)	−0.107 (−0.437)	0.140 (0.585)	−0.055 (−0.211)	0.024 (0.088)	0.081 (0.284)
Rel. income cohort 18–24	−0.436 (−1.139)	−0.089 (−0.293)	−0.193 (−0.647)	0.012 (0.075)	0.023 (0.079)	0.130 (0.706)						
Rel. income cohort 25–34							−0.410 (−1.933)	−0.602* (−2.810)	−0.218 (−1.050)	−0.277 (−1.263)	−0.435* (−2.997)	−0.328 (−1.320)
Rel. cohort size 15–24	−0.762 (−1.606)	−0.063 (−0.130)	−0.261 (−0.995)	−0.317 (−1.348)								
Rel. cohort size 20–29					0.143 (0.568)	−0.147 (−0.467)	−0.111 (−0.521)	−0.090 (−0.354)	0.083 (0.505)	0.183 (0.911)		
Rel. cohort size 30–39											0.830 (1.595)	0.802 (1.573)
Female emp. 20–24	−0.178 (−0.526)	−0.223 (−0.543)	−0.037 (−0.154)	−0.059 (−0.296)	−0.119 (−0.517)	−0.139 (−0.602)						
Female emp. 25–29							0.193 (1.123)	0.434** (2.448)	0.204 (1.194)	0.365** (2.234)		
Female emp. 30–34											−0.363 (−1.173)	−0.310 (−0.952)
$\bar{R}^2$	0.727	0.651	0.338	0.399	0.364	0.401	0.629	0.546	0.655	0.594	0.263	0.268
$N = 88$												

NOTE: Twelve age-specific fertility equations represent different model specifications.
t-statistics are in parentheses and computed on the basis of heteroskedastic-consistent standard errors. * significant at .01 level. ** significant at .05 level.

school graduates, both at ages 25–34. This variable could allow for the fertility impact of the rates of return on education. The *rel. income 18–24* and *25–34* variables are the ratios of men's mean real incomes in a specified age group to such incomes at ages 25–34 and 35–44, respectively. This is a relative income variable discussed in the relevant literature (Oppenheimer, 1982). The *rel. income cohort 18–24* and *25–34* variables are the ratios of men's mean real incomes at specified ages in 1980 to men's mean real income at ages ten years older in 1970 in a given state. This is a proxy for the individual current income relative to that of the family of origin. The *rel. cohort size 15–24, 20–29*, and *30–39* variables are the ratios of the size of the male cohort of specified ages to male cohorts ten years older in a given year. This is a relative labor supply variable with possible negative impacts on relative incomes and fertility (Easterlin, 1973, 1980). The *female emp. 20–24, 25–29*, and *30–34* variables are female employment-to-population ratios at specified ages.

The *dynamic rel. inc. 1, 2*, and *3* variables (tested for 1980 only, due to limitation of comparable data) in Table 2 are devised to test the impact of relative opportunities of children, via relative incomes of their parents who belong to different cohorts and age groups. All comparisons are with men's mean incomes in constant dollars. Form 2 is the ratio of men's income at ages 18–24 in 1980 to men's income at the same ages in 1970. This is supposed to approximate the expenditures available for newly planned children of young parents relative to the expenditures that were available for an older group of children, that is for competitors. Form 1 takes men's income at ages 18–24 in 1980 and relates it to the square root of the product of men's income at ages 18–24 in 1970 and at ages 25–34 in 1980. Form 3 applies the same procedure to incomes of men aged 25–34 in 1980 relating them to men aged 25–34 in 1970 and 35–44 in 1980. This variable is meant to account for simultaneous competition of young parents with the same cohort of older parents in the latter's income dynamics. This is the competition for the economic future of respective cohorts of children. Forms 1 and 3 of the dynamic relative income variables also approximate the influence of earnings seniority in dynamic perspective.[10]

Commenting on Tables 1 and 2, I shall focus only on the three main variables whose influence was posited earlier. These are social security income, public education expenditure, and various indicators of relative income over generations. All these variables are meant to estimate the influence of interfamily transfers and relative opportunities of children in the competition between families. (Other independent variables did not show consistent influences, although some findings are interesting.) In 20 equations, coefficients of these main variables have predicted signs and are significant at the 1 percent or 5 percent levels, except for some regressions at ages 30–34. Negative coefficients of the social security income and public education expenditures and positive coefficients of my dynamic relative income variables (relating opportunities of own children to those of others) were highest at ages 15–19 and declined gradually at ages 20–24 and 25–29. At ages 30–34 coefficients were low and often not statistically significant.

If one is to trust these regressions, both social security transfers and public education expenditures per pupil have a strong negative effect on fertility at ages up to 30. High economic position of parents and children of preceding cohorts relative to given cohorts of earners also has a very strong negative relationship to fertility (or, conversely, as presented in the tables, own incomes relative to those of predecessors and competitors in reproductive dynamics have a strong positive relationship to fertility).

One of the most important features of these equations is the consistency with which the postulated effects of interfamily transfers and relative opportunities affect the age-specific pattern. The effects increase from older to younger ages of fertility at a steady pace. Fertility elasticities are especially high at ages 15–19, high at ages 20–24, and moderately high at ages 25–29, except for expenditures on public education. On the average, high elasticities at prime fertile ages imply in the cross-section that, for example, a 10 percent increase in social security benefits (holding earned incomes constant) may induce a 6–9 percent decline in fertility. The same 10 percent increase in public education expenditures per pupil may induce a 3 percent decline in fertility. Declining relative incomes of young men have an even stronger effect, with the average of about a 10 percent decline in fertility in response to a 10 percent decline in dynamic relative incomes. A time series of this kind is probably too short to be robustly tested. If, however, cross-sectional findings can be taken at face value, they suggest that a significant portion of the below-replacement decline may be accounted for by the interfamily transfers of incomes and their effects on child opportunities as seen by parents.

An additional illustration based on the US cross-sectional data

It was said earlier that under interfamily transfers one would expect fertility to be higher at younger ages in the areas with lower transfers and higher at older ages in the areas with higher transfers. The latter is possible if older parents are better-off in terms of opportunities for their children relative to those of younger parents than without transfers. From this perspective one can look at the overall fertility rates at ages 20–24 and 30–34 in the US states with relatively high and relatively low interfamily transfers. Those are Northeastern states and Southern states, respectively.[11] Table 3 shows that, with a very few exceptions in some age groups in some states, fertility among whites at ages 20–24 is higher in the South and at ages 30–34 was higher in 1980 in the North.[12] The regional average rates were 90.7 per thousand in the North versus 126.1 per thousand in the South at ages 20–24 and 55.5 per thousand in the South versus 62.7 per thousand in the North at ages 30–34. Such an age-specific reversal of relative regional fertility cannot be observed from the 1940 data listed in columns 1–2. This seems to be rather a recent phenomenon. It may be indicative that at ages 20–24 fertility was the lowest in 1980 in such states as New York, New Jersey, Massachusetts, and Connecticut and was the highest at ages 30–34 in the same states. There may be, of course, numerous

TABLE 3 Fertility rates per 1,000 women among whites at ages 20–24 and 30–34, US Northeastern and Southern states, 1940 and 1980

	1940		1980	
	Age 20–24	Age 30–34	Age 20–24	Age 30–34
Northeast	100.9	81.1	90.7	62.7
Connecticut	89.0	79.8	76.4	64.2
Maine	155.8	86.4	122.1	50.3
Massachusetts	93.7	87.0	74.6	62.7
Michigan	146.1	85.1	110.9	58.9
New Hampshire	136.5	85.2	108.1	56.7
New Jersey	87.6	73.3	79.8	69.2
New York	88.9	75.8	86.1	68.0
Pennsylvania	117.1	78.9	94.2	59.3
Rhode Island	90.7	84.6	86.6	55.5
Vermont	157.4	102.8	104.5	59.5
South	160.1	94.5	126.1	55.5
Alabama	160.5	99.9	116.7	47.3
Arkansas	178.8	101.9	134.6	45.4
Delaware	117.1	76.3	98.9	55.4
Georgia	150.2	92.8	111.9	52.2
Kentucky	183.4	113.6	123.5	50.1
Louisiana	157.9	85.4	130.1	59.5
Mississippi	153.7	95.4	128.3	52.8
North Carolina	154.6	101.0	97.9	46.8
Oklahoma	163.9	85.5	136.3	49.3
South Carolina	164.0	101.9	107.3	49.6
Tennessee	160.9	100.6	109.5	46.8
Texas	159.6	88.8	151.0	72.9
West Virginia	180.6	105.7	125.4	46.7

SOURCES: 1940: US National Center for Health Statistics, Robert D. Grove and Alice M. Hetzel. *Vital Statistics Rates in the United States 1940–1960*. Washington, D.C.: US Government Printing Office, pp. 150–161.
1980: Births: US National Center for Health Statistics, *Vital Statistics of the United States*, Vol. 1, *Natality*, 1980, Washington, D.C.: US Government Printing Office, 1984. Women: US Bureau of the Census, *Census of Population: 1980, Detailed Characteristics, State Summaries*, Washington, D.C.: US Government Printing Office.

other economic and cultural reasons for this pattern, which reflects, among other things, postponement of births. The pattern is, however, consistent with the findings in the regressions in Tables 1 and 2 where I controlled for many other possible influences.

United States time series plots

The same social security and public education expenditure variables that were used in regression equations in Tables 1 and 2 can be plotted against the same age-specific fertility variables for the United States as a whole over time. Figures 1, 2, and 3 present such time series plots for the period 1960–83.[13] For presentational purposes I reversed the ratios used in the regression tables. Here men's mean real incomes at ages 25–34 were divided by social security

FIGURE 1 Marital fertility at ages 15–19, relative social security benefits, and relative public education expenditures, United States, whites, 1960–83

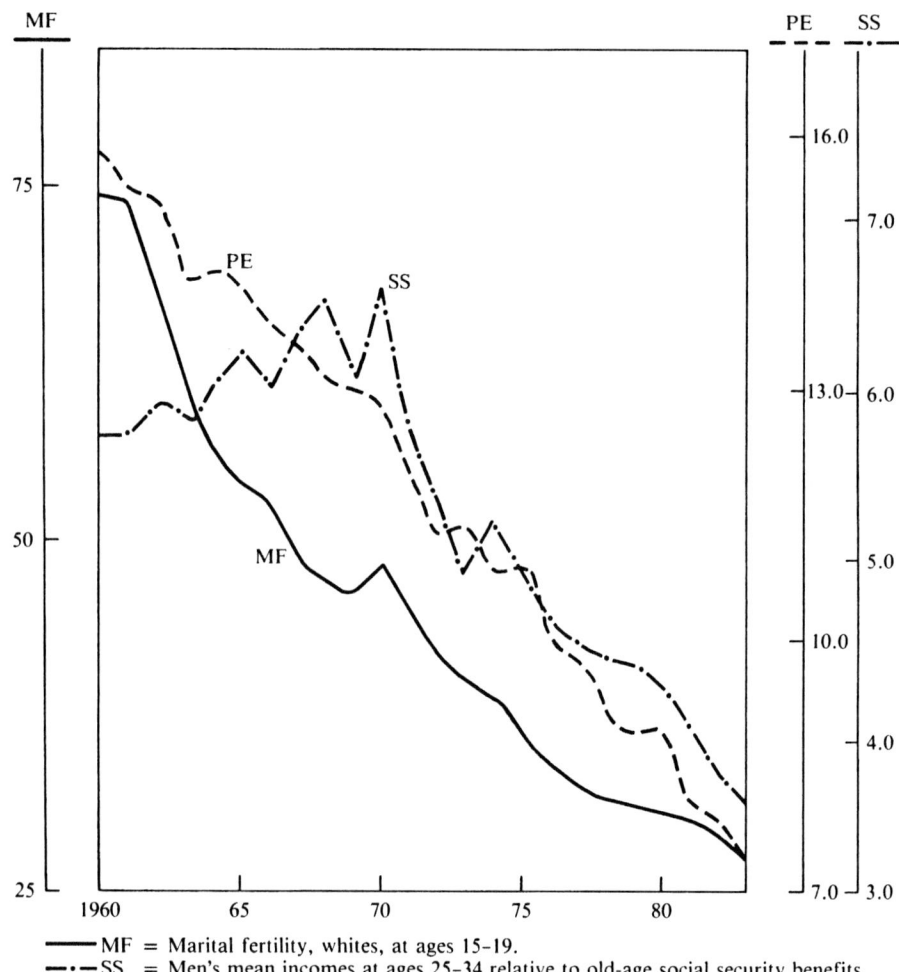

———— MF = Marital fertility, whites, at ages 15–19.
—·— SS = Men's mean incomes at ages 25–34 relative to old-age social security benefits.
– – – PE = Men's mean incomes at ages 25–34 relative to per pupil public education expenditures.

NOTE: Income, social security, and public education measures are from one year earlier.
SOURCES: See note 13.

benefits or by public education expenditures. Marital fertility rates for whites at ages 15–19, 20–24, and 25–29 are used (marital births are related to all women in a given age group, excluding out-of-wedlock mothers). The same rates for blacks (not shown) indicate similar patterns since the late 1960s. Fertility was plotted with a one-year lag with respect to economic variables; the dates relate to fertility. All three plots show a reasonably close relationship

FIGURE 2 Marital fertility at ages 20–24, relative social security benefits, and relative public education expenditures, United States, whites, 1960–83

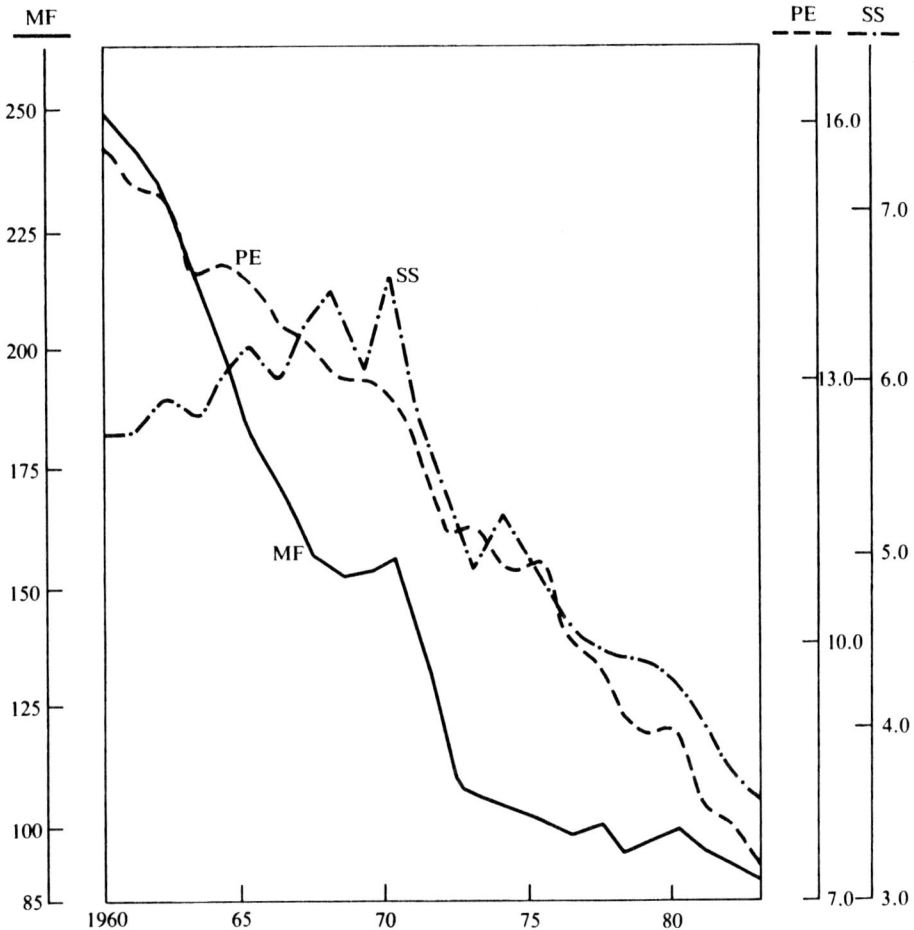

NOTES: For definitions of MF, SS, and PE, see Figure 1. Income, social security, and public education measures are from one year earlier.

SOURCES: See note 13.

in trends in declining men's incomes relative to social security incomes and public education expenditures, and in declining fertility rates at ages 15–19, 20–24, and 25–29. Since real incomes actually increased until 1973, the trend shows an interesting fit with a small fertility rise in 1969–70. Other annual fluctuations in incomes relative to social security transfers match annual fertility fluctuations. Consistent increases in public education expenditures (decline in incomes relative to public education expenditures) match a general declining trend in fertility.

FIGURE 3 Marital fertility at ages 25–29, relative social security benefits, and relative public education expenditures, United States, whites, 1960–83

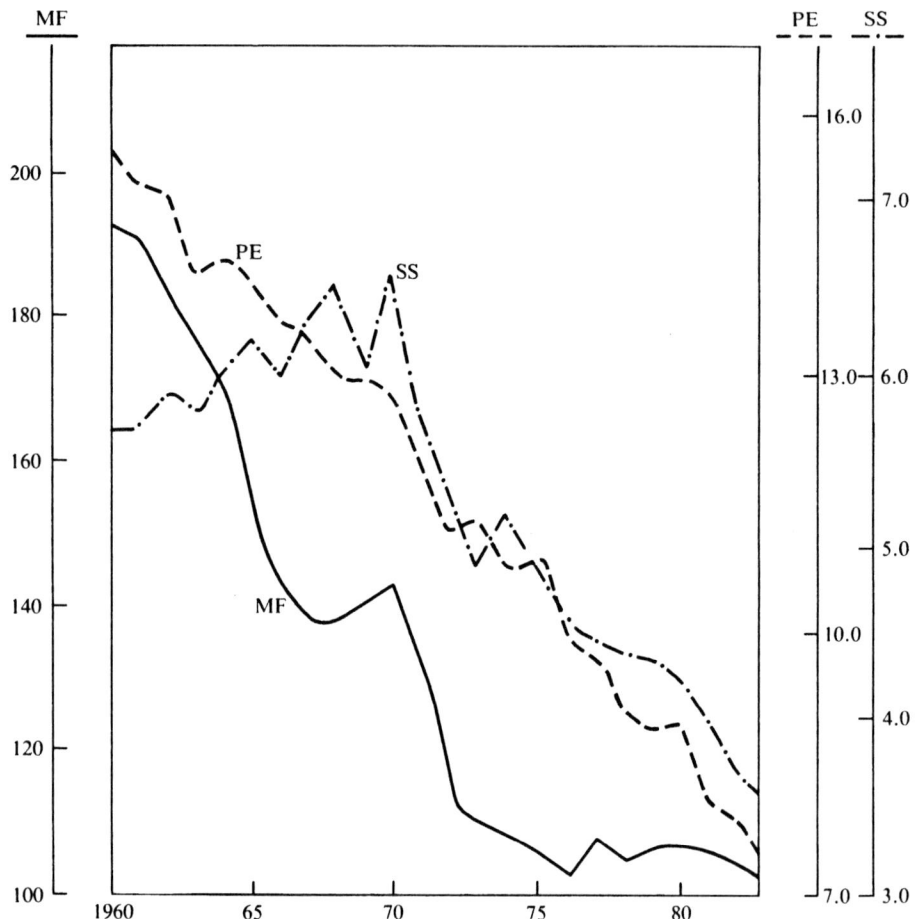

NOTES: For definitions of MF, SS, and PE, see Figure 1. Income, social security, and public education measures are from one year earlier.

SOURCES: See note 13.

Evidence from the Soviet Union

I have discussed elsewhere interpretations of below-replacement fertility among white populations of the Soviet Union along the lines of the present article (Bernstam, 1986 and forthcoming). Nothing similar to the US statistical tests presented above can be performed with the available Soviet data. However, we have one unique opportunity to look directly at two segments of the Soviet population that are highly similar as to their socioeconomic characteristics except for the role of interfamily transfers in their welfare. Both segments are rural and consist, roughly, of 85 percent farm workers and 15 percent managers and civil servants (USSR Central Statistical Administration, 1984). Both populations are dispersed without a definite spatial pattern across the same areas in their respective Union Republics. Both segments have more or less the same ethnic and cultural composition.

Legally, however, the populations are very different. One is categorized as state farm workers, the other as collective farm members. State farms are larger in size but are no different from collective farms in technology and type of agricultural work in the white areas of the Soviet Union that we are discussing. The real difference is that the state farm population are employees of the state while the collective farm population are members of cooperatives. Workers on state farms thus have always had the same legal rights as urban workers, including identification cards (Soviet internal passports), right of movement, educational opportunities, social security coverage, and wages based on seniority. Their schools were built and subsidized by the state. Collective farmers did not have the same legal rights as urban workers and state farm workers until very recently. They did not have social security coverage until 1964, no meaningful coverage until 1971, and no sufficient social security benefits until 1974 (Bernstam, 1986; McAuley, 1979). They did not have identification cards until 1976 and thus lacked right of free movement outside their villages, a restriction that, among other things, restricted opportunities for higher education of their children. Their school construction was often self-financed and most local schools went up to only the eighth grade. Their incomes were dependent on crops and productivity and were not subject to seniority schedules; many payments were in kind. Without social security and expanded public education, their interfamily transfers were not extensive. In terms of children's opportunities, they were more or less confined to local collective farms. The general environment was thus not highly competitive. Often collective farms were transformed into state farms, with concomitant changes in the socioeconomic setting. Things have changed very significantly since 1964 and especially since the mid–1970s when collective farms rapidly converged with state farms in all respects, including social security, public education, monetary payments, and seniority wage schedules.

The unique piece of evidence I mentioned is the sample survey of rural Soviet families conducted in 1984. This sample contains data on the proportions of families with different numbers of children younger than 16 years among all families with children by Union Republics, and by state and collective farm settings. To be sure, all these children were born in the period since 1968, by which time differences with respect to SS-PE-ES arrangements between the two institutions had largely dissipated. The change was gradual, though, until the mid–1970s. Table 4 presents data that I calculated from this 1984 sample. The table shows that the previously lower-transfer, less competitive settings, that is, the collective farms, had in 1984 higher mean numbers of children and higher proportions of families with children of higher order. This is true for all Soviet republics with below-replacement fertility, except Lithuania, where

TABLE 4 Selected measures of fertility among rural Soviet families in state farm and collective farm sectors, USSR and six republics with fertility below replacement, 1984

	Mean number of children aged 0–16[a] per family	Percent of families with more than 3 children	Percent of families with more than 4 children
USSR			
State farms	2.027	22.8	10.6
Collective farms	2.238	29.8	15.8
Republic			
Russian			
State farms	1.713	12.8	3.6
Collective farms	1.806	16.9	5.3
Ukrainian			
State farms	1.616	9.9	2.0
Collective farms	1.729	14.7	4.2
Byelorussian			
State farms	1.783	14.6	3.7
Collective farms	1.802	18.4	6.2
Lithuanian			
State farms	1.860	18.2	6.6
Collective farms	1.853	20.9	5.6
Latvian			
State farms	1.645	11.4	1.9
Collective farms	1.756	15.1	4.4
Estonian			
State farms	1.715	12.3	3.2
Collective farms	1.895	20.0	3.2

[a]Children born during 1968–84.
SOURCE: Calculated from *Vestnik Statistiki*, No. 12, Moscow, 1985, pp. 73–74.

one can observe no significant differentials. The differences are small, probably because for most of the period the two sectors were converging. However, this is a natural experiment for the same type of fertility effect—that of interfamily transfers—observed in the United States.

For the USSR as a whole the difference between the two sectors in terms of the mean number of children per rural family is 10 percent. The national difference is larger than in the republics with white population because the differential between the two sectors is higher in the nonwhite republics with high fertility. The story of these republics is also relevant to the arguments presented in this article because they have been experiencing rapid fertility decline, pronounced since the mid–1970s when collective farms joined in the rest of the country's competitive setting. High fertility levels in nonwhite republics were suggested earlier to be due to their land and livestock entitlements for young households, which reduce competition between the families. The movement in the opposite direction, toward fertility decline, is influenced by life cycle interfamily transfers. Table 5 presents the Coale-Trussell indices of parity-specific control at consecutive age groups for two nonwhite republics, the Kazakh SSR and the Uzbek SSR. For the Uzbek SSR I was able to obtain the data for the indigenous rural population.

The Kazakh SSR had already experienced rapid fertility decline and moderately high values of the Coale-Trussell m in the late 1950s because in the mid–1950s, during the Virgin Lands program, state farms were introduced throughout Kazakhstan, replacing collective farms (Bernstam, 1986 and forthcoming). There are very few cultural or other noneconomic differences between Kazakh and Uzbek. If anything, the Kazakh population was historically poorer and more backward; it was a nomadic population, while the Uzbek population was sedentary, more developed and better educated. State farms were not introduced to the Uzbek population, and it had negative indices of parity-specific control until the mid–1960s. After social security and other interfamily transfers were extended to collective farms in 1964 and expanded in 1971 and 1974, parity-specific control started to increase among the rural indigenous Uzbek population. The most important feature of Table 5, however, is that in both the Kazakh SSR and the Uzbek SSR this parity-specific control exhibits what may be called a counter-transitional pattern. Control was not started by older women who wanted to complete their family size after having reached

TABLE 5 Indices of parity-specific fertility control (the Coale-Trussell m), indigenous rural population of the Uzbek SSR, and total population of the Kazakh SSR (selected years)

Age	Uzbek SSR 1959	1963	1966	1975
25–29	−0.119	0.164	0.695	0.697
30–34	−0.123	−0.081	0.042	0.455
35–39	−0.024	−0.033	0.167	0.094
40–44	−0.274	−0.237	−0.074	0.086
45–49	−1.030	−0.832	−0.674	−0.461
	Kazakh SSR 1959	1966	1975	1979
25–29	0.740	1.239	1.399	1.403
30–34	0.630	0.878	1.100	1.045
35–39	0.470	0.691	0.908	1.002
40–44	0.384	0.479	0.860	0.865
45–49	−0.199	−0.457	0.616	0.699

SOURCES: Data for the Uzbek SSR is calculated from: 1959: V.A. Borisov. *Perspektivy Rozhdaemosti*. Moscow: Statistika, 1978, p. 55; 1963: I.R. Mulliadzhanov. *Narodonaselenie Uzbekskoi SSR*. Tashkent: Uzbekistan, 1967, p. 107; 1966, 1975: M.K. Karakhanov. *Nekapitalisticheskii Put Razvitiia i Problemy Narodonaseleniia*. Tashkent, 1983, p. 139; Data for the Kazakh SSR is derived from: *Narodonaselenie Stran Mira*. Moscow, 1984, p. 42. *Naselenie SSSR. Chislennost, Sostav i Dvizhenie Naseleniia. 1973*. Moscow, 1975, p. 137; Marital schedules for both republics are from: *Itogi Vsesoiuznoi Perepisi Naseleniia 1970 goda*. Moscow: Statistika, 1972, Vol. 2, p. 264.

a certain birth order. Control was started by younger families who experienced a decline in relative opportunities of their children due to life cycle interfamily transfers. The table shows that in both republics the level of control decreases over age. This is the same pattern we observed in the US regressions with respect to the age-specific fertility impact of social security, public education expenditure, and earnings seniority.

The new life cycle service system?

The argument in this article has been that interfamily transfers in the highly competitive and economically mobile environment of modern societies may cause additional fertility reduction on the margin. This margin may make the difference between replacement and below-replacement fertility. Interfamily transfers, such as social security, public education expenditures, and earnings seniority on the labor market, affect both relative incomes of parents and relative prices of children. They may reduce opportunities of younger families relative to those of middle-aged families. This way the transfers shift the marginal rate of substitution of the quality of children for their quantity toward favoring lower fertility. This means fewer children with higher per child expenditures.

Paradoxically, the modern SS-PE-ES system reminds us of the old European life cycle service system, but with the opposite fertility effect. In the old system, transfers from the unmarried very young to the newly married couples of about 30 years of age helped to promote moderately high numbers of moderately high quality children. In the Present SS-PE-ES system, a new life cycle service pattern seems to have emerged. Transfers from unmarried and married young individuals to middle-aged families may contribute to the production of small numbers of high quality children. The individual and societal effects of this new system seem to be mixed, and they deserve a further and more sophisticated analysis.

Appendix: The model of the race between children

Individuals form a family of their own, h, on the market where there are many other families of the aggregate, j. Parents in family h derive utility from their own consumption of the composite good, Z, from the number of their children, N, and from the future economic position, opportunities, and success of each of their children, S. This latter argument can also be considered as the output of the quality of children. Therefore, parents maximize

$$U_h = f(Z_h, N_h, \bar{S}_h) \quad (1)$$

subject to the production function

$$\bar{S}_h = g(\bar{Q}_h, \bar{R}_h, \bar{S}_j) \quad (2)$$

where $\bar{Q}_h$ is the total quantity of the quality inputs per child (e.g., number of hours of education or the size of land given to children), $\bar{R}_h$ is the per child biological endowment and family background, and $\bar{S}_j$ is the average success of children of other parents on future markets. The latter argument can also be considered as the average quality output of other children. It is itself a function of the amount of quality inputs in other children, $\bar{Q}_j$, of these children's biological endowments, $\bar{R}_j$, of the quality-unit prices for these children, p_j, and of full income of their parents, I_j. Thus

$$\bar{S}_j = y(\bar{Q}_j(I_j, p_j), \bar{R}_j) \quad . \tag{2a}$$

The budget constraint for (1) is given by

$$I_h = p_z Z_h + N_h p_h \bar{Q}_h \quad , \tag{3}$$

where I_h is full income of the family, p_z is the unit-price of Z and p_h is the price of quality-unit inputs for own children. Eq. (3) can be rewritten as

$$I_h = p_z Z_h + N_h p_h g^{-1}(\bar{S}_h, \bar{R}_h, \bar{S}_j) \quad . \tag{4}$$

A special case can follow as

$$Q_h = g^{-1}(\bar{S}_h, \bar{R}_h, \bar{S}_j) = \bar{S}_h^\alpha \bar{S}_j^\beta \bar{R}_h^\gamma \quad , \tag{5}$$

where $\alpha > 1$ signifies diminishing returns and $\alpha < 1$ signifies increasing returns.

Putting (5) into (4), one can maximize

$$U_h = f(Z_h, N_h, \bar{S}_h) \tag{6}$$

subject to

$$I_h = p_z Z_h + N_h p_h \bar{S}_h^\alpha \bar{S}_j^\beta \bar{R}_h^\gamma \quad . \tag{7}$$

Let us assume that Z_h is fixed. Take the total derivative of (7) with respect to N_h and $\bar{S}_h$. Then

$$0 = p_h \bar{S}_h^\alpha \bar{S}_j^\beta \bar{R}_h^\gamma dN_h + \alpha p_h N_h \bar{S}_h^{\alpha-1} \bar{S}_j^\beta \bar{R}_h^\gamma d\bar{S}_h \tag{8}$$

and

$$\frac{d\bar{S}_h}{dN_h} = -\frac{1}{\alpha} \frac{\bar{S}_h}{N_h} \tag{9}$$

For the first order conditions, maximize

$$U_h = f(Z_h, N_h, \bar{S}_h) - \lambda(I_h - p_z Z_h - N_h p_h g^{-1}(\bar{S}_h, \bar{R}_h, \bar{S}_j)) \tag{10}$$

The first order conditions are then given by

$$\begin{cases} \dfrac{\partial f}{\partial Z_h} - \lambda p_z = 0, \\[6pt] \dfrac{\partial f}{\partial N_h} - \lambda p_h g^{-1}(\bar{S}_h, \bar{R}_h, \bar{S}_j) = 0, \\[6pt] \dfrac{\partial f}{\partial \bar{S}_h} - \lambda N_h p_h \dfrac{\partial g^{-1}}{\partial \bar{S}_h} = 0, \\[6pt] I_h = p_z Z_h - \lambda N_h p_h g^{-1}(\bar{S}_h, \bar{R}_h, \bar{S}_j). \end{cases} \tag{11}$$

It follows that the equilibrium conditions are

$$\lambda = \frac{\partial f}{\partial Z_h} \bigg/ p_z$$

$$= \frac{\partial f}{\partial N_h} \bigg/ \left\{ p_h g^{-1}(\bar{S}_h, \bar{R}_h, \bar{S}_j) \right\} \tag{12}$$

$$= \frac{\partial f}{\partial \bar{S}_h} \bigg/ \left\{ N_h p_h (\partial g^{-1}/\partial \bar{S}_h) \right\} \quad .$$

It is clear that the shadow price of the number of children, that is $p_h g^{-1}(\bar{S}_h, \bar{R}_h, \bar{S}_j)$, depends on the average success of other children, $\bar{S}_j$.

Figure A-1 depicts the indifference curves and budget constraints of the family h under conditions of changing average success of other children. First, suppose Z_h is fixed. With the initial magnitude of $\bar{S}_j$, called $\bar{S}_{j1}$, family h will have N_1 number of children of the average quality $\bar{S}_{h1}$ and the equilibrium will be at point e_1 on the budget line AB. When $\bar{S}_j$ increases, so that $\bar{S}_{j2} > \bar{S}_{j1}$, and Z_h is still fixed, the new budget line for h is moved to EF. If Z_h is not fixed and an additional portion of it can be sacrificed for children at the expense of parents' consumption, the budget line under conditions of $\bar{S}_{j2} > \bar{S}_{j1}$ will be CD. If income elasticity of per child expenditures, $p_h \bar{Q}_h$, is higher than income elasticity for numbers, the level of $\bar{S}_{h1}$ can be retained. It will logically be retained if the same level of success per child is imperative for parents. Since $\bar{S}_j$ is the function of, among other things, I_j (see equation 2a), income elasticity of *own* per child expenditures is, in fact, a response to effective increases in incomes of *other* parents. (Conversely, if $\bar{S}_j$ is unchanged while I_h increases, the number of own children should increase revealing *own* income elasticity for numbers.)

If Z_h is fixed, the number of children moves to N_3 and if part of Z_h can be sacrificed, the

FIGURE A-1 Interaction between quality and quantity of children with changing average quality of children of other families: Indifference curves and budget constraints of the average family

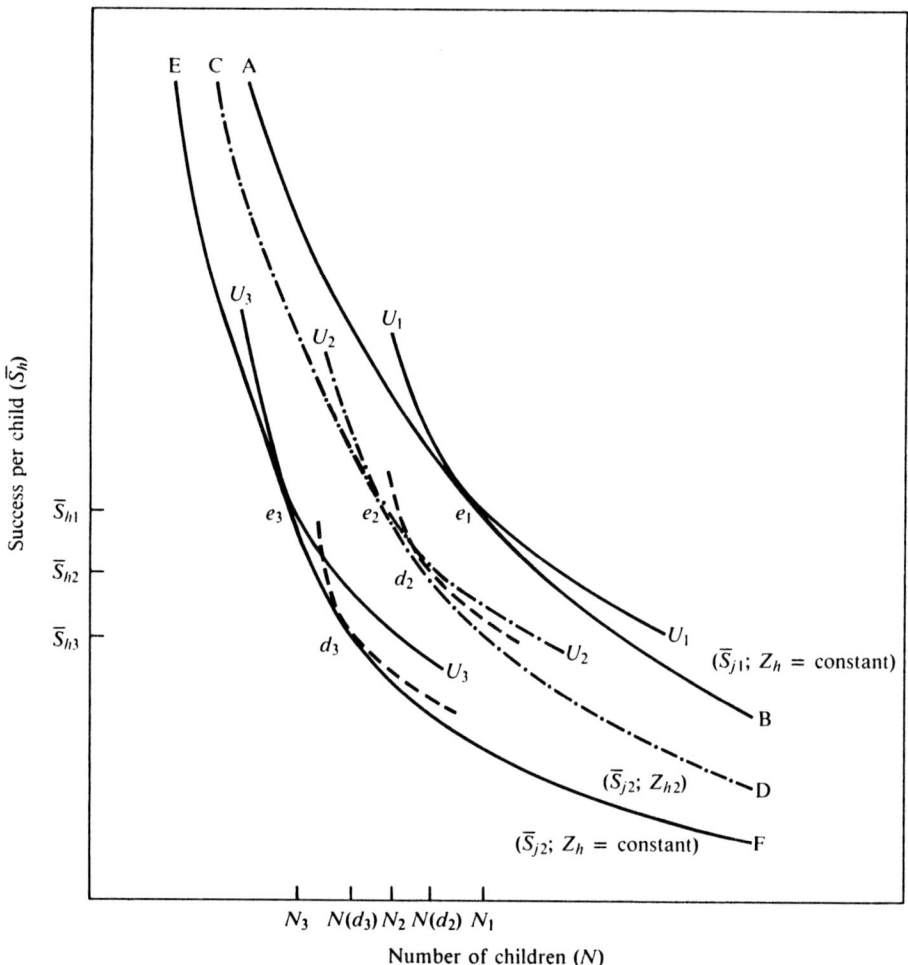

number of children moves to N_2. The equilibrium points are given by e_3 and e_2, respectively. If income elasticities for expenditures per child and numbers of children are equal, the number of children moves to $N(d_3)$ when Z_h is fixed. The number moves to $N(d_2)$ when an additional expenditure for children is substituted for a part of parental consumption. The main implication is that, whatever the solution, own per child expenditures are increased and fertility is reduced when opportunities of other children increase.

Notes

Warren C. Sanderson of the State University of New York at Stony Brook generously reduced my ignorance in comprehending some of the intricacies of the model. Gary S. Becker,

Yoram Ben-Porath, Masanori Hashimoto, Robert T. Michael and Sherwin Rosen provided insightful comments on previous presentations of the theory and illustrations. John P. Holland provided invaluable assistance.

1 This framework is similar in operation to the Chicago social interaction and quality-quantity interaction analysis of fertility decision-making (Becker and Lewis, 1973; Becker, 1974; Becker and Tomes, 1976; Ben-Porath, 1976; Ben-Porath and Welch, 1980; Becker, 1981, chapters 5, 6 and 7). But it also introduces an additional argument into the own production function when the success of own children depends on the success of the children of other parents. The competitive approach is also similar to some of the "reference group" literature that emphasizes an external inducement of incremental child costs (Okun, 1958; Davis, 1963; Turchi, 1975; Leibenstein, 1976). The difference with this literature is that here tastes are invariant as in Stigler and Becker (1977). There are no external social influences, and only price signals are present with regard to the market opportunities of competing children. The same difference holds with respect to the "relative income" literature (Easterlin, 1973, 1980; Oppenheimer, 1982). With this my approach is similar in comparing incomes of different age groups—but only as determinants of opportunities of other children relative to one's own.

2 On the combined fertility effect of transfers see Becker, 1981; Willis, 1983; Bernstam, 1986 and forthcoming. On social security behavioral effects see Barro, 1974; Willis, 1980; Hohm, 1975; Davis, 1979; Davis and van den Oever, 1981; Soderstrom, 1983; Swidler, 1983; Parsons, 1984; Preston, 1984; Ricardo-Campbell, 1984. On earnings seniority see Pettengill, 1980, 1981; Ricardo-Campbell, 1985.

3 Friedman and Friedman (1981) summarized the relevant evidence from the United States. Also, in the Soviet Union, utilization of the best types of higher education is concentrated among higher educated and more privileged classes (Samoilova, 1975).

4 Hohm (1975) found a strong negative fertility effect of social security coverage and social security benefits relative to average earnings in an international cross-section for 67 countries in the early 1960s. Swidler (1983) tested the impact of social security on fertility in the United States time series. He found fertility elasticities with respect to social security benefits, taken separately and in combination with coverage, to be negative, low, and statistically significant.

5 Only ordinary least squares estimates are presented here. Instrumental variables test was also conducted assuming female employment and incomes of young workers relative to incomes of their fathers 20 years ago to be endogenous. This test showed results consistent with the OLS test, with somewhat higher elasticities of transfer variables. The functional form is log-linear. The technique used is heteroskedastic-consistent standard error estimation (White, 1980, 1982) which makes it possible to account for different sizes of states without applying arbitrary weighting. Several observations were dropped for some states where data on blacks were missing.

6 The data are derived from US National Center for Health Statistics (1975, 1984) and from US Bureau of the Census (1970, 1980).

7 US Bureau of the Census (1970a, p. 122, 1981, p. 154).

8 US Department of Health and Human Services, Social Security Administration (1982, p. 195).

9 US Department of Health and Human Services, Social Security Administration (1970, p. 34; 1982, p. 74).

10 The dynamic relative income variables include current incomes and incomes ten years ago by race in the same state. It was impossible to devise comparisons of 1970 with 1960 because only data for nonwhites, not for blacks, were listed in the 1960 census. Therefore, Table 2 covers only the year 1980, which corresponds to the 1970 data. Also, since most variables, except social security participation, are race-specific, and incomes are highly collinear with race, the race dummy was not used. Several other control variables were also collinear and were dropped; and so was relative income by education in columns 7–8 in Table 1. Due to repetitiveness of tests, t-ratios cannot be taken with full confidence.

11 See evidence in the sources cited in notes 7 and 8.

12 Similar and even more pronounced results can be obtained for blacks if one excludes out-of-wedlock fertility as a separate production function.

13 Fertility data are obtained from *Vital Statistics of the United States*, annual volumes. Social security incomes are obtained from US Department of Health and Human Services, Social Security Administration (1985, p.158). The public education expenditures per pupil are given in *Statistical Abstract of the United States*, annual series. Incomes are derived from *Current Population Report*, Series P-60, annual issues.

References

Barro, Robert J. 1974. "Are government bonds net wealth?," *Journal of Political Economy* 82, no. 6: 1095–1117.
Becker, Gary S. 1974. "A theory of social interactions," *Journal of Political Economy* 82, no. 6: 1063–1093.
———. 1981. *A Treatise on the Family*. London, Cambridge: Harvard University Press.
———, and H. Gregg Lewis. 1973. "On the interaction between the quantity and quality of children," *Journal of Political Economy* 81, no. 2: S279–288.
———, and Nigel Tomes. 1976. "Child endowments and the quantity and quality of children," *Journal of Political Economy* 84, no. 4: S143–62.
Ben-Porath, Yoram. 1973. "Short-term fluctuations in fertility and economic activity in Israel," *Demography* 10, no. 2: 185–204.
———. 1975. "First-generation effects on second-generation fertility," *Demography* 12, no. 3: 397–405.
———. 1976. "Fertility response to child mortality: Micro data from Israel," *Journal of Political Economy* 84, no. 4, Pt. 2: S163–178.
———, and Finis Welch. 1980. "On sex preferences and family size," in *Research in Population Economics*, vol. 2. Greenwich, Conn.: JAI Press, pp. 387–399.
Bernstam, Mikhail S. 1986. "The demography of Soviet ethnic groups in world perspective," in *The Last Empire: Nationality and The Soviet Future*, ed. Robert Conquest. Stanford: Hoover Institution Press, pp. 314–368.
———. Forthcoming. "Trends and economic conditions of Soviet population and labor force dynamics, 1959–2000," in *The Future of the Soviet Empire*, ed. Henry S. Rowen and Charles Wolf, Jr. New York: Oxford University Press.
———, and Peter L. Swan. 1986. "The production of children as claims on the state: A comprehensive labor market approach to illegitimacy in the United States, 1960–1980," *Hoover Institution Working Paper Series. Working Papers in Economics.* E–86-1.
Blekher, Feiga. 1979. *The Soviet Woman in the Family and in Society*. New York: John Wiley and Sons.
Cook, Maria Sophia Lengyel, and Robert Repetto. 1982. "The relevance of the developing countries to demographic transition theory: Further lessons from the Hungarian experience," *Population Studies* 36, no. 1: 105–128.
Davis, Kingsley. 1963. "The theory of change and response in modern demographic history," *Population Index* 29, no. 4: 345–366.
———. 1979. "The continuing demographic revolution in industrial societies," in *The Third Century: America as a Post-Industrial Society*, ed. Seymour Martin Lipset. New Delhi: Kalyani Publishers, pp. 37–64.
———, and Pietronella van den Oever. 1981. "Age relations and public policy in advanced industrial societies," *Population and Development Review* 7, no. 1: 1–18.
Demeny, Paul. 1972. "Early fertility decline in Austria-Hungary: A lesson in demographic transition," in *Population and Social Change*, ed. D.V. Glass and Roger Revelle. New York: Edward Arnold, pp. 153–172.

Easterlin, Richard A. 1973. "Relative economic status and the American fertility swing," *Family Economic Behavior: Problems and Prospects*, ed. Eleanor Sheldon. Philadelphia: J.B. Lippincott Company, pp. 170–223.

———. 1980. *Birth and Fortune: The Impact of Numbers on Personal Welfare.* New York: Basic Books.

Friedman, Milton, and Rose Friedman. 1981. *Free to Choose.* New York: Avon Publishers.

Hajnal, John. 1982. "Two kinds of preindustrial household formation system," *Population and Development Review* 8, no. 3: 449–494.

Hohm, C. F. 1975. "Social security and fertility: An international perspective," *Demography* 12, no. 4: 629–644.

Inkeles, Alex. 1986. "Rethinking social welfare: U.S. and U.S.S.R. in comparative perspective," *Hoover Institution Working Paper Series. Working Papers in Economics.* E–86–34.

Leibenstein, Harvey. 1976. "The problem of characterizing aspirations," *Population and Development Review* 2, no. 3/4: 427–431.

McAuley, Alastair. 1979. *Economic Welfare in the Soviet Union.* Madison: The University of Wisconsin Press.

Okun, Bernard. 1958. *Trends in Birth Rates in the United States since 1870.* Baltimore: The Johns Hopkins Press.

Oppenheimer, Valerie K. 1982. *Work and the Family: A Study in Social Demography.* New York: Academic Press.

Parsons, Donald O. 1984. "On the economics of intergenerational control," *Population and Development Review* 10, no. 1:41–54.

Pettengill, John S. 1980. *Labor Unions and the Inequality of Earned Income.* Amsterdam, New York: North-Holland.

———. 1981. "The long run impact of a minimum wage on employment and the wage structure," in *Report of the Minimum Wage Study Commission*, vol. 6. Washington, D.C.: US Government Printing Office, pp. 63–104.

Preston, Samuel H. 1984. "Children and the elderly: divergent paths for America's dependents," *Demography* 21, no. 4: 435–457.

Ptukha, M. V. 1960. *Ocherki po Statistike Naseleniia.* Moscow: Gosstatizdat, 1960.

Ricardo-Campbell, Rita. 1984. "Social Security Reform," in *To Promote Prosperity*, ed. John H. Moore. Stanford: Hoover Institution Press, pp. 91–123.

———. 1985. *Women and Comparable Worth.* Stanford: Hoover Institution Press.

Samoilova, E. 1975. "Vliianie obrazovaniia i professionalnoi zaniatosti roditelei na sotsialnye peremeshcheniia molodezhi," in *Demograficheskie Aspekty Zaniatosti.* Moscow: Statistika, 1975, pp. 84–93.

Soderstrom, Lars, ed. 1983. *Social Insurance. Papers Presented at the 5th Arne Ryde Symposium, Lund, Sweden, 1981.* Amsterdam-New York: North-Holland.

Stigler, George J., and Gary S. Becker. 1977. "De gustibus non est disputandum," *American Economic Review* 67, no. 2: 76–90.

Swidler, Steve. 1983. "An empirical test of the effect of social security on fertility in the United States," *The American Economist* 27, no. 2: 50–57.

Turchi, Boone A. 1975. *The Demand for Children: The Economics of Fertility in the United States.* Cambridge: Ballinger Publishing Company.

United States Bureau of the Census. 1970, 1980. *Census of Population: 1970, 1980. U.S. Summary; State Summaries.* Washington, D.C.: US Government Printing Office.

———. 1970a, 1981, 1984, 1985. *Statistical Abstract of the United States. 1970, 1981, 1985, 1986.* Washington, D.C.: US Government Printing Office.

United States Department of Health and Human Services, Social Security Administration. 1970, 1982, 1985. *Social Security Bulletin. Annual Statistical Supplement, 1970, 1981, 1984–85.* Washington, D.C.: US Government Printing Office.

―――. 1984. *Social Security Programs throughout the World—1983*. Washington, D.C.: US Government Printing Office.

United States National Center for Health Statistics. 1975, 1984. *Vital Statistics of the United States, 1970, 1980*. Vol. 1: *Natality*. Washington, D.C.: US Government Printing Office.

USSR Central Statistical Administration. 1984. *Chislennost i Sostav Naseleniia SSSR. Po Dannym Vsesoiuznoi Perepisi Naseleniia 1979 goda*. Moscow: Finansy i Statistika.

White, Halbert. 1980. "Using least squares to approximate unknown regression functions," *International Economic Review* 21, no. 1: 149–170.

―――. 1982. "Maximum likelihood estimation of misspecified models," *Econometrica* 50, no. 1: 1–25.

Willis, Robert J. 1980. "The old age security hypothesis and population growth," *Demographic Behavior: Interdisciplinary Perspectives on Decision-Making*, ed. Thomas K. Burch. Boulder, Colorado: Westview Press Inc., pp. 43–69.

―――, 1983. "Life cycles, institutions, and population growth: A theory of the equilibrium interest rate in an overlapping generations model," *Hoover Institution Working Paper Series. Working Papers in Economics*. E-83-15.

INTERPRETATION

The Family That Does Not Reproduce Itself

Nathan Keyfitz

Mean family size in the industrial nations is less than the 2.1 children per couple needed for the population to remain constant over the long run. The countries of Western Europe have a mean family size of about 1.61 children per couple, with West Germany as low as 1.42; Japan is at 1.71; Europe as a whole at 1.90; the United States at 1.85 (United Nations, 1985). That at least is the implication of present birth rates.

Austria, largely Roman Catholic, has over the centuries faced attacks by Turks, Russians, French, and Germans, any one of which could have terminated its national existence, and it survived them all. Now, if its net reproduction rate of 0.76 continues, its population will decline by one-quarter in each generation once its age distribution stabilizes. Already the number of births is less than the number of deaths. The damage that external enemies could not do its own young couples are doing.

To see the difficulty of theoretical explanation, think of asking a man or woman of 1885 for a forecast of our late twentieth-century childbearing. When told of the great wealth of 1985, most inhabitants of earlier ages would have said that we would bear more rather than fewer children. Here was the chance to attain the goal of all earlier humanity—our individual perpetuation through our children. In the face of past scarcities of food and other resources and past difficulties of maintaining a home, children were an incalculably greater burden than they are now; yet fertility was high then while now it is low.

It is easy enough, after one realizes that the late twentieth century has turned its huge resources to other ends than childbearing, to invent models that will account for the low level of births. We can refer to earlier ignorance of birth control; we can say that the traditional family had to be big so that the parents could be supported in their old age and that children are no longer needed as a source of support; we can say that women's wages are so high that they cannot afford the time for childbearing; we can say that women have been liberated so that they are free to act like men. This article asserts that all these assertions are true, and so also are other considerations, and that the interplay of causes is what now needs study.

Levels of causation

The decline of births is related to contraceptive use, frequency of intercourse, and other variables that are immediate, or "proximate," causes of fertility (Davis and Blake, 1956). Some scholars (e.g., Bongaarts and Potter, 1983) modestly portray their work as dealing with the proximate causes only. Others dealing with birth control claim more. For instance, William Pratt and colleagues (1984) call their work "Understanding U.S. fertility." Understanding in terms of proximate causes, impeccable in its own terms, is less than satisfying in a wider perspective. The deeper problem centers on decisionmaking—specifically on whether or not to have a child.

That decision is less and less constrained by physical and biological circumstances. On the one side, increasingly effective means of contraception enable parents to have as few children as they want. On the other side, couples who seem infertile can be more effectively treated than in the past. The options have never been wider, and our problem is to determine why choices are made at the low end of the increasingly wide range that is biologically available. The more completely the biological has come under control, the more we are prompted to seek extra-biological causes of change.

At the level of choices, William Butz and Michael Ward (1979) and James Smith and Ward (1984) take up economic variables, saying for example, "Our estimates indicate that an increase in women's wages decreases the number of their children" (Smith and Ward, p. xxi); and in turn, as they see it, "the most important determinant of women's work during this century was the increase in their wages" (p. xx). They also find that "smaller families reduce the demands on women's time, freeing women for greater participation in the market" (p. xxi). The observed strong temporal associations suggest that economic causes are operating in the system.

Underlying the proximate causes are economic causes, and I will argue that below these is a further layer: political-social changes. Past high fertility was associated with the authority of the man within the family and the fact that women were sufficiently hemmed in so that their time was not worth much outside the household. Husbands had the major part in decisionmaking. As the authority structure within the household collapses, so does fertility. Assigning women to raising children, even if the children were nothing but a prestige symbol (and they were often more than that, especially for rural families), was a way of using women's time in those historical epochs when social arrangements made that time worth very little in the marketplace.

None of these three levels of explanation contradicts the others. Certainly the immediate influence on the birth rate is contraception, for the first time controlled by women (using the pill, foam, diaphragm) rather than by men (using the condom or withdrawal). Certainly women's employment outside the home often lies behind the use of contraception. The democratization of decisionmaking within the couple, part of the third level of explanation mentioned above, is supported by the work opportunities offered to women. On the view here developed, it is indeed work opportunities for women that lower the birth rate, but they do so by freeing women from the dictatorship of men. A complete causal model, which no one is yet in a position to present, would involve elements at these three levels.

Women seek work and careers, so they use various contraceptive instruments. But there are unanswered questions in this determination of proximate causes by economic causes. Why do women take jobs now when before World War II they stayed home, even though the real incomes of their husbands were then one-third as large as they now are? "We work because we need the money" is a common statement; but did not people need money in the 1920s? This is not the only field where the reason given by the actor cannot be accepted as definitive by the scientific observer.

Unfortunately the progression from proximate cause to ultimate causes is also a progression from plentiful data to very little data. There are more data on proximate causes than on underlying causes; as among the latter there are more on economics than on social structure. What data exist on social structure tend to be qualitative and anecdotal. Yet the lack of data is not intrinsic, and persistently asking the questions can provide a stimulus to gathering the data.

An activities approach

Is childrearing work or pleasure?

The opportunity cost of time is an important variable in accounting for fertility. Women indeed think about what they could be earning in the time they would spend looking after children, and this indeed influences their decision on whether to have children.

Yet we know of other activities that would not usually be seen as having an opportunity cost: watching television, constructing a model railroad, playing computer games, vacation travel. The opportunity cost of the three-hour average time per day spent watching television in the United States adds up to something like a trillion dollars per year, enough to pay off the national debt in two years. Applying the argument used for the opportunity cost of a child, people ought to find television increasingly expensive in terms of opportunity costs as wages rise, and they should be able to afford less of it.

Why is such an argument perfectly silly with respect to television and perfectly reasonable with respect to childrearing? If we could answer that question we would be closer to understanding why the birth rate is so low.

The argument of this section is a comparison of the activity of childrearing with other uncompensated activities that occupy people's leisure on the one hand, and with paid work on the other hand. We will suggest that both leisure and work—regarded simply as activities and in abstraction from their cost or the return to them—become more attractive as time goes on.

So also, to be fair, does childrearing become less of a burden. Disposable diapers, readymade formulas and baby food, television that acts as an electronic governess, earlier kindergarten, all of these lighten the load. But such advances are outstripped by the increasing attractiveness of both leisure and paid work.

The pleasures of modern life include air travel at excursion fares that couples can readily afford—especially if they have no children—the automobile and the highway system that permit easy displacement over distances up to a few hundred miles, convenience foods and restaurants, video games. For the high-fertility epoch that ended in the 1930s, practically none of these were available, though they had begun to appear in the brief high-fertility period of the 1950s.

One can sort out the technological benefits now available to the average couple according to the degree of their compatibility with having children. Of the series, television may well be the most compatible—having children to care for cuts less into the time available for that—though children reduce the degree of concentration that is possible, something that television producers take into account in setting the coherence of their programs and the demands on their audience. The automobile lends itself to family travel, though in the typical instance not without some friction. Air travel, living in hotels, eating in restaurants are all handicapped by the presence of children, and one can be impressed by the relative scarcity of young children on airplanes; the parent who is tied to them typically does not travel. If the passengers on a large commercial airplane were taken as a population, demographic calculations based on its age distribution would show a very low rate of reproduction.

Women in offices rather than factories

To proceed to work activity, consider a well-run office where morale is high and the tasks not excessively repetitive. Compare this with the factory that was the chief alternative to homemaking for the nineteenth-century woman. Relatively free from the arduousness and repetitiveness of the factory and the feudal subordination of domestic service, clerical work has agreeable social elements combined with tolerable and limited duties. Many a clerical worker finds his or her friends at work; some find their first husband or wife; others find a new spouse to replace the old one. The office may well be preferable hour for hour to looking after children, and so preferred to childrearing even if the latter could be confined to an eight-hour day, and even if childrearing were paid the same wage as office work.

Staying home and looking after children does permit a degree of autonomy for the housewife, yet it lacks crisp challenges and interpersonal relations. The home is a lonely place in which to spend seven days a week. Childrearing cannot possibly lead to promotion; the end of the trail comes 20 years later when the child leaves home and the mother is just where she started and 20 years older. The fact that children leave home earlier, often becoming mere friends or semi-strangers to their parents, helps to give the impression of pointlessness to the work that has been put into raising them.

The relative earnings of couples of childbearing age determine their wish to bear children—as Richard Easterlin (1980) shows in what is the standard explanation among demographers of at least the American baby boom and current low fertility. The Easterlin effect emerged clearly and unambiguously in the 1950s, and the drop in fertility in the 1970s accords with it. Yet there is a great deal of noise in the system: technical change that makes both leisure and paid work more attractive activities; introduction of new consumer goods; the play of fashion, are all exogenous to the Easterlin scheme. What are to other disciplines deep and essential causes are noise when seen from the vantage point of a crisp hypothesis like Easterlin's. The effect cannot be expected to emerge above the noise on every repetition of the two-generation cycle that it specifies.

Considerations of the quality of work life versus domestic life parallel the effect of wages. Women's wages are not yet equal to those of men. A part of the reason is the tendency of women to enter noncareer jobs, as the contingencies of childrearing and their husbands' careers dictate; the process of liberation has gone only part way. As women become freer in relation to husbands and children, their wages will rise against those of men. Progress can be expected in this direction. Will it be associated with an even lower birth rate?

Quite aside from any possible tendency for pay to equalize between the sexes is the availability of a kind of work that is acceptable to women, as reflected in the numbers of women employed. Female white-collar workers in the United States rose from 12 million to 28 million in the years 1960 to 1980, while female blue-collar workers rose only from 4 to 6 million (US Bureau of the Census, 1982–83, p. 386). Surely what has drawn women into the labor market, with heavy consequences for childbearing, is the relative availability of congenial office work.

The progress of women in work is associated with increased education. Women have always completed elementary and secondary school in slightly higher proportions than men, but the fractions going on to college and completing college have been decidedly less (Smith and Ward, 1984, p. 39). The correlation of college attendance with low fertility is strong. Education generates a taste for activities other than tending a baby; at the same time it qualifies one for better paying jobs.

A recent survey commissioned by the Austrian Ministry of Health asked women what was good about having children; the answer most frequently checked was the sense of being needed by the child. But the sense of being needed is also found at work. The more educated and skilled the woman, the more she is needed once she is installed in an office or other organization.

What activity is childrearing similar to?

Work as an activity is a variable requiring study quite apart from the income it brings. I have no data on the distastefulness of the activities of childrearing in comparison with office work, say, or with serving hamburgers. Yet if we are to know why people have tended to give up having children in favor of these and other activities, we need some knowledge of this kind: how do people perceive the actual motions, hour against hour, of preparing food for a child, dressing the child, entertaining the child, compared with the other things they might be doing in that time? Compared, that is, with the actual motions that one goes through in a typical office day on the one hand, or with modern leisure pursuits on the other.

Such an activities approach (as against the production-of-commodities approach of the following section) is suited to a society where the future is heavily discounted. Parents still identify with their children and gain a kind of immortality through them, and they also derive some clear benefits of a social and even material character from having children; yet at the time the child is conceived these are all far in the future. What dominates in the foreground is the work of bringing up the child. If the process of making a decision is heavily weighted by the next two or three years, and parental activities in the early years of the child's life are contrasted with the pleasures of alternative activities in this exciting world of consumption and the no-longer-painful world of work, then the alternative can be expected to win out. We need to study attitudes toward these several activities.

This view that people choose among activities is also appropriate to the degree that more and more of our income goes into services, that is, nonmaterial commodities, or into goods that have a brief usefulness. The inheritance of such items is of little importance. No one saves in order to bequeath an automobile to his son or daughter, or even a house; we live with rapid turnover of material goods. Fewer and fewer of us own businesses (for instance farms) that we can pass on, and even those who do and have a child will probably find the child unwilling to take over. The son or daughter will seek an independent career, one not requiring parental financing once the college years are past. The bequest motive, establishment of a hereditary fortune, does not have the significance for us that it did for a Victorian enterpriser building an independent business.

Further pushing the couple to choose among activities rather than according to pay are compression of the after-tax salary range, the backstopping by welfare and social security, and the lesser importance of a unit of marginal difference of income as incomes rise. No one is going to starve; people can survive on welfare if they do not work at all; not only the choice of job, but the choice between working and not working, come to depend increasingly on the appeal of these several activities, as judged by the individual. Fortunately not everyone has the same preferences. It does not take much extrapolation beyond our present condition to see most people as having about the same income, and hence making a choice of kind of work based on the appeal to them of the activity proposed rather than on the compensation offered.

So far I have presented childrearing as an activity and have compared it with other activities, first of leisure, then of work. It is not easy to separate commodities from the activities involved in making and using them, but I have tried to do just this.

More observation is needed, then, of childrearing compared with contemporary work and leisure, all regarded as activities in disregard of the products that result. Comparison with the past would show a shift in respect of convenience and attractiveness away from childrearing.

A recent report of the German Federal Institute for Population Research entitled "Children or consumption?" expresses regret that babies come second in attractiveness to other goods. We leave activities and proceed to a discussion of how on the one hand children have changed, and how on the other goods have changed.

The child as commodity

If parents do not spend their money and time producing children, they can apply both money and time to the purchase and use of a dazzling array of other goods. Money can buy cars and weekend cottages. The child may well be a joy to have around, but so are many other things whose consumption competes with having children.

If the child is not a consumption good but an investment, the investor in children increasingly runs into the question of appropriation. Without doubt an entity of enormous value is produced by the labor of parents. But to whom does it belong? The answer to this question involves the nature of the child today and 50 years ago. If the child is brought up as an instrument, and to respect and support its parents, then indeed it can be an investment, and when we think of the high fertility of the Third World this aspect of intrafamily discipline comes first to mind.

There are two features of industrial society that make such discipline obsolete. The first is that the child becomes his or her own person at a very early age. Traditional childrearing, of which a main aim was to inculcate respect for parents, is not possible today, because the child is in large part no longer formed by the parents; it is formed by television, by schools, by peer groups in the street.

The second is that the parents are provided for in other ways; they do not want to depend on their children in old age, but on their own savings and on the state. They do not need to appropriate the child, and they could not do so even if they wanted to.

Extrafamilial forces and the qualities of the child

Some of the theory presented by John Caldwell (1982) on the effects of education at the youngest ages can be applied to the qualities of children in low-fertility countries. Education takes the child out of the home for long hours each day at an impressionable age; it gives him or her standards of conduct that are alien, often incomprehensible, to the parents; it is not only an expenditure in itself, but it adds other expenditures to those initially intended by the parents; it gives the child a status in the home that is in some respects superior to that of the parents.

The child on whom more is expended will turn out to be "better" in the sense of being more productive in later life (Becker and Lewis, 1973; Schultz, 1974; Sanderson, 1974). The child who attends Groton and Harvard will earn several times as much as the child who goes to a public school in the Bronx and then drops out. The greater expenditure produces a child of higher quality in the sense that it is more valuable, but we raise the question, "More valuable to whom?" and suggest the answer: "Certainly more valuable to the child himself or herself, possibly more valuable to society, but not more valuable to the parents of the child." And it is the parents who decide whether that child will be born or not. Gary Becker (1960) and Robert Willis (1973) have stressed the amount of expenditure on the child as a measure of quality. I add to that a suggestion that we look closer at qualities, what the child is like qualitatively, and we will find the modern child very different from the child of high-fertility regimes in many respects, including that he or she desires freedom from outside control.

Can the parents, knowing all this, decide to have the child and to determine its upbringing, including the kind and amount of expenditure on it, with a view to making it an object that will be a continuation of themselves? Hardly; they are constrained by social pressures that form both the child and themselves as parents. They cannot decide to keep it out of school; they cannot decide to dress it other than in the way children are dressed; they cannot even easily withstand the pressures to let it watch television. What few options in upbringing they may have they are often not skilled or determined enough to apply.

An option that couples do have is whether or not to conceive the child. After the child is conceived they can still decide to abort it, but once it is born the important decisions are out of their hands.

This dynamic that is loosed with the birth of the child is of course partly in the laws protecting children against their parents in various ways, but the legal constraints on what parents can do are trifling in comparison with the social constraints. Perhaps if they knew more about raising children they could counter many of the social constraints and produce a child more in line with their own preferences, keep the evolution of the child from getting out of hand. But in the nature of the case the new parent is not a skilled parent. A depressingly common question asked by parents after their children have grown up is, "What did we do wrong?"

How many children one is going to want depends on the kind of children expected. Will they be like ourselves, and obedient to our wishes to boot? Will they help us in need? Or will they be rebellious and independent, concerned with their own activities, needing us little and helping us little? In earlier ages children were largely brought up within the home and could be formed to whatever model the parents wished. The imperfect controls that today's parents exercise and the resulting uncertainties are well described by Paul David in this volume.

In a high-fertility regime new parents had already learned how to handle children. Older brothers and sisters could not only watch what their parents did to control the younger ones, but could themselves practice during the plentiful opportunities they were given to take charge of their younger siblings. And what does skill in raising children amount to if not forming them according to the ideals of the parent generation? When families become so small that children do not learn from observing the way that parents handle siblings, the skill is no longer passed on, and hence the children produced are not according to the parents' taste and parents cease to want them and families become even smaller—a clear example of positive feedback.

Once control of the children passes to outside agencies, whether it be schools or television, and upbringing is out of parents' hands, then the very different objectives of the outside agencies compete with those of the parents. Especially if parents' time with children is limited because both have jobs, the outside agencies overlay their own strong effects on the parents' weaker ones and obscure them.

Identification of parents with their children is essential to even a moderate level of fertility. That identification can be called altruism, and it has been defined as the parents' obtaining positive utility from the individual utilities of their children.

Altruism can indeed provide for the continuance of the race in the absence of flows of income from children to parents. The idea of altruism is important, but we need to know more about it: when and why does it come into existence; does altruism apply to parents only with respect to their children, or with respect to other kin as well and even to friends and neighbors (or for that matter to the university one attended as an undergraduate); how can it be both strengthened and focused more directly on children; will it be weakened or strengthened with further economic progress? Endowing a chair at Harvard provides scope for altruism with less trouble than raising a child.

In short, the existence of altruism is unquestioned, and the definition is unobjectionable; yet the research starts rather than ends here. And we must above all guard against attributing to altruism what people do because of hidden social compulsions. A wife's loyalty to her husband is indeed admirable, but if things are so arranged that she would starve to death if she left him then altruism is an incomplete description of her behavior.

Counting the images on the television screen, the schools, the play groups on the street, the church in those cases where it is a factor, the books that the child reads insofar as they are not selected by the parents, the proportion of waking time subject to outside-the-home influences as against parental influence, all of these must increase in proportion as economic development goes forward. The factors in this removal of parental control over the child's environment are in part wealth as such, in part increased schooling, increased labor force participation of mothers, spread of technology—for instance in the form of television, records, books, home computers.

Thus my argument so far is that childrearing as an activity is less able to compete in attractiveness either with work or with leisure, and the child as a product is of insufficient value to the parents to cause them to give up alternative commodities.

All this seems to prove too much, for there have been periods—during most of human history up to the 1950s, and still in less developed countries—when childbearing and childrearing went on at very high quantitative levels. Almost never did parents produce all the children they could have produced, but they produced enough to keep the population increasing despite high death rates. We need to consider the decisionmaking process both in times of high fertility and now.

Decisionmaking within the family

A long sequence of events is set in train by the act of having a child, a sequence largely unalterable for the succeeding 20 or so years. Few other individual decisions have the power to carry so much in their train. One can start on a trip and if the circumstances do not accord with expectations one can simply go home. The only other branching points for the individual that approach the fatefulness of having a child are choosing an occupation and choosing a spouse, but even these are not irrevocable.

Part of the problem of producing a child as a commodity is indivisibility. If parents could commit themselves a day at a time, they might be more willing to try; in fact they have to commit a major part of their lives. All of this influences intrafamily decisionmaking.

During most periods of history women were subordinate to men; they were in a prison from which breaking out was possible only for the few of exceptional talent. If we examine the means by which society channeled women's activities, we will see why there could be high fertility in most past ages, and how in contrast low fertility—perhaps even lower than we have seen anywhere so far—is the ultimate natural outcome of gender equality.

In an age when the only alternative for married women to staying home and having children was going on the street or working a 60-hour week in a factory, women could have little input into the couple's decisions to have children or anything else. In extreme patriarchal societies the man could in effect say, "Do as I command or starve." The employment market may everywhere still be biased against women, but at least developed countries have a market offering tolerable employment. A woman can leave her husband and get a job with acceptable work that will keep her alive, permit her to own a car, travel, watch television, have friends. The credible threat of leaving democratizes decisionmaking within the family.

Those promoting gender equality were innocent of any wish to cause population decline; with hindsight we can see that women's equality has indeed had an effect in this direction. Included in the context is the continuing disinclination of men to take an equal part in the raising of children; as Harriet Presser points out in this volume, many surveys have shown that in the two-worker household the wife averages very much more time with the children than the husband, even though her job may take as many hours as his. After divorce four times as many children remain with their mothers as with their fathers.

Acceptable jobs for women have increased their weight in domestic decisionmaking. Women's liberation gave them the moral right to decide whether or not to have a child, and the technology of the pill, the IUD, and sterilization put in their own hands the physical means to implement that right.

Gender roles

A feature of earlier high fertility was the inculcation of differentiated gender roles starting long before marriage, indeed in the cradle. The traditional husband did not need to tie down his wife bodily; she was tied down by the way that girls were raised from infancy. The commodity, "child," that was produced was wholly different for boys than for girls. It is an aspect of human plasticity that the girl—taught to play with dolls, protected against rough sports, oriented to attracting a man as the start of her real adult life, promoted by her kin as properly oriented to wifehood and motherhood—typically became a wife and mother and was neither competent nor happy in any other role. Teaching her a profession was carefully avoided; instead she was taught some art that would initially attract a husband, and later entertain him. For the majority of women escape was impossible against the many constraints imposed not so much by their husbands as individuals—though the husbands certainly acted their part—as by the expectations of neighbors, relatives, friends, churches, community groups, sewing circles; and celebrated in weddings, birthdays, and other family and community events. One was constantly reminded of the difference between the sexes by clothing, vocabulary, and the various forms of physical and moral protection of girls that boys were not supposed to require.

Thus no consideration of the child as a product can fail to note that boys and girls were highly differentiated products. Everything went together from the start in forming the child and the subsequent adult. A society that is consistent can produce the kind of human it needs. And, at least with respect to the role of women, the traditional society was nothing if not consistent.

Think then of the condition of a recently past age in which women are totally subordinate, where their only hope is marriage. Once they are married their time is at the disposal of their husbands. What should the husband do with that essentially free time? In the country a part of it can go into labor on the farm, a part of it is available for raising children. Children enhance the prestige of their father, in due course provide him with various services, continue the farm enterprise after he retires, perpetuate the family line after his death and so give him a vicarious immortality.

Within this command system all of agricultural production took place, and much of other production, as Kingsley Davis (1984) has described. For the farseeing parent, children were a crop, rather like wheat, except that the time for their reaping was not months but 12 or more years. Between the patriarchal command system and the self-contained production system the way to high fertility was clear. A tight ship was necessary for effective combat in sailing-ship days, and a tightly run household, in which wife and children were disciplined and childrearing was integrated with production, helped the household business. The traditional family fitted the circumstances in which it existed: there was much work to be done merely to survive; the family was not only an economic unit, but was also a unit for the defense and protection of its members. Rural fertility in America and Europe remained high after the cities had fallen well below the traditional family size.

The urban household prior to World War II had evolved, in Davis's (1984) scheme, beyond the point where it was a production unit; there was no integration of childrearing with earning, but there was a clear division of labor between husband and wife. The husband was the breadwinner; the wife did not work outside the home; her time was not worth very much to her husband because there was no worthwhile job for her to take. I ask again, what should the husband, having the authority, with a wife at home who was in something like the relation of a servant to him, give his wife to do? Preparing his meals and ironing his shirts was not full-time work. What could be more natural than to give her the dignity of motherhood and set her to raising children?

In the late twentieth century we are so used to the freedom and self-determination of individuals that it is hard to see how the traditional authority of the husband within the family was maintained. Greater physical strength of the man was no significant part of the answer. The secret was a convergence of many elements in the culture and the society: starting with the inculcation of appropriate gender roles in childhood—reading sentimental stories like *Little Women* and its sequels, in which even tomboy Jo ends up as a contented wife and mother, acquiring the "womanly" arts and avoiding rough sports as the proper way for girls to behave—and going on to absence of independent occupations in adulthood, not to mention social disapproval at all stages by both men and women for the girl who acted like a boy or the woman who tried to live as a bachelor. What from our point of view seems like a vast conspiracy surrounded the individual female to remind her of her role and force her to play it. That conspiracy was weakening even before World War II, and in recent decades it has been increasingly difficult to maintain.

The word "conspiracy" may sound overly dramatic, but it is a not inaccurate way of describing how the various elements mentioned above combined to maintain women in a position where their time was available for reproduction and for not much else. It was not a conspiracy on the part of men to dominate women, though that was the result, but a conspiracy of both sexes. From an early age a girl was taught to look forward to marriage, an expectation that could only translate into finding a man who would support her for the rest of her life. To make sure that she would concentrate on this goal of finding a man, college attendance or professional education that might have made her independent was withheld.

Women who did go to college followed decorative courses that would make them more cultured mothers: literature, romance languages, and the arts rather than engineering or medicine. Those who did manage to secure training for a career were discouraged by all possible means from practicing it. And those who did practice it were by no means held up as an ideal—think of the spinster schoolteacher as portrayed in literature, a scarcely less pathetic figure than the semislave governess of the Victorian era. Work outside the home was only encouraged for the (hopefully few) years between school and marriage. And once a woman was married, she was locked in by laws that made divorce difficult and by attitudes toward the divorcée that few would have cared to face even if the legal obstacles had been easier to surmont.

While in fact the woman had to find a man and do his will or be socially degraded, even go hungry, that is not the way it looked to those involved. The brutal facts were dressed up; the man was working for his wife and family, not to dominate, but to protect them. If one can trust Victorian novels, a prison was constructed into which most women were eager to enter, and from which few sought to escape.

Spread of the high-fertility, male-dominant society

High fertility may or may not have been the conscious object of all of this, even though the configuration of practices certainly promoted fertility. As among competing ethnic groups, those with high fertility increased their numbers while those with lower fertility grew more slowly—or actually declined, given the high death rates of earlier times. This spread of the high-fertility cultures did not need to be planned by anyone; it was a selection effect that came about through the facts of arithmetic. Intertribal competition and evolution spread high-fertility cultures, characterized by the nearly universal subjection of women.

Thus, sheer arithmetic worked at second remove to make male dominance universal. The spread of Islam's strong support of males and its high fertility is an aspect of this that persists into the present. We can see a simple causation here, with a culture of male dominance promoting high fertility, and that high fertility in turn causing an increase in the population that carried the culture of male dominance. Why are there so few societies around the world in which women dominate? Our answer is that with prevailing mortality such societies would have died out through having too few children. In short, male dominance could well have been functionally necessary for high fertility, and high fertility arithmetically necessary for the continuance of societies.

To generalize the proposition: if it is desired to have something produced by people acting "voluntarily," then fence off a part of the adult population, thus preventing them from engaging in the other work of the society, so that there is virtually nothing else they can do. In classical India, shoes were less expensive because a caste of leatherworkers was not permitted to work at anything else. The main application of interest here is the fencing-off of women that kept them from gaining a livelihood by any means other than childbearing. The economics of caste applies to motherhood as well.

I have argued that the societies that constrain women will increase and so increase the numbers that bear their culture; those that do not will contract. But the point could well be applicable *within* societies as well; to the extent that individual families have their own culture, the ones that "protect" their women will spread while those that lack this feature will contract. So there will be a selection feature at the family level as well as at the tribal level, always favoring male dominance insofar as that restricts women to childbearing.

One of the aspects of present trends that remain unexplained concerns the distribution of children. The argument of this article, like that of others in this volume, tells us that under modern conditions there will be few children. What will require additional hypotheses to explain is the present prevalence of the two-child family. Instead of family size declining steadily and uniformly toward zero, as much of my argument would make it seem to do, it tends to move toward two, and the special position of the two-child family still demands explanation. I can offer nothing in this direction except to agree with Harriet Presser's statement, in this volume, that couples do want some descendants, though not necessarily enough to reproduce the population (Vaupel and Goodwin, 1986).

Population policy

Will it be possible to tie policy to a forward movement of history, one that might be called professionalization? This is characterized by the limitation of responsibility, the shortening of hours, the application of specialized knowledge, preferably in a specialized place.

The physician of 50 years ago was a servant to his patients; he was subject to house calls 24 hours a day; he was unspecialized and responsible for any kind of health contingency. His consulting room was usually in his home; this tended to limit his private life, so that even taking a holiday was difficult. Today, he is on duty a limited number of hours; he is specialized in a certain branch of medicine; he has an office that is not part of his home; he makes no house calls. A reversion to the previous way of practicing medicine would seem to him like reversion to domestic service.

The wife and mother is still largely in that earlier stage. Her influence on the child may be reduced, but her attention can never be far from it. She is responsible for all contingencies, 24 hours a day; her life outside childrearing is secondary. Would parenting be more acceptable if it moved in the same direction as the practice of medicine or office work: toward the limiting of responsibility? Better day care and attractive nursery schools from the age of one or two years, child care outside the home for parents who want to take a vacation, prompt and convenient medical services that could be depended on in emergencies—all these would professionalize motherhood in the sense that medicine is professionalized.

Does this mean that economic incentives can be disregarded? By no means. Children's allowances, in Canada, France, Sweden, and elsewhere, have tended to be set at the level that at best covers the marginal additional cost of a child. (One Swedish mother I know uses her allowance to provide pocket money to her children.) There is a large gap between that and the opportunity cost of the wife's time. Closing it would entail a greater expense than electorates so far are willing to pay. If the United States needs 4 million births per year and if we pay mothers $10,000 per year for five years of their time, on the average, for each birth, that totals $200 billion per year; even confining the payment to third and later children has not been seriously considered.

Whether money and privileges stimulate fertility depends on the level of income and facilities in the community in question. It is worth contrasting the energetic measures for promotion of fertility in East Germany with the absence of such measures in West Germany, or their relative ineffectiveness in France. During the past decade there was a clear and sharp rise in the East German birth rate, though not sufficient to attain replacement-level fertility and probably not permanent. The measures taken have included payments to mothers for not working while they look after their children and, in particular, the provision of housing. It would make little sense to provide housing in France or West Germany, where the market is more or less adequately supplied. Similarly, where salaries are already high, it would be both expensive and less effective to offer couples money to have children. The East German measures have worked because money and housing mean a great deal to couples there.

For advanced countries in general the two obvious lines of policy are money and the professionalization of motherhood. Something has been done on both—family allowances and day-care centers are respective examples—but either it is not enough or these are ineffective measures for increasing fertility, however desirable they may be on other grounds.

More money enables people to buy more goods and so seems to increase their taste for them. Helping to professionalize motherhood by providing schooling and other facilities could make the children seem less the mother's own. Both ways of helping mothers are socially beneficial, but their contribution to fertility is uncertain. It could be negative.

If all this makes the low-fertility problem seem even more difficult, then I have made my point. Our aim should be a theoretical description in which low fertility appears as stubborn as our experience is proving it to be in real life.

References

Becker, Gary S. 1960. "An economic analysis of fertility," in *Demographic and Economic Change in Developed Countries: A Conference of the Universities-National Bureau Committee for Economic Research*. National Bureau for Economic Research, Special Conference Series, no. 11. Princeton, N.J.: Princeton University Press.

———, and H. Gregg Lewis. 1973. "On the interaction between the quantity and quality of children," *Journal of Political Economy* 81, no. 2, Part II (March/April): S279–S288.

Bongaarts, John, and Robert G. Potter. 1983. *Fertility, Biology, and Behavior: An Analysis of the Proximate Determinants*. New York: Academic Press.

Butz, William P., and Michael P. Ward. 1979. "Will US fertility remain low? A new economic interpretation," *Population and Development Review* 5, no. 4 (December): 663–688.

Caldwell, John C. 1982. *Theory of Fertility Decline*. New York: Academic Press.

Davis, Kingsley. 1984. "Wives and work: The sex role revolution and its consequences," *Population and Development Review* 10, no. 3 (September): 397–417.

———, and Judith Blake. 1956. "Social structure and fertility: An analytic framework," *Economic Development and Cultural Change* 4, no. 4 (July): 211–235.

Easterlin, Richard A. 1966. "On the relation of economic factors to recent and projected fertility changes," *Demography* 3, no. 1: 131–151.

———. 1973. "Relative economic status and the American fertility swing," in *Family Economic Behavior: Problems and Prospects*, ed. Eleanor Bernert Sheldon. Philadelphia: J. B. Lippincott Company, pp. 170–223.

———. 1980. *Birth and Fortune: The Impact of Numbers on Personal Welfare*. New York: Basic Books.

Herrstrom, Staffan. 1985. *Die familienpolitik in Schweden vor den Wahlen von 1985*. Paper no. 335. Stockholm: Svenska Institutet.

Pratt, William F., William D. Mosher, Christine A. Bachrach, and Marjorie C. Horn. 1984. "Understanding U.S. fertility: Findings from the National Survey of Family Growth, Cycle III," *Population Bulletin* 39, no. 5 (December): 3–40.

Sanderson, Warren C. 1974. "Economic theories of fertility: What do they explain?" NBER Working Paper Series, no. 36. New York: National Bureau of Economic Research.

Schultz, Theodore W. (ed.). 1974. *Economics of the Family: Marriage, Children and Human Capital*. A conference report of the National Bureau of Economic Research. Chicago: University of Chicago Press.

Smith, James P., and Michael P. Ward. 1984. *Women's Wages and Work in the Twentieth Century*. Report R-3119-NICHD. Santa Monica, Calif.: The Rand Corporation.

United Nations. 1985. *World Population Prospects: Estimates and Projections as Assessed in 1982*. New York.

United States Bureau of the Census. 1982–83. *Statistical Abstract of the United States*, 103rd Edition. Washington, D.C.: US Department of Commerce.

Vaupel, James, and Dianne Goodwin. 1986. "The division of labor." Working Paper. Laxenburg, Austria: International Institute for Applied Systems Analysis.

Willis, Robert J. 1973. "A new approach to the economic theory of fertility behavior," *Journal of Political Economy* 81, no. 2, Part II (March/April): S14–S64.

Perspective on Nuptiality and Fertility

Charles F. Westoff

One of the most dramatic sociodemographic changes in the United States and in other Western countries in the past quarter-century has been the postponement of marriage. Figures 1 and 2 show the proportions of women in selected European countries and the United States who are single at ages 20–24 and 25–29, respectively. Between 1960 and 1985, the proportion of US women aged 20–24 who have never married has doubled, from 28 to 58 percent; at ages 25–29 the proportion of single women has risen from 10 to 26 percent (US Bureau of the Census, 1985). The trend toward postponing marriage has been apparent throughout the reproductive ages; even the conservative Bureau of the Census has now accepted the likelihood that the proportion of persons going through life without ever marrying will increase. It would thus appear that marriage may simply be going out of style, although historical comparison reveals that the demographic situation is not dissimilar to that of the late nineteenth century (see Figure 3). At the beginning of the century, the proportions of women never married (Taeuber and Taeuber, 1971, p. 285)—52 percent at ages 20–24 and 28 percent at ages 25–29—were, on the surface, little different than they are now (Rodgers and Thornton, 1985, p. 272). The modern decline in age at marriage began around 1940, accelerated over the following 20 years, and began its reversal around 1960. Have we simply returned to the nineteenth century pattern of marriage, or are new trends in the making?

There are several reasons for interpreting the recent trend toward marriage postponement in quite different terms. The amount of premarital sexual activity is undoubtedly an order of magnitude greater than that around the turn of the century. This seems likely not only because of the obvious changes in attitudes and in the status of women (in education and employment, for example) but also because of the technological innovations in contraception and later the

FIGURE 1 Percent of women aged 20–24 who are single, selected Western European countries and the United States

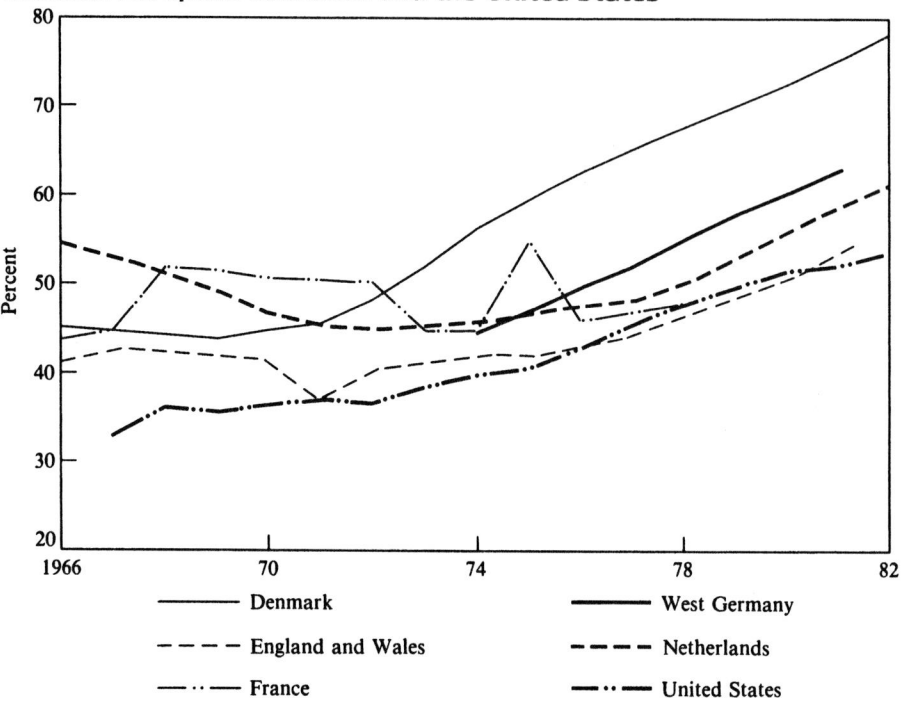

SOURCES: United Nations, *Demographic Yearbook*, 1976, Tables 25 and 41; 1982, Tables 24 and 40.

increasing availability of legal abortion—in short, a veritable revolution in fertility regulation. In this context, the high rates of premarital teenage pregnancy in this country can be viewed as the result of an enormous increase in the amount and duration of exposure to risk (at younger ages and for more years). Pregnancy, when it does occur, is no longer an automatic prelude to marriage.

Another social change that sharply differentiates contemporary marital behavior from that of earlier decades, as well as from the nineteenth century, is the rapidly increasing popularity of informal cohabitation. This institution, which developed first in the Scandinavian countries, has become quite pervasive there in recent years. The proportion of Swedish women aged 20–24 who are living together in so-called paper-less unions is estimated in 1981 at 44 percent and constitutes three-quarters of all unions at those ages. In fact, a comparison of US and Swedish data reveals fairly similar proportions of young couples living together, but in Sweden the bulk are not formally married. In both societies, the sense of "commitment" to enduring unions seems to have diminished considerably, a conclusion that is consistent with the experimental nature of informal cohabitation and its frequent dissolution (Blanc, 1985) as well as with the more conventional inference from the high divorce rate.

FIGURE 2 Percent of women aged 25–29 who are single, selected Western European countries and the United States

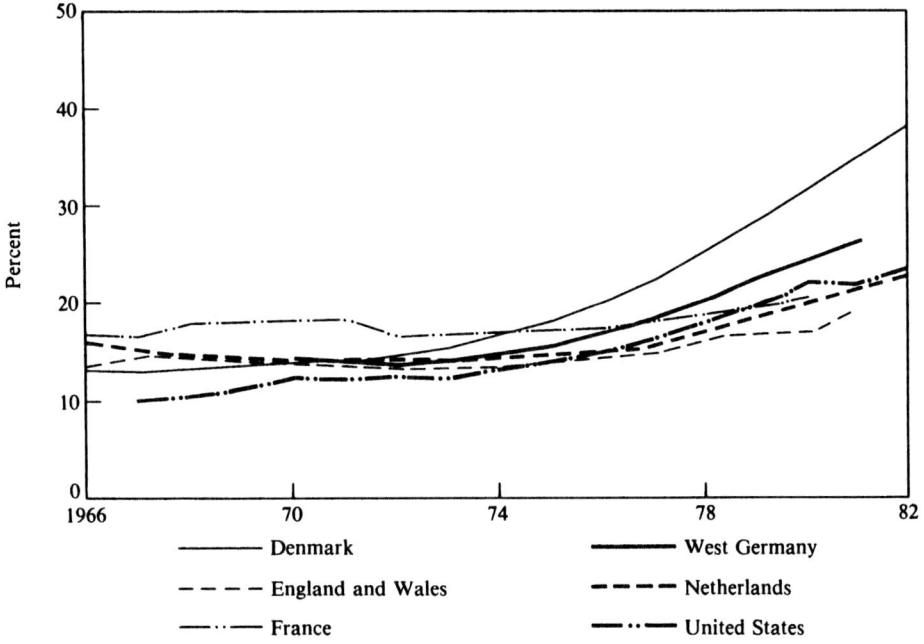

SOURCES: United Nations, *Demographic Yearbook*, 1976, Table 41; 1982, Table 40.

This new institution has become an object of sociological inquiry with many questions and few answers. The impression that emerges from the Swedish experience is that such unions, whatever their durability, are experimental in nature and as such are low-fertility arrangements (Hoem and Rennermalm, 1985). We do not have direct evidence on such matters for the United States, but inferences from Census household-composition data suggest that nearly 2 million couples were living together outside of formal marriage as of 1983 (Glick, 1985, p. 210). The practice is becoming sufficiently institutionalized that the Census Bureau is even contemplating the addition of a category to the marital status question in the 1990 Census to capture such arrangements.

The other index of marriage that is included conventionally in any analysis of nuptiality is the rate of dissolution. As is well known, the divorce rate in the United States is the highest of any country in the West (Figure 4), for reasons not readily understood. Curiously, this issue has received less scholarly attention than it would seem to deserve. Current experience implies an ultimate dissolution rate approaching one of every two marriages. The conventional sociological wisdom has increasingly dismissed this high divorce rate as an indicator of the weakening of the family or even of marriage, asserting that it merely reflects disenchantment with particular partners and that the divorced simply go on to marry another person—a kind of change-partners-and-dance

FIGURE 3 Percent of women who are single at ages 20–24 and 25–29, United States, 1890–1985

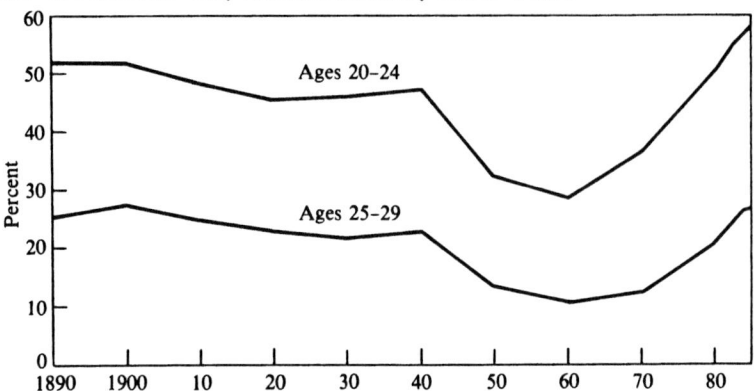

SOURCES: Taeuber and Taeuber (1971, p. 284); Current Population Reports, *Marital Status and Living Arrangements: March 1983*, Series P-20, No. 389, p. 2; US Bureau of the Census, *Population Characteristics*, "Marital status and living arrangements: March 1984," Table B, p. 2 and *Population Characteristics*, Series P-20, No. 402, October 1985, Table 4, p. 8.

routine. Such a facile interpretation ignores the fact that many women are left with little prospect of remarriage given the demographic nature of the marriage market (Goldman, Westoff, and Hammerslough, 1984). As men grow older their pool of available potential mates increases; as women age, their market shrinks. This is a consequence of two phenomena: men's preference for younger women and, at the later ages, women's greater survival. Since this age preference phenomenon would seem to have economic roots, it could eventually change as women's economic standing increases.

What do these trends imply for the future of marriage? It seems premature at best to conclude that the institution is on the way out. After all, it has been around for many centuries. But it seems reasonably clear that it is changing in important ways. Several propositions seem plausible:

— Marriage will become less nearly universal than it has been in recent cohorts, and it will occur at later ages than ever.

— Informal cohabitation will increase both before and between marriages but will not function as a true substitute for marriage.

— The divorce rate will continue at a high level, although if cohabitation (read long live-in engagement) becomes very common along with the postponement of marriage, it may moderate and eventually decrease. A countervailing view expressed by Andrew Cherlin (1981) is that since cohabitation is based on the principle of mutual gratification, it may not lead to lower divorce rates. Evidence from a study of Swedish and Norwegian data indicates that divorce rates are in fact higher rather than

FIGURE 4 Number of divorces per thousand married couples, selected Western European countries and the United States

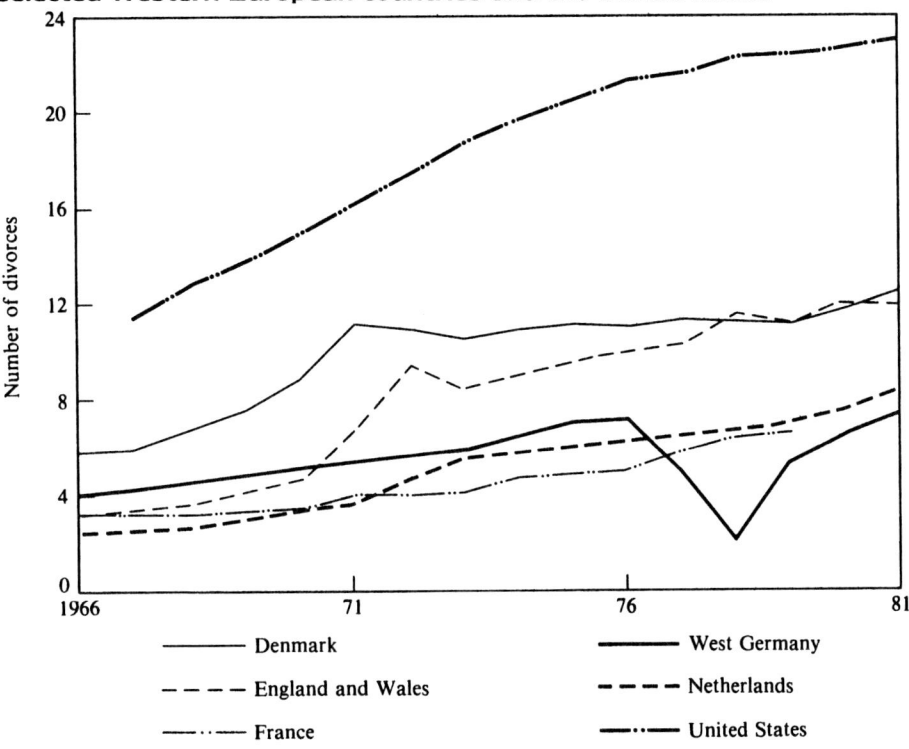

SOURCES: United Nations, *Demographic Yearbook*, 1968, Table 35; 1976, Tables 25, 33, 41; 1982, Tables 24, 32, 40.

lower for couples with premarital cohabitation experience, thus supporting the hypothesis of self-selectivity of persons with lower potential for commitment (Blanc, 1985, pp. 75–79).

Several important sociological changes underlie these demographic prognostications. Probably the most important force underlying the weakening of marriage is the growing economic independence of women caused by their increasing participation in the work force—a social change typical of Western countries (Figure 5)—and their slowly increasing earnings relative to those of men. Economic explanations are basic to understanding the roots and persistence of marriage in general. In essence, marriage can be viewed traditionally as an economic exchange system in which men offer their support and status in exchange for the childbearing and domestic services of women. What happens to this foundation when women become less economically dependent on men? It seems clear that the basis for marriage becomes seriously eroded. To sharpen the point: imagine a society in which men and women are genuinely equal economically, with similar proportions as plumbers, bank presidents,

FIGURE 5 Percent of women aged 15–49 in the labor force, selected Western European countries, Australia, and the United States

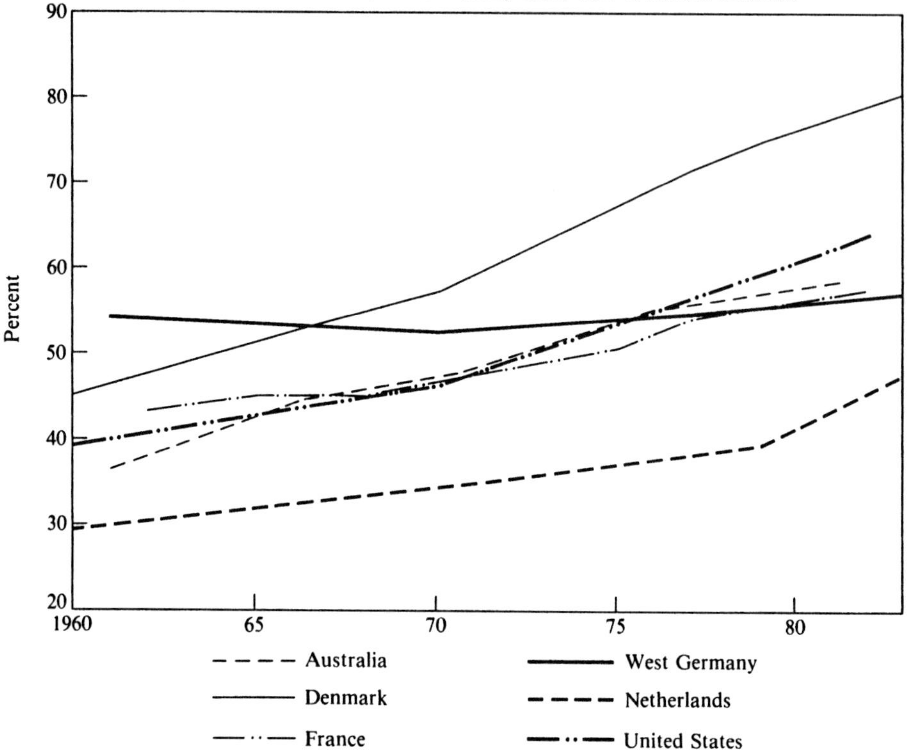

---- Australia   ——— West Germany
——— Denmark   ---- Netherlands
—··— France   —··— United States

SOURCE: International Labour Office, *Yearbook of Labour Statistics*, Table 1.

professors, and secretaries, and with men and women earning the same income associated with such activity. What then is the point of marriage once the cultural habits—those sets of expectations about the naturalness of marriage—are commensurately weakened? Of course, there is the remaining economic argument that two incomes are better than one, but this objective can be served without formal marriage. The primary remaining function that marriage would serve would be the legitimation of offspring or, to continue the economic metaphor, the private ownership of children. However, when we observe the trends in childbearing in Western countries, even this function, the most basic of all biosocial functions, seems increasingly questionable.

This view of marriage is shared by some, but not all, observers. Robert Schoen and his colleagues have assembled a statistical portrait of marriage and divorce in the United States beginning with the birth cohorts of 1888–92 and extending to synthetic cohort estimates for 1980. They conclude:

> The present results are consistent with the view that a fundamental change in the traditional concept of marriage is underway. . . . Recent economic changes

have undermined the social and economic forces that maintained the institution of marriage. . . . The "marital union" of the past may be giving way to the "marital partnership" of the future, which will accommodate informal as well as formal marriages, less dependence between spouses, greater egalitarianism, lower fertility, and higher levels of divorce. (Schoen et al., 1985, pp. 112–113)

Kingsley Davis seems a little less certain about the future of marriage. He points out that age at marriage cannot rise indefinitely, that the rising proportion of married women in the labor force (which influences marriage, divorce, and fertility) will soon reach its upper limit, and that "the divorce rate also seems to have a limit, but the limit is indeterminant and very high" (1983, pp. 40–41). John Modell concludes from a historical evaluation that the "record, however, is one of resilience and persistence" (Modell, 1986, p. 182). This theme is also sounded by Willard Rodgers and Arland Thornton, who write: "although recent changes in family life and values may represent dramatic changes from the past that could be registered in even further declines in marriage, there is also considerable evidence that Americans continue to value marriage" (1985, p. 277).

As Thomas Espenshade recently concluded, projections of the future of marriage "depend on whether one subscribes to linear or to cyclical theories of social change. Linear theories anticipate that the future will be a continuation of the recent past, whereas cyclical theories expect marriage to rebound over the next decade . . ." (1985, p. 239).

Fertility

It is difficult to reach any conclusion from an examination of recent fertility trends in the industrialized countries other than that childbearing is becoming less popular. In fact, period fertility rates are well below replacement in most countries and are still headed down in many (Figure 6). In the United Kingdom and in France, the current total fertility rate (TFR) is around 1.8. In the Netherlands, the rate has dropped from 2.4 in 1971 to around 1.5 in 1982. In West Germany, which is now experiencing population decline, the estimated rate for 1984 is below 1.3, the lowest in Europe. Other low and still declining rates are apparent in Austria (1.5), Switzerland (1.5), Italy (1.6), Denmark (1.4), Sweden (1.6), and Norway (1.7). In the Catholic countries of Spain and Portugal, the total fertility rate seems to be collapsing, from rates close to 3.0 at the beginning of the 1970s to around 2.0 by the early 1980s. The case of Ireland is even more dramatic. This orthodox Catholic population had by far the highest fertility rate in Western Europe in 1970 at 4.0 births per woman. By the end of 1982, it had dropped to 2.9 and seems destined to join its neighbors in another few years. The legislature in that country has even managed to legalize over-the-counter sales of male contraceptives.

These low fertility levels were reached even earlier in the socialist Eastern European countries (a well-known example of the demographic irrelevance of

FIGURE 6 Total fertility rates in industrialized countries since 1971

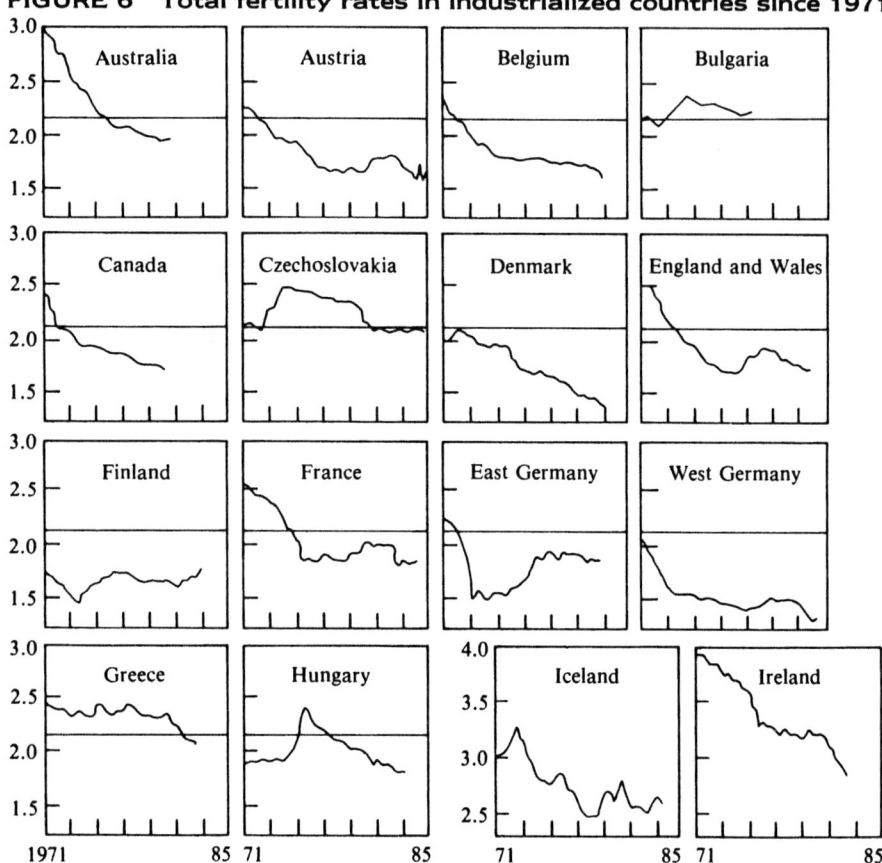

types of economic systems). Some of these, such as Czechoslovakia, Hungary, Romania, and more recently East Germany, managed to increase their fertility in the mid-1970s, presumably by government intervention, but in most instances the recovery has been short-lived. Only Poland contrives somehow to maintain above-replacement fertility, at around 2.4.

Canada is down close to 1.7 (with French Catholic Quebec even lower at 1.4). Australia and New Zealand have experienced declines of about one-third in their total fertility rates since 1970 and are already below replacement and still headed down. The fertility rate in the United States has declined sharply after the prolonged baby boom of the 1950s and 1960s and has appeared to level off at about 1.8 since the mid-1970s.

What is to be made of all this? Do the explanations lie in the contemporary economic scene, or in the use of new birth control methods, or in the increased availability of abortion, or in recent changes in the status of women? Demographers are far better at measuring what is happening than at explaining it in nondemographic terms, but it seems to me that the explanation is in a sense only the modern manifestation and continuation of what has been happening for a century or more. Some very fundamental changes have occurred in

FIGURE 6 (continued)

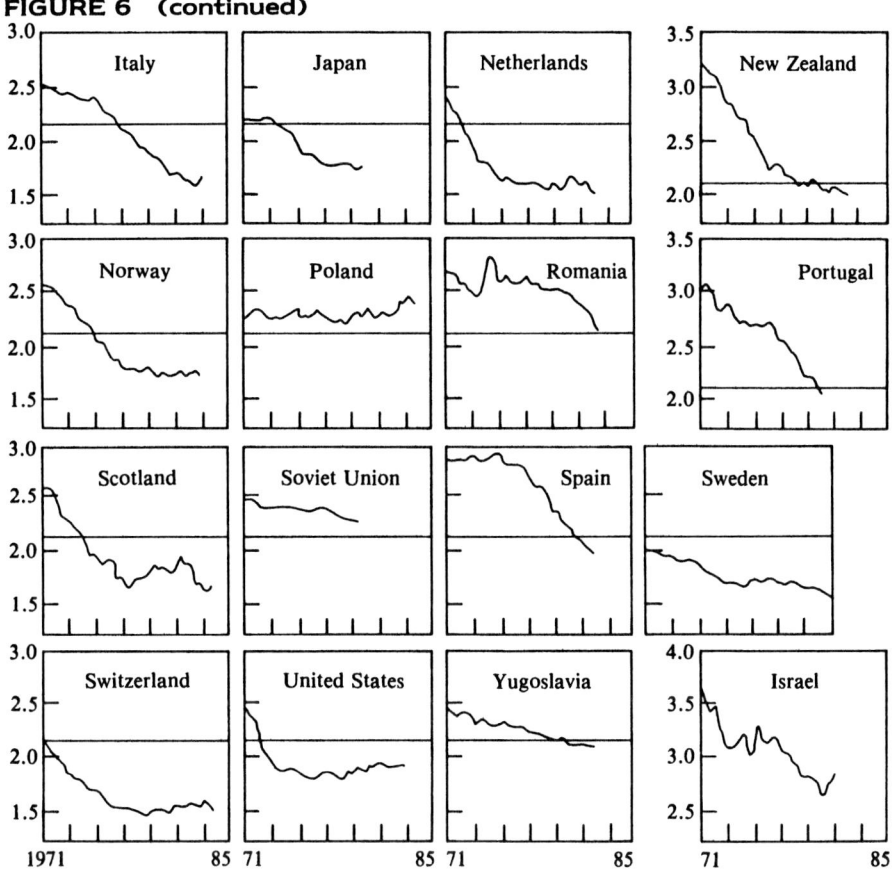

SOURCE: INED, Paris. Estimates as of 5 April 1985.

Western civilization in the last 100 years or so, in themselves probably triggered by even more basic economic transformations in earlier times. At the root have been economic changes that radically altered the economic value of children from producer to dependent. Along with the forces that transformed labor-intensive agrarian economies into urban industrialized systems, the child not only became less useful, but also required ever-increasing investment in education as the demand for greater skills developed.

New laws and customs related to children and women eventually rationalized the changing status of both, as the economic value of women's work outside the home became increasingly realized with expanding economies and the rise of mass education. Traditional religious values began to change with the forces of modernization, which also contributed to the redefinition of the proper place for women and of the sacrosanct nature of marriage. Individualism, with an emphasis on competitive success in the marketplace, emerged and joined forces with materialism and its modern counterpart, consumerism.

This version of the story is probably the standard explanation for the historical onset of the decline of fertility. The supporting evidence, however, is far from incontrovertible. Both historically and in contemporary developing countries, there are all too many cases in which birth control has spread and fertility has declined without any accompanying or preceding economic transformation. The main determinants appear instead to have been education, region, language, and other cultural variables that support a theory of diffusion of ideas without any basic economic explanation. This position is well argued by John Cleland and Chris Wilson (1985) in a recent paper, based on an evaluation of the implications for transition theory of World Fertility Survey data.

Whatever the admixture of causes, the birth rate in the United States, which had been dropping throughout the nineteenth century, continued its decline, reaching a low in the 1930s. Then came economic recovery from the Depression, World War II, and a baby boom that pushed fertility back up to a high not witnessed for half a century. More importantly, the level of births remained high long beyond anyone's expectations. As social scientists look back on this phenomenon, they can explain what happened demographically, but they remain uneasy with the sociological explanations. People married in large numbers at young ages and had two or three children quickly. The proportion of women of this generation having at least two children reached a high of 82 percent (close to a maximum), up from 55 percent in the preceding generation (Ryder, 1979, p. 361). There was clearly no return to the larger families of earlier generations, but rather a near-universal franchise on marriage and the two-child norm.

Contrast that situation with the current picture. American women now in their mid-20s may well match or even exceed the historic high of childlessness of 22 percent recorded by the 1908–09 birth cohorts. David Bloom and James Trussell (1984) estimate that between 20 and 25 percent of the most recent cohorts will remain childless. Given the postponement of marriage and childbearing, the proportion of American women who will have only one child is already increasing significantly. That proportion has ranged historically from a high of 23 percent in the cohorts 1902–08 to a low of 9.5 percent for the 1932 cohort. When they reach the end of their reproductive ages in 15–20 years, close to half of the cohorts of today's young women appear likely to have either no children or only one child.

Much of this change, it is worth noting, has occurred without any apparent change in the norms about childlessness or one-child families. The annual series of data on fertility expectations collected in the Census Bureau's Current Population Survey shows hardly any change in the proportions of young women (aged 18–34) expecting to remain childless or to have only one child—10.6 percent (US Bureau of the Census, 1983, 1976, 1973). Demographic analysis, even allowing for considerable forecasting error, suggests an ultimate proportion childless about twice that expected by the women themselves. As George Masnick put it, referring to expectations about childlessness and only children: "Expectations seem to address norms about motherhood and only children more directly than likely behavior" (1981, p. 177). This is a good example of a more general sociological proposition—that changes in behavior precede changes in norms. Women still expect to have children—mostly two, of course—an attitude that persists even among women who reach their late 20s without any children. Over 60 percent of all childless women aged 25–29 expect two or more births in their lifetime (US Bureau of the Census, 1983, Table 8). Childlessness—and perhaps to a lesser extent having an only child—is a status that women tend to back into as the "costs" (age, job considerations, lifestyle) of making the actual decision to have a child loom larger. In addition, of course, there is the ever-increasing possibility of involuntary sterility as women approach the later years of childbearing.

Perhaps this picture is only a caricature of the college-educated career woman whose dilemmas about "finding a man" and having a child late in life have become the subject of popular journalism in the past few years. The typical American woman, although she is clearly marrying at a later age than did her mother during the decade of the baby boom, still has children and still has them during her 20s, on average at age 26 (as of 1980). American women continue to have a lower age at maternity than is common in most European countries. The postponement of childbearing into the 30s is far from universal in the United States, but judging from the experience of other countries, the United States seems to be pointed clearly in that direction.

The picture of fertility described here also seems to imply that conscious decisionmaking largely governs the reproductive process. Most of history must have witnessed little conscious intervention in the spacing or limitation of births, but there has been a veritable revolution in this area of human decisionmaking. Although large proportions of pregnancies still occur unintentionally in Western countries—the 1982 National Survey of Family Growth estimates that 29 percent of all pregnancies in the United States were unplanned during the preceding five years—the fraction of births reported by women as unwanted, that is, those births that would theoretically never occur if contraception were perfect, has dropped steadily in the United States from 20 percent in 1961–65 to 13 percent in 1971–75 to 7 percent by 1978–82 (Pratt et al., 1984, p. 31). This impressive improvement in the control of fertility has occurred because of better and more effective contraception—the pill, IUD, and especially surgical sterilization (which has become the leading method of contraception in the United States) and has been facilitated by the availability of legal abortion. This is not to say that the "perfect contraceptive society" has finally arrived. There are high rates of unintended teenage pregnancy in the United States (in sharp contrast, for example, to very low rates in such countries as the Netherlands, Sweden, and France), and the high rate of induced abortion in the United States bears ample testimony to the significant incidence of contraceptive failure and to the failure to use contraception. The demographic impact of this reduction in unwanted fertility has been considerable. With further improvements in contraceptive technology and with the inevitable reduction of the teenage birth rate, the fertility rate could be reduced possibly by another 10 percent or so, perhaps even more.

The important point is that American couples are showing many signs of wanting fewer children and that even if the current decline in the quantity and change in the tempo of childbearing do not continue, such as they show signs of doing in some other countries, the level of fertility can be expected to drop further merely as a consequence of the reduction of the unintended component.

The future

But will these patterns continue? Are there reasons to believe that society will change in ways to encourage higher fertility? One's confidence in answering such a question is chastened by the recent experience of the baby boom. At the end of World War II, we all would have predicted a short-lived boom of marriages and births and then a resumption of the historical decline or a stabilization of fertility at low levels, certainly not the still partly incomprehensible phenomenon that did occur.

A recent appraisal concludes that "a close look at the historical record . . . suggests that in some ways the 1970s were more consistent with long-term trends in family life than were the 1950s" (Cherlin, 1981, p. 7). Viewing the situation somewhat differently, however, Richard Easterlin (1980) has predicted another baby boom in the 1990s, when the relatively small birth cohorts of the 1970s come of age and experience the economic advantages of small numbers. His theory, based empirically on a negative association between the size of a cohort and its own fertility in the next generation during twentieth century US history, has been extensively reviewed and intensively examined, and it is not necessary to review all of the arguments here. The one important, indeed crucial, element of the theory, however, is the assumption that the woman's role in the marketplace is a derivative of the man's; that is, with large cohorts and consequent competitive disadvantage, women work to supplement husbands' incomes or to support themselves because marriage is delayed for the same economic reasons that men find good jobs more difficult to obtain. Conversely, in good times, marriage and childbearing need not be postponed, and women are not pressed into the supplementary breadwinner role. The basic implication seems to be that women are programmed primarily as wives and mothers and that satisfaction of these roles is periodically frustrated by economic conditions, which in turn are influenced by cohort size. The argument does not allow for changes in the status, attitudes, and interests of women who may be refocusing their lives around the same occupational and nonfamilial interests traditionally associated with the male world. It is possible, of course, that this is a characterization of only a minority of educated women and not an accurate description of the large bulk of women currently in the labor force.

In any event, granting the large element of uncertainty in such prediction, the weight of history of all Western countries seems to lean heavily in the direction of continued low fertility. Few if any of the presumably relevant historical determinants of low fertility have changed. The only possible exceptions are the constraints to availability of abortion and an apparent surge of religious fundamentalism in the United States. The abortion controversy seems likely to be around for some time to come. There may be increasing roadblocks to easy availability, but it seems unlikely that any sweeping changes in the situation will occur.

Contrary to the impressions generated by the media, the American population is evidently not drifting toward fundamentalist religious beliefs. According to trend data from public opinion polls, the proportion of the population with fundamentalist beliefs (defined as believing that the Bible was divinely inspired, and/or reporting having had a "born-again" experience, and/or engaged in proselytizing) has remained unchanged, at about 20 percent, for the past 15 years or so. The religious revival that has commanded attention in recent years is evidently the result of the increasing political activity and visibility of this segment of the population. This political activism coincided with the controversial Supreme Court decision on abortion, regarded by many as the intrusion of politics into the moral domain, and was legitimized by the occupancy of the White House in 1976 by a born-again Christian, Jimmy Carter. Since that date, there has been a substantial increase in the political participation of this part of the electorate.

The significance of these trends for the future of marriage and fertility is probably not great, but the increase in political influence of this kind of conservatism may indeed retard the decline in unintended fertility by making abortion more difficult to obtain or by impeding the provision of contraceptive services to teenagers or the adoption of sex education in local school systems. Although the main goal of much of this political action is to reverse the Supreme Court decision on abortion, the alternative of providing contraceptive services and information to teenagers appears to be an unacceptable solution to many actively opposed to abortion. One study suggests that the underlying attitude is one of opposition in general to premarital sexuality. This is in sharp contrast to attitudes and behavior in Western Europe. In Sweden, for example, where the liberalization of the abortion law was widely debated prior to passage in 1975, there was great concern that one undesirable result would be an explosion of teenage abortions. The response by the government was to include as part of the legislative package a program to establish 32 youth clinics around the country to provide contraceptive counseling and services along with other health services, which would also be integrated with the institutionalized sex education programs in the schools. A wide publicity campaign was also undertaken. The results were dramatic. The abortion rate among Swedish teenagers not only failed to rise with the new easy access to abortion, but between 1975 and 1981 it actually declined by a third (by 50 percent among girls under 18). The birth rate for teenagers under 17 is now virtually zero in that country. An important part of the picture is that the abortion rate for adults remained unchanged or increased somewhat, which further corroborates the direct results of the youth clinic program. In 1975, the teenage abortion rate in Sweden had been the same as in the United States; while it has since declined there by 33 percent, it has risen in the United States by 43 percent. What makes this contrast even more striking is that recent survey data in the two countries indicate that Swedish teenage girls begin sex even earlier (one year younger on average) than American girls, which means longer exposure to risk in the teenage years. The United States is the only Western country (with data on both births and abortion) in which the teenage pregnancy rate (defined as the sum of the birth rate and the abortion rate) has actually increased in the past decade or so. Since the teenage birth rate decreased during the decade by some 20 percent, the increase in the abortion rate had to be substantial.

The United States is in an anomalous international position in terms of adolescent fertility. Although the country's overall fertility is in the middle range of contemporary Western levels, its teenage fertility is extremely high by these international standards. American teenage fertility is 70 percent higher than the average teenage fertility in the rest of the developed world. Among teenagers under 18, the contrast is even more dramatic, showing the United States with a rate at ages 15–17 three times the average of the other countries. (Although the rate for black teenagers is two to three times that of whites, the US rate for whites is still very high by international standards.)

As noted above, the teenage birth rate is declining as a consequence of increasing abortion rates rather than by any reduction in pregnancy rates, but it will take a long time for it to reach European levels. Adult fertility remains low in all Western countries, and, as we have seen, there is little on the horizon to suggest that it will increase substantially in the future. This means that sooner or later, governments will undoubtedly enter the picture in an effort to stimulate growth. This has already happened in some countries in Eastern Europe.

Conclusions

The future of marriage and fertility translates ultimately into the future of the family and of the population, a not unimportant consideration for any society. In the Western world today, we see a general picture of change, resuming a process begun over a century ago that features an apparent diminution of the functional importance of marriage and a general decline of fertility in virtually all Western countries to levels well below replacement.

One's interpretation of these changes determines the prognosis. We have seen late marriage and low fertility in earlier decades, only to be followed in some countries by a sharp reversal of trend and a prolonged plunge into early marriage and childbearing at young ages. Perhaps we are simply at the threshold of repetition of that cycle. Perhaps, as Easterlin suggests, the cohorts reaching the ages of marriage and parenthood during the next decade may react to the opportunities afforded by smaller numbers by marrying earlier and having more children. Or perhaps unpredictable changes in lifestyle will occur, making marriage and parenthood more fashionable. Although the element of fashion cannot be ruled out, my guess is that enough radical changes have occurred in recent decades—including changes in women's status, cohabitation, high marital dissolution rates, developments in contraceptive technology, and legal abortion—which, when combined with historical forces that have been driving birth rates down for a century or more, strongly suggest a future of low rates of reproduction in the Western world. The United States fits squarely within this picture, although its high teenage birth rate differentiates it sharply from the general Western pattern. My guess, however, is that even this anomaly will largely diminish by the end of the century.

The big question that already confronts some European countries and that will confront many others in short order if current trends continue is that of impending population decline. West Germany, with its total fertility rate in 1984 estimated at 1.27, is already experiencing more deaths than births. Several other countries have also reached that turning point. The United States has considerably more time before it faces this problem because of the demographic legacy of the baby boom and the volume of immigration, although the preliminary symptoms of an aging population exist. How countries will react to this new challenge remains to be seen. Special commissions will undoubtedly be appointed to study the question, and increasing government subsidies will be offered to encourage marriage and childbearing. International labor migration will doubtless be relied upon to an increasing extent. In the final analysis, however, there is no insurance on the future of many nation-states.

References

Ariès, Philippe. 1980. "Two successive motivations for the declining birth rate in the West," *Population and Development Review* 6, no. 4 (December): 645–650.

Blanc, Ann Klimas. 1985. *The Effect of Nonmarital Cohabitation on Family Formation and Dissolution: A Comparative Analysis of Sweden and Norway*. Doctoral dissertation, Department of Sociology, Princeton University.

Bloom, David E. 1984. "Putting off children," *American Demographics* 6, no. 9 (September): 30–33, 45.

———, and James Trussell. 1984. "What are the determinants of delayed childbearing and permanent childlessness in the United States?," *Demography* 21, no. 4 (November): 591–611.

Carmichael, Gordon. 1984. "Living together in New Zealand (data on coresidence at marriage and on de facto unions)," *New Zealand Population Review* 10, no. 3 (October): 41–54.

Cherlin, Andrew J. 1981. *Marriage, Divorce, Remarriage*. Cambridge, Mass.: Harvard University Press.

Cleland, John, and Chris Wilson. 1985. "Economic theories of the fertility transition: An iconoclastic view," manuscript.

Darrow, Morton. 1984. *The State of Families: 1985*. New York: Family Service America.

Davis, Kingsley. 1983. "The future of marriage," *Bulletin of the American Academy of Arts and Sciences* 36, no. 8 (May): 15–43.

——— (ed.), in association with Amyra Grossbard-Schechtman. 1986. *Contemporary Marriage: Comparative Perspectives on a Changing Institution.* New York: Russell Sage Foundation.

Easterlin, Richard A. 1980. *Birth and Fortune: The Impact of Numbers on Personal Welfare.* New York: Basic Books.

Espenshade, Thomas J. 1985. "Marriage trends in America: Estimates, implications, and underlying causes," *Population and Development Review* 11, no. 2 (June): 193–245.

———. 1986. "The recent decline of American marriage: Blacks and whites in comparative perspective," in Davis (1986), pp. 53–90.

Glick, Paul C. 1985. "American household structure in transition," *Family Planning Perspectives* 16, no. 5 (September/October): 205–211.

Goldman, Noreen, Charles F. Westoff, and Charles Hammerslough. 1984. "The demography of the marriage market in the United States," *Population Index* 50, no. 1 (Spring): 5–25.

Hoem, Jan M., and Bo Rennermalm. 1985. "Modern family initiation in Sweden: Experience of women born between 1936 and 1960," *European Journal of Population* 1, no. 1 (January): 81–112.

Kain, Edward L. 1984. "Surprising singles," *American Demographics* 6, no. 8 (August): 16–19, 39.

Masnick, George S. 1981. "The continuity of birth-expectation data with historical trends in cohort parity distributions: Implications for fertility in the 1980s," in *Predicting Fertility,* ed. G. E. Hendershot and P. J. Placek. Lexington, Mass.: Lexington Books, pp. 169–181.

Modell, John. 1986. "Historical reflections on American marriage," in Davis (1986), pp. 181–196.

Pratt, William F., William D. Mosher, Christine A. Bachrach, and Marjorie C. Horn. 1984. "Understanding U.S. fertility: Findings from the National Survey of Family Growth, Cycle III," *Population Bulletin* 39, no. 5 (December): 3–40.

Rodgers, Willard L., and Arland Thornton. 1985. "Changing patterns of first marriage in the United States," *Demography* 22, no. 2 (May): 265–279.

Ryder, Norman B. 1979. "The future of American fertility," *Social Forces* 26, no. 3 (February): 359–370.

Schoen, Robert, William Urton, Karen Woodrow, and John Baj. 1985. "Marriage and divorce in twentieth century American cohorts," *Demography* 22, no. 1 (February): 101–114.

Spanier, Graham B. "Cohabitation in the 1980s: Recent changes in the United States," in Davis (1986), pp. 91–111.

Statistics Sweden. 1984. "Fertility survey in Sweden, 1981: A summary of findings," *World Fertility Survey,* No. 43 (April): 9.

Taeuber, Irene B., and Conrad Taeuber. 1971. *People of the United States in the 20th Century.* Washington, D.C.: Bureau of the Census, US Government Printing Office.

Thornton, Arland, and Deborah Freedman. 1983. "The changing American family," *Population Bulletin* 38, no. 4 (October): 3–42.

United States Bureau of the Census. 1973. *Population Characteristics,* "Fertility expectations of American women: June," Table 3, p. 19.

———. 1976. "Fertility of American women: June 1976," Table 4, p. 14.

———. 1983. "Fertility of American women: June 1983," Table 8, p. 22.

———. 1985. "Households, families, marital status and living arrangements: March," Table 3.

Westoff, Charles F. 1983. "Fertility decline in the West: Causes and prospects," *Population and Development Review* 9, no. 1 (March): 99–104.

Wulf, Deidre. 1982. "Low fertility in Europe: A report from the 1981 IUSSP meeting," *International Family Planning Perspectives* 8, no. 2 (June): 63–69.

Comment: Shigemi Kono

In Japan the feminist movement has not been influential; labor force participation by married women, while increasing, has been lower than in the United States and Western European countries; the oral contraceptive has been banned for medical reasons;[1] and the divorce rate is lower than in the West and is rising more slowly. Why, in spite of conditions such as these that presumably would tend to favor higher fertility, has the Japanese total fertility rate recently been between 1.7 and 1.8, well below replacement level?

Actually, there are good reasons for the current low fertility in Japan. It is in large part a response to that country's resource-scarce environment. Today, the Japanese population, at some 120 million, numbers about half that of the United States in an area smaller than the state of California. Japan produces practically no oil and little iron ore, and it imports much agricultural produce from such countries as the United States, Canada, and Australia. A scarcity of resources relative to population has figured in Japanese history since the 1860s, when massive efforts to industrialize began.

Distinguishing Japan and the surrounding East Asian region from other parts of Asia is the pervasive and deeply rooted doctrine of Confucianism. The role of Confucianism in Japan is probably comparable to that of Protestantism in Europe at the dawn of industrialization, as depicted by Max Weber. Confucianism emphasizes the ethical value of hard work, asceticism, frugality, and regularity in the daily conduct of life.

What happens when the scarcity of resources and the ethic of hard work collide? The answer is fierce competition within the society. This has led to the emergence of a quasi-meritocracy with an overemphasis on educational attainment. This in turn has contributed to declining fertility. After World War II, Japanese fertility fell sharply. Between 1960 and 1974 the rate was relatively stable at a level slightly higher than replacement, but after 1974 it declined to its current unprecedentedly low level. (It is noteworthy that 1974 was the year of the "oil shock": the Arab oil embargo reinforced the psychological resource-scarcity syndrome in Japan.)

In a resource-scarce but advanced society, fierce competition permeates every corner of life. Rigorous entrance examinations for ranking universities and for large and prestigious corporations become common. Resource scarcity narrows the chances for a better quality of life. Demographic responses to such an environment are to delay marriage and reduce family size.

I shall briefly elaborate on three features of modern Japan that are relevant to the current fertility picture: the postponement of marriage in response to scarce resources and narrow life chances; tough entrance examinations for admission to high schools and universities; and the emergence of a mass-consumption culture.

Postponement of marriage

Age at first marriage in Japan has become one of the highest, if not the highest, in the world. According to 1984 vital statistics, the mean age at first marriage was 28.1 years for males and 25.4 years for females. For females this represents a rise from a mean age of 23.0 years in 1950 and 24.3 years in 1974. Although the divorce rate is lower in Japan than in many Western countries, the very high age at first marriage effectively shortens the reproductive span of married couples. According to the 1985 census, the proportion of the population aged 20–24 who were currently married was only 17.9 percent for females and 7.4 percent for males. Even in the age group 25–29, only 67.7 percent of females and 38.7 percent of males were currently married.

Since fecundability starts declining after age 30 and by age 35 is reduced to three-fourths of the fecundability level attained at ages 20–27, late entry into married life, in a setting inimical to premarital births, acts as a biological depressant to fertility. It keeps some Japanese couples from achieving their desired or expected fertility (Atoh et al., 1983).[2] According to national fertility surveys in 1977 and 1982, Japanese couples expected to have 2.2 children on average; in both years actual fertility was below replacement (ibid.).

Late marriage in Japan is due to the interplay of economic and social factors. Housing is extremely costly, and young men are not expected to marry until they are capable of maintaining new households without financial assistance from their parents. In addition, marriage in Japan is a very costly event: wedding ceremonies are elaborate and expensive; before the start of marriage the groom must make financial arrangements to set up a new home, and the bride must bring a dowry in kind if not in cash. Normally, a bride is expected to bring to the new home all the necessary furnishings—including major household appliances and furniture.

Competitive entrance examinations for school admission

Another important factor conducive to low fertility in Japan is the exceedingly rigorous competition for admission to ranking schools such as the University of Tokyo. It is an ordeal not only for the applicants but also for their families. The advantages of success are great, the costs of failure severe. One lucky enough to gain acceptance to a prestigious school wears a badge of honor for the rest of his life. A graduate of a ranking university is usually promoted faster than others and benefits professionally from membership in a network of alumni who hold key positions in government and business. Sometimes, prestigious corporations send notices of job openings only to ranking universities. Actually such universities do provide the highest quality education and training to their students. Those achieving exceptional marks in the highest ranked civil service examinations are usually graduates of law schools of top universities.

Japanese society is not a land of continuing opportunity for people who seek a good career or success in life. Once a young man or woman fails to pass an employment examination to enter government or a prestigious corporation as a career officer, he or she is not given another chance. In the government service, only career officers who enter their positions with top-notch test scores are permitted to become directors.

The ordeal of educational competition begins when young children start preparing for examinations in primary school and even in kindergarten. In order to get into a good university, one has to enter a good senior high school, and to get into a good senior high school, one has to enter a good junior high school, and so on. In Tokyo at 10:30 P.M. on Friday, suburban trains are filled with primary school pupils aged around 10 who are just returning from well-known *juku* (after-school cram sessions) located in the central district.[3] Some of them are already asleep, but the strong ones are rehearsing what they have just been taught. To foreigners it is an eerie scene.

In a national sample survey conducted by the Office of the Prime Minister in 1985, about 80 percent of the approximately 10,000 respondents aged 20 years and over felt that the social hierarchy and professional mobility pivot around employees' academic careers, particularly the stature of the universities from which they graduated (Office of the Prime Minister, 1985). A graduate of an outstanding school like the University of Tokyo can not only get a good job in government or in a respectable large corporation, but can also reach a high step on the hierarchical ladder.

This characterization of the academic career-centered system of promotion and upward mobility in Japan still requires statistical substantiation, but an important point is that it is entirely consistent with public perception. Hence, it is natural for anyone with above-average intelligence and some career ambition to try to get a ticket for the super-express in his life course. Thus, severe and ruthless examinations become the style of life in Japan. Under such circumstances, children become financially and psychologically expensive. Once modern methods of family planning and abortion have become available to every household, no one wants a large family. In Japan the ideal number of children (the number the average couple would like to have if circumstances permitted) is three, but the expected family size is two. In the most recent national fertility survey conducted by the Institute of Population Problems in 1982, one question asked why the couple did not attempt to have their ideal family size. The four most frequent answers from couples with wife aged 20–35 were as follows: (1) the cost of education is too high; (2) raising children requires a lot of money; (3) raising children imposes heavy physical and psychological burdens on the parents; (4) present house or apartment is too small for an ideal family size (Atoh et al., 1983). The answers did not identify burdens from the strain of preparing for school entrance examinations since the questionnaire was not structured to ask such a question, but the implication would be clear.

According to a survey conducted in 1984 by the Tokyo Metropolitan Government, households in Tokyo now pay an average of 20 percent of their monthly expenditures to send their children to preparatory schools or after-school cram sessions, or to hire private teachers at home, in order to provide the children with the knowledge and skills to pass the examination for ranking junior high or senior high schools (Tokyo Metropolitan Government, 1984). Such extracurricular activities cost the average household in Tokyo approximately US$360 per month, including tuition fees, commutation cost, books, and so on. Unless children are exceptionally bright, they cannot pass an entrance examination for admission to ranking schools without having been sent to preparatory schools or after-school cram sessions.

Advent of the mass consumption society: Reinforcing the fertility decline

A major characteristic of Japan is its homogeneity in race, religion, language, and even social class. Once every few years leading newspapers in Japan, such as Asahi Newspapers, repeat a public opinion poll asking "to which social class according to the grouping of 'upper,' 'middle,' or 'lower' do you think you belong?" Each time, more than 80 percent of interviewees respond that they belong to the "middle" class.

It is well known that income differentials among Japanese workers are the smallest among the industrial market economies. Superimposed on Japan's small territory and its homogeneity in language, social class, taste, and life styles has been the Western-based mass consumption culture, involving universal television ownership and an enormous volume of advertisement of consumer goods and services in every household. Thus, every other home in the neighborhood and every other colleague at the office serves as the reference group of the "middle class." Japanese couples are confronted by innumerable "musts" that they need to buy to maintain their middle-class status and prestige. Already the two-child norm has become a household word in Japan. Under the circumstances, having more than two children has fallen totally out of fashion and having more than two adolescents at home strenuously preparing for examinations for admission to high schools and universities seems out of the question. In short, the low birth rate is a natural consequence of the social and economic conditions just described.

Notes

1 It has been reported, however, that the Ministry of Health and Welfare may lift the ban within the next few years.

2 The average ideal family size reported by survey respondents was 2.6 children per couple, while the average expected fertility was 2.2 children (Atoh et al., 1983).

3 According to the results of a survey released by Japan's Fair Trade Commission on 19 February 1986, half the country's junior high school pupils attend *juku*. The report pointed out that the number of such pupils attending these cram sessions has tripled over the past ten years. About 23 percent of the parents responded that expenses for their children's attendance at *juku* represents a great financial burden, while nearly 50 percent said that such expenses were a slight financial burden (*The Japanese Times*, 20 February 1986).

References

Atoh, Makoto, et al. 1983. *Results of the Eighth National Fertility Survey I: Births and Marriages among the Japanese*. Tokyo: Institute of Population Problems, Ministry of Health and Welfare.

Kono, Shigemi, et al. 1984. *Bio-Demographic Analysis of Fertility*. Tokyo: Institute of Population Problems, Ministry of Health and Welfare. January.

Office of the Prime Minister, Public Relations Office. 1985. *Public Opinion Survey on Education Issues (Academic Career)*. February.

Tokyo Metropolitan Government, Living and Culture Bureau. 1984. *The Survey on the Expenditure for Education*. June.

Changing Values and Falling Birth Rates

Samuel H. Preston

In an earlier article in this volume, I presented evidence on trends since World War II in fertility, marriage, divorce, family size orientation, and contraception in the five major non-European industrialized countries. The immodest aim of the present article is to explain these trends, especially the decline in fertility. No brief analysis can hope to do full justice to this complex subject. My approach is to set forth an explanatory framework and to sketch in examples of how this framework aids in the interpretation of the monumental events that have occurred. I believe that, by emphasizing the changing social construction of parenthood, the framework fills a gap left by more conventional approaches.

In seeking explanations of the decline in fertility in these countries, it is first useful to recognize that the changes were extraordinarily pervasive, extending through all social strata. This feature has been vividly demonstrated for the United States by Ronald Rindfuss and James Sweet (1977) and Sweet and Rindfuss (1983). Rises and declines in fertility were quite uniform across standard socioeconomic categories (e.g., race, educational attainment, region, husband's income). For example, between 1970 and 1976, the number of children below age three for currently married white women declined by 22–26 percent in each of the seven husband's income classes (in 1960 dollars) above $1000–1999. The overall decline was 23 percent (Sweet and Rindfuss, 1983: Table 4). Adjustment for other measurable factors has little effect on this uniformity. Makoto Atoh (1985) has performed a similar demonstration for Japan, showing that a small family has become prevalent within all social and economic strata of Japanese society. Somewhat larger proportionate declines can be noted for the rural and more poorly educated population, but the differences are not large.

In short, compositional changes are not able to account for much of the postwar changes in fertility in these countries. Couples are evidently responding to very generalized phenomena that are felt within all major groups. What are these phenomena? The principal possibilities can be grouped into three clusters: economic factors; contraceptive technology; and a system of values.

A strong case for the importance of economic factors has been made by Gary Becker (1981), Jacob Mincer (1984), and Richard Easterlin (1980) in a series of well-known works that have been elaborated by many others. The importance of contraceptive technology has been stressed above all by Charles Westoff and Norman Ryder (e.g., 1977). Values are seldom mentioned in discussions of fertility change, although Ron Lesthaeghe (e.g., 1983) has been attempting to move European discussion in this direction. In my view, consideration of all three factors is necessary for a complete understanding of recent fertility change in these countries—and in most times and places. Since values have been relatively underplayed, I will focus discussion in this area and nest the consideration of economic and contraceptive factors within such a discussion. The discussion does not pretend to be complete or original; it is based upon relatively standard sociology with a functionalist cast (e.g., Davis, 1955).

A sociological theory of fertility in industrial societies

Let us begin with the assertion that societies place values on social acts: acts that affect the well-being of persons other than the members engaging in them. Acts that benefit others are rewarded, while detrimental acts are punished. The set of values attached to social acts is a value system. This system is reflected in legal codes, in institutions, and in interpersonal applications of esteem and rebuke—key indicators of an individual's long-term access to society's resources. The value system is the means by which societies "internalize the externalities" of social acts. By its indifference to them, the value system also defines acts that are not social, acts whose consequences are perceived to fall entirely on the actors. As societies develop administratively, more and more of the rewards and punishments become formally encoded, to the point where some members may confuse legality with morality.

The value system and its institutional, legal, and interpersonal manifestations are among the factors that influence behavior; in a loose sense, at least, they enter the utility functions that individuals use to weigh the merits of alternative behavior. Value systems encourage people to act in ways that they would not otherwise have acted, and adherence to a particular value system entails sacrifice of some other good, often of immediate material gratification. Individuals are continually faced with making choices that are more or less consistent with the predominant value system. The outcome of these choices across members of a society establishes a set of behavior patterns. If these patterns diverge sufficiently from a particular value system, that system erodes because its strength resides in widespread acceptance and enforcement. Individuals recognize that a value system has lost salience and adjust their behavior accordingly. In this reciprocal fashion, the values of a group influence individual behavior and individual behavior influences group values.

Value systems are constructed and deconstructed over long stretches of time. Within most societies, several competing value systems can be found, usually evolved in different ecological and historical settings. The pervasive role of the media in modern industrial societies allows much more rapid change in values than was previously possible, and greater homogenization. The media transmit images of novel behavior and provide a wide-reaching forum for those whose responsibility is to interpret social acts and assign value to them. In this role, the clergy have increasingly been replaced by social scientists and political leaders. The modern-day priests play an important independent role in value shifts, but people can also choose the priests who minister to their own interests.

Childbearing and childrearing are social acts in all societies. Children eventually become independent of parents, and it is critical that they be raised to be productive citizens. The number of children born will, in the aggregate, determine population size, a matter of significant social concern. In western societies over the past 300 years, social values attached to childbearing and childrearing can be summarized under the doctrine of "responsible parenthood." Parents (rather than, for example, the extended family) were directly responsible for childrearing. Marriage and childbearing were to occur only when means for raising a family appeared relatively secure. Parenthood was an elevated status, as in all societies, and lifestyles alternative to parenthood were proscribed (e.g., Blake, 1972). But in the matter of parenthood, more was not always better. When children threatened to disturb the social order or to make claims on group resources, their birth was discouraged. Great emphasis was placed on raising children who would contribute to the social good. Relative to many other cultures, obligations of western parents to young children were stressed above obligations of parents toward their own parents.

Long-term economic growth increased the value of skilled and well-educated workers, just as the development of complex democracies required better educated citizens. Private incentives for parents to invest the socially desirable amount in their children were weak because, in the absence of strong values attached to filial piety (observed, for example, in much of Asia), they did not recoup the bulk of the investment. In the course of modern economic growth, social values were reorganized to emphasize the importance of producing high-quality, well-educated children, even at the expense of reduced fertility; the eugenics movement in the late nineteenth and early twentieth centuries is a formal manifestation of this emphasis. Legislation required what parents would not always yield voluntarily, and compulsory school legislation swept through western countries in the late nineteenth century. The changing values and their legal correlates clearly served to raise the costs of children to parents, but did not undermine the basic doctrine of responsible parenthood. In Peter McDonald's (1984) apt characterization, fertility declined in large part so that women could better pursue motherhood.

But long-term economic growth not only affected the quality/quantity tradeoff within the role of responsible parent; it also increased the incentives to abandon the role altogether. Higher incomes, product diversification, and urbanization presented a vast array of consumption possibilities—for relationships as well as for goods and services—whose pursuit was increasingly constrained by the time and money demands of responsible parenthood. Short periods of unusual economic change could evoke the expected reaction: periods of rapid growth would permit earlier marriage and higher fertility, while periods of decline would encourage parents to restrict childbearing in order to provide adequately for children already born. As Andrew Cherlin (1981) documents effectively, fertility levels during the Depression and in the 1950s do not require separate explanations but can be seen as reflecting the same type of response to very different stimuli. But the long-term patterns of economic change, by raising the socially constructed "costs" of children and the opportunity costs of pursuing a lifetime of responsible parenthood, produced a century of nearly uninterrupted fertility decline.

Recent changes in family and fertility in English-speaking countries

With the stage thus set in spartan furnishing, let us try to focus more specifically on fertility change during the period 1950–85, and particularly on the rapid decline since the 1960s. The century of fertility decline should caution against invoking interpretations unique to the period, just as its universality in western countries should discourage nation-specific explanations. Indeed, one of the main factors at work during the period, a rapid increase in wages and real per capita incomes, was evident in earlier periods as well. But two other factors were relatively peculiar to the period and appear to be important in understanding its unusually rapid fertility decline. We will first discuss these two factors and then conclude this section with a discussion of economic growth.

The population/environmental issue

I have argued that social values attached to responsible parenthood were highly influential in directing people's lives toward making childbearing and child-rearing investments. Motherhood was sanctified to such an extent that it was an oft-repeated joke to say that a politician was in favor of it. Sometime in the 1970s, this joke lost its punch. Some of the change is probably attributable to the growing concern that having children may be a socially damaging act. Whether or not many people came to believe in the extreme version of this doctrine, the doctrine itself was well known, spread with sober earnestness by a problem-oriented media. Since the value attached to parenthood was socially constructed and depended on widespread and largely unquestioning assent, it was highly vulnerable to well-articulated dissent. The more embracing doctrine of responsible parenthood was in fact sufficiently adaptable that substantial changes in the volume of childbearing could be justified within its confines; to some, it could even justify childlessness ("it would be irresponsible to bring a child into this world"). It was principally the traditional numerical implications of the doctrine that were vulnerable to a number-based attack.

After 15 years of popular attention to the population "explosion" in developing countries and rapid growth in the developed world, Paul Ehrlich's *The Population Bomb* was published in 1968, followed by scores of personal appearances on television. Meadows et al.'s *Limits to Growth* appeared in 1972 and received an immense amount of attention in scholarly and popular circles. These books, and others, argued that the human race was propagating itself toward extinction. While growth rates were fastest in poor countries, growth in affluent countries could be even more damaging because of the vastly greater resource charges per person. Besides, we were all part of one community, spaceship earth. Ecosystems were unstable, the more so as they became simplified through human interference. The prospect of collapse loomed larger and larger, although it was difficult (and unnecessary) to predict when it would occur.

Did this doctrine affect fertility? If the view of reproduction presented here is basically correct, it must have. Some empirical support is provided by Rindfuss's (1972) review of data from the 1965 and 1970 National Fertility Studies. The proportion of women (currently married and below age 55 in 1965; ever-married and below 45 in 1970) saying that "United States population growth is a serious problem" grew from 57 percent in 1965 to 69 percent in 1970. There was surprisingly little class variation in responses. In 1970, 62 percent of women who had not completed high school agreed with the statement, as did 71 percent of women who attended college. Perhaps more important, the women agreeing with it had substantially smaller intended family sizes, as well as much larger reductions in these intentions between 1965 and 1970, a period of rapid fertility decline (see Table 1).

TABLE 1 Mean additional number of children intended according to expressed concern for population growth: women under age 30, by parity

	1965	1970
Parity-one women		
Concerned	1.51	1.18
Intermediate	1.82	1.64
Not concerned	1.93	2.00
Parity-two women		
Concerned	0.69	0.40
Intermediate	0.94	0.72
Not concerned	0.87	1.16

SOURCE: Rindfuss, 1972: Table 5.

Women unconcerned with population growth actually registered an increase in the number of additional children intended during this period, while those most concerned had a substantial decline. ("Concerned" women consider both US and world population growth to be a serious problem; "Intermediate" women consider world growth to be serious but not US growth; "Not concerned" consider neither US nor world growth a serious problem.) For all ages of women in the two surveys, the mean desired family size among those concerned with population growth declined by 0.29; for unconcerned women it rose by 0.13.

Skeptics will argue that concern over population growth simply provided a rationalization for women whose personal circumstances led them to want smaller families. This position would deny importance to the socially constructed values attached to childbearing. Even if it were valid, however, the population/environmental movement provided for some a more convenient rationale for their behavior than would otherwise have been available, and the value system presented few alternatives. It thus reduced the social costs of lowered fertility and had a direct antinatalist effect even as a rationalization. But one must ask why rationalizations would be necessary unless there were palpable social expectations about the behavior in question.

John Caldwell (1981) and Wendy Cosford et al. (1976) cite the debate over the population explosion and environmental preservation as one of the major phenomena affecting Australian fertility during the 1960–80 period. Caldwell refers to a 1971 Melbourne Survey in which 87 percent of respondents felt that population growth should be discouraged in poor, crowded countries. Twenty-nine percent believed that Australians should be discouraged from having more than two children. Almost two-thirds knew of arguments relating population growth to pollution. According to Cosford et al., the hazards of rapid population growth had become a standard lesson in schools, churches, and the media. No attempt was apparently made to relate individual views on this matter to desired or intended fertility. But Caldwell notes that "By the late 1960's, the use of contraception was almost a moral priority, a very different position from the private and somewhat guilty practice which was typical in the early decades of the century and persisted until after the Second World War" (1981: 31). Cosford et al. argue that the ideological changes associated with the population/environmental movement legitimated the very small and even childless family and all but silenced protests from the perhaps more pronatalist older generation.

Improved contraceptive technology

The availability of superior contraceptive technology can affect fertility without altering value systems. Except among Catholics, the practice of contraception within marriage was already widespread and essentially value-neutral in the 1950s. The substitution of more efficient for less efficient means would clearly be expected to lead to reduced fertility among couples trying to prevent or delay the next birth. Such substitution became possible with the introduction of the pill and IUD in the early 1960s and with the later legalization of abortion. In the United States, the reduction of unwanted fertility was probably a major factor in the decline in marital fertility between the 1960s and 1980s, as noted in my earlier article in this volume.

Among traditional Catholics, however, the introduction of these improved methods of birth control dramatically raised the cost of adherence to a value system in which the use of abortion and artificial contraception was strictly proscribed. Couples seeking to avert a birth were enjoined from using a simple, cheap, safe, and highly effective method. This proscription, reaffirmed in a Papal Encyclical in 1968, was integral to a value system that idealized large families.

We would predict that, as the costs of adherence to a particular value system rise, behavior increasingly departs from the ideal and eventually erodes the legitimacy of that value system. This prediction is consistent with events in the Catholic communities of the English-speaking countries. Catholic birth control practice in the United States changed dramatically. In 1955, half of all Catholic contraceptive practice was periodic abstinence (rhythm); the figure had fallen to 12 percent by 1982 (Mosher et al., 1985). A comparison of National Fertility Surveys found that the proportion conforming to church doctrine on birth control (by using no method or the rhythm method) among Catholic women married 15–19 years declined from 67 percent in the marriage cohort of 1936–40 to 16 percent for the marriage cohort of 1956–60 (Jones and Westoff, 1979). Catholic fertility declined far more rapidly than non-Catholic fertility. During the peak years of the baby boom, the Catholic total marital fertility rate was .9 to 1.1 children higher than the non-Catholic rate (Mosher et al., 1985). This differential declined to .26 in 1977–81 and actually reversed in sign (to −.02) when Hispanics are excluded from the calculation. An enormous differential of .84 children in the total marital fertility rate by frequency of communion had declined to .05 in 1971–75 and to insignificance in 1977–81 (Jones and Westoff, 1979; Mosher et al., 1985). Many observers have also argued that the Papal Encyclical, a reassertion of traditional church teachings and authority in the area of birth control, actually had the effect of undermining that authority not only in the area of birth control and fertility but in other areas as well.

The story is likely to be similar in the other English-speaking countries, although data on religious fertility differences are much less abundant there. Fertility in predominantly Catholic Quebec fell much faster than in Canada as a whole. In 1959, Quebec's crude birth rate of 28.3 per thousand exceeded the all-Canada rate of 27.4; nine years later, it had the lowest fertility of any province and by 1972 the birth rate stood at 13.8 per thousand, half the level of 1958 (Beaujot, 1978). Three-quarters of Quebec women below age 35 interviewed in a 1971 fertility survey disagreed with the Roman Catholic Church's ban on all artificial means of contraception (Beaujot, 1978). Cosford et al. (1976) note the faster decline of Catholic than non-Catholic fertility in Australia. I would contend that the far more rapid drop in Catholic fertility can be best understood by reference to a value system that became increasingly inappropriate in the face of technical change, rather than by reference to individual characteristics of Catholics (see also Jones and Westoff, 1979).

The other value change encouraged by the contraceptive revolution was probably more far-reaching but had more ambiguous fertility consequences. As in most other areas, the institution of monogamous marriage in Western Europe evolved for many purposes. Central among them was the opportunity it provided for licit sexual activity in a context wherein fiscal and socializing responsibility was clearly assigned for the predictable consequences of such activity, children. The social logic of this arrangement was threatened by any advance in contraceptive technology, but the threat was greatest when the techniques were coitus-independent. When a method required unique implementation for each act of intercourse, and especially the cooperation of both partners, the risk of contraceptive failure was greatest outside of a stable sexual union. With the pill and IUD (and abortion), no such risk differential existed between stable and unstable unions.

With the contraceptive changes, the social value of confining sex to marriage was clearly reduced. If a couple were adequately protected, who could obejct to sex between mutually consenting adults? Sex became less a social act and more a purely private one, and the institution contrived to govern access to it predictably began to erode. Rates of entry into marriage declined sharply and rates of exit grew, aided by legal changes reflecting an altered value system. The number of persons of opposite sex cohabiting without marriage rose sharply. That this tendency reflects not only individual calculation of gains and losses but also widespread social acceptance is reflected in a 1981–82 Australian Institute of Family Studies national survey. Among the 18–34-year-old respondents, 76 percent of females and 80 percent of males agreed that "It is alright for a couple to live together without planning to get married." Only 40 percent of males and 47 percent of females felt that "If you live together there is a lot of social disapproval" (Carmichael, 1984).

Time series data of a different sort are available from the valuable study *The Inner American,* which reported the results from identical questionnaires applied to representative samples of American adults in 1957 and 1976 (Veroff et al., 1981). Interviewers asked, "Suppose all you know about a woman was that she did not want to get married. What would you guess she was like?" The proportion answering with negative characteristics (e.g., "selfish, immature, peculiar") declined from 53 percent to 34 percent between these years, with similar results for male and female respondents. Although many factors besides improved contraception were undoubtedly involved in the reduced disapproval of nonmarriage, the role of contraceptive change was probably very important.

The fertility effect of the change in marriage prevalence resulting from contraceptive change is difficult to predict but is likely to be downward. The increased attractiveness of informal unions and, possibly, of sequential partners, would clearly reduce the average degree of commitment of partners to one another. Without such commitment, having a child is a risky business, at least for a woman. The legal guarantees of marriage, in Becker's (1981) terms, enhance the return to investment in marriage-specific capital, especially in the form of childbearing. The declining prevalence of persons residing in this risk-reducing institution could be expected to lower average levels of fertility.

Sustained economic growth

Between 1950 and 1980, real gross domestic product per capita grew by the factors 1.481 in New Zealand, 1.898 in Australia, 1.778 in the United States, 2.092 in Canada, and 7.402 in Japan (Summers and Heston, 1984). These rates were rapid by historical standards. The mean annual growth rate in US real gross domestic product per capita between 1890 and 1950 was .0172, compared with the mean rate of .0192 in the 1950–80 period (Summers and Heston, 1984; US Bureau of the Census, 1975, Table F1-5). The near doubling of per capita gross domestic product in this 30-year period brought with it expanded horizons for consumption, for leisure pursuits, and for personal relationships. All of these effects can be summarized in Becker's terms: the increased wage rate raised the value of time and led to substitution away from activities requiring a great deal of time, such as childrearing and spouse-attending. Opportunities grew for personal interaction and for joint consumption of goods and services among people sharing similar tastes. Why limit the sphere of personal interaction to one's children and parents, whose traits are only marginally under one's direct control, or even to one's spouse, whose behavior patterns were imperfectly predictable from traits revealed before marriage?

As they had been doing for a century, men and women grew increasingly restive under the yolk of responsible parenthood and monogamous matrimony. While most attention has gone to the female side of the ledger, Barbara Ehrenreich (1984) makes a strong case that a massive male rebellion against family strictures has also occurred. Male restiveness with the dullness and exploitative character of marriage and family relations was reflected in popular works such as *The Man in the Grey Flannel Suit* (Sloan, 1955) and *On the Road* (Kerouack, 1957) and in scholarly works such as *The Organization Man* (Whyte, 1956). It reached the popular mind most vividly, Ehrenreich argues, in *Playboy* and the Playboy Philosophy, which ingeniously focused on severing the powerful link that had existed in the public's eye between nonperformance of traditional male roles and homosexuality. Perhaps because it was more novel, similar questioning of the traditional female role has been more widely publicized. *The Feminine Mystique* (Friedan, 1963), *The Women's Room* (French, 1955), *The Second Sex* (de Beauvoir, 1953), and other works advanced the case that women's lives were unjustly constrained by the sexual division of labor implied by traditional versions of responsible parenthood.

The Inner American makes clear that males and females alike considered parenthood and marriage to be more restrictive in 1976 than in 1957. An open-ended question in both years asked, "How is a woman's (man's) life changed by having children?" Certain responses were categorized as "restrictive" (e.g., you give up your freedom, you have to think of somebody else). The proportion of respondents giving nothing but restrictive responses rose between these years from 29 to 45 percent for males and from 31 to 44 percent for females (Veroff et al., 1981: 215). A similar question about marriage, "How is a woman's (man's) life changed by being married?" produced a similar result. The proportion of men giving all restrictive responses rose from 43 to 60 percent between 1957 and 1976, while the female proportion rose from 46 to 58 percent (1981: 174). There is no obvious reason why the objective restrictions of marriage and parenthood should have increased during this period; in fact, higher incomes and legal changes (e.g., divorce laws) should have permitted some relaxation of restrictions. But, relative to the expanded opportunities that presented themselves, the institutions appeared more restrictive than ever.

Not only is the increase in perceived restrictiveness noteworthy, but so also is the fact that the male increase was slightly larger than the female. This result clearly supports Ehrenreich's argument. A national survey of 1981–82 also found Australian-born males mentioning the restrictions imposed by children (loss of freedom, effects on social life, effects on finances) more frequently than females (Khoo, 1984: Table 16). But males could work their way out of family entanglements without massive change in role identity. Somewhat later marriage, somewhat more nonmarriage, somewhat higher rates of transfer between partners, and somewhat less attentiveness to child support could produce the desirable alterations. But the bulk of males' adult lives was already spent outside the home, as a result of a much earlier wage-driven social transformation.

For women, on the other hand, a major overhaul of role identity was needed. To take advantage of higher earnings prospects and the greater possibilities for independence these afforded, women needed to alter the sexual division of family labor that had existed for a century or more. That this process has begun in earnest is too obvious to require documentation.

As people responded to the new incentive structures, behavior changed and these alterations, in turn, changed the perception of the social values attached to performance of family roles. The value changes accelerated the process of social change. A massive shift occurred in the value attached to the role of housewife and mother. Helen Glezer (1984) reports the results of Melbourne surveys of married women aged 18–34 that asked women whether they agreed with the statement, "Whatever career a woman may have, her most important career role in life is that of becoming a mother." In 1971, 78 percent agreed with the statement, compared with only 46 percent in 1982 (1984: Table 2). With the statement, "A woman is only really fulfilled when she becomes a mother," 68 percent agreed in 1971 and 30 percent in 1982. In a multivariate analysis of factors influencing women's sex role attitudes that pooled observations for the two years, Glezer finds that "date of observation" is by far the most important predictor of the response, having twice the standardized beta coefficient of women's own labor force participation. This result certainly supports the notion that people respond to a social climate of attitudes and values as well as to their own material circumstance.

Arland Thornton and Deborah Freedman (1982) document a similar change among a cohort of Detroit mothers giving birth in 1961. In 1962, 84 percent of these women agreed that "almost all married couples who can ought to have children." By 1980, only 43 percent of them supported that view. They present similar data from European countries. Thornton et al. (1983) provide abundant detail on the individual-level factors associated with these and other attitude changes in the United States.

While I have chosen to discuss these changing attitudes and the value system they reflect primarily in the context of economic change, it is evident that the other factors described above are also likely to be involved.

The other "economic" factor noted above as an explanation of long-term family trends was the rising "cost" of (i.e., expenditure on) children. This concept should be distinguished from the "price" of children, which has probably increased no more rapidly than other prices, on average. For next to nothing, parents could be raising the ill-clothed, ill-housed, and often sickly children of the eighteenth century. They are not. Why are they undertaking to provide the enormous material resources now "required" for childrearing when they recoup so little of the material benefit therefrom? Two possible explanations are altruistic instincts (see Becker, 1981) and social values ("responsible parenthood"), both emphasizing the importance of raising children well equipped to compete in the modern world. This equipment includes, of course, ever-increasing levels of education. These hypotheses are not necessarily mutually exclusive, since social values would presumably serve to direct whatever altruistic instincts existed. Nevertheless, altruism does not require the intervention of values and can equally well account for rising investments of parents in children. The relative virtues of these two explanations cannot be assayed here, but it is worth noting that sociobiological studies of altruism stress the contribution that altruistic behavior makes to the propagation of one's genes in the gene pool of the next generation. "Instinctive" altruistic behavior emerges to increase the *quantity* of "descendants"; evolutionary theory would not predict the emergence of behavior that reduces the quantity over the long term of surviving offspring or relatives, whatever the effect may be on quality. Of course, instincts can readily go awry in a complex world very different from the one in which they evolved. In any event, it should be reassuring for both approaches as explanations of fertility decline that parental aspirations for child quality are inversely related to achieved and intended fertility. Thornton (1979: Table 8) shows that the average number of children intended by US women below age 40 in 1975 with very low aspirations for child quality (education, lessons, maternal time input) was .40 higher than for those with very high aspirations. This difference increased to .47 when other factors were controlled.

One of the most concrete ways in which changing value systems have affected fertility in the countries under review was the liberalization of abortion laws. These changes were "exogenous" to the individual couple, but they were hardly exogenous to the value system. They reflect most fundamentally a social devaluation of the fetus. "Unwanted" fetuses posed greater threats to the orderly adult lives of the parents, who petitioned for relief. They also threatened to add to perceived population pressures and to reduce the average "quality" of children being born. The social case for preventing their birth became compelling. The liberalization of abortion laws doubtless sped the decline in aggregate fertility, reflecting very directly the activity of value systems in fertility change.

Other ideological explanations of fertility change

Lesthaeghe (1983) has made a powerful case that ideational systems are strongly implicated in family and fertility change in Western Europe. He traces the fertility decline in Europe principally to the spread of secular individualism, the "pursuit of personal goals devoid of references to a cohesive and overarching religious or philosophical construct" (p. 415). Strikingly high aggregate-level correlations among indicators of religious, political, and family behaviors support his position.

Caldwell (1981) has similarly described fertility decline in Australia largely in terms of spreading individualism and the egalitarian aims it promoted. In the family arena, he argues, this philosophy was first directed toward relations between the generations, and then toward relations between the sexes. A recent, already influential volume by Robert Bellah et al. (1985) has refocused attention on the individualistic bases on which Americans make decisions. "We insist, perhaps more than ever before, on finding our true selves independent of any cultural or social influence, being responsible to that self alone, and making its fulfillment the very meaning of our lives" (1985: 150). Although pertinent to countries in a very different setting, John Cleland's (1985) conclusion from the comparative analysis of World Fertility Survey data is relevant here as well:

> Taken *en masse,* the results [of the WFS] are more consistent with an ideational theory of change based on the spread of new aspirations or new attitudes towards family formation or birth control, than with a structural theory, which emphasized changes in the economic roles of family units or of children. (p. 243)

The role of ideational change in western countries—especially increasing individualism—appears to be central to the process of postwar fertility decline. Americans clearly adopted a different stance toward marriage and childbearing in 1976 than in 1957. They were more inclined to justify their behavior in terms of its consequences for personal development, and less inclined to justify it on grounds of fulfilling or adhering to valued social roles (Veroff et al., 1981). If men and women should be freed from social constraints and expectations in the family sphere, it follows that their personal and professional opportunities should be equalized and arbitrary restrictions removed. Unquestionably, many more people in the 1960s and 1970s chafed at the strictures of traditional responsible parenthood and the sexual division of labor that it implied. The assignment of traditional roles based on sex, a characteristic over which one has no control, came increasingly to be seen as unjust and unfair.

These ideological changes were extremely important. But where did they originate? According to Lesthaeghe (1983: 412), the changes were largely autonomous, representing natural extensions into new spheres of the egalitarian and utilitarian thought originating in the Reformation and Enlightenment. A similar view emerges from Caldwell's discussion. This view may well be correct. But such a development would also be predicted by the explanatory schema sketched above. Individualism can be seen not so much as a doctrine embodying social value itself as the negation of social value. The spread of individualism increases the domain of behavior within which socially neutral values are assigned. The rhetoric of individualism, first legitimated within the political domain, is conveniently available to justify the dismantling of earlier values when they are no longer serviceable.

In a sense, individualism rushes into a vacuum. It has not spread inexorably through all spheres of modern life. Although women's assignments to restrictive sex roles have come to be seen as increasingly unjust, fewer people now than two decades ago are railing at the arbitrary manner in which social class of origin or race constricts an individual's life chances. No one is arguing that crime should not be punished because such punishment unduly encumbers the perpetrator in his pursuit of happiness; penalties are becoming stiffer, not weaker. Rather than being removed from the domain of public interest, a wide variety of personal behaviors toward the environment *became* social acts during the 1960s and 1970s, with palpable legal and informal sanctions attached.

In short, growing individualism in a particular area can be seen as a response of value systems to changed conditions, rather than as an autonomous force. Such is the view taken here, but in terms of individual behavior the two approaches yield identical predictions; examining behavior alone, an analyst could not distinguish between a situation in which the social *value* of acts was diminished and one in which individuals adopted a new *ethical* system that increasingly discounted whatever social values were present. It is only when we examine attitudes and sanctions addressed toward other people's behavior that the two can be distinguished. We have reviewed several attitudinal surveys that show very substantial changes in attitudes toward other people's family and fertility behavior, suggesting that the values themselves have shifted. Even here, however, one could argue that the ethical system maintained antihypocrisy codes such that people would not expect of others what they did not want expected of themselves. What is becoming less doubtful is that, if we are to understand social change, the things at work inside people's heads, whether they are called ideas or social values or habits of thought, need analysis as much as the objective conditions that lie outside. In an era when social values related to childbearing and marriage are much diminished in salience, there is a temptation to assume that they were never strong. Such an assumption would almost certainly be seriously misleading in the study of family change.

This is not to deny the merits of an economic approach to studying fertility change. Economists' predictions about the direction of change have in general been on the mark, and their modes of reasoning have shed a good deal of light on the basis for private decisions. But it is doubtful whether the observed pace of fertility decline could be produced by the cumulation of millions of private decisions made with constant utility functions under marginally altered economic circumstances. Nor does such reasoning shed much light on the international distribution of fertility decline (Mincer, 1984). Social values—malleable and discretionary as they may be—have probably functioned as critically important accelerators of the changes that drew much of their impetus from utilitarian motives. Their role should not, in fact, surprise economists, who have predicted (and verified) that institutions would develop to internalize the externalities arising in such activities as bee-keeping and orchard-tending (e.g., Willis, 1985); why not also in the far more fundamental area of species propagation?

Much is omitted from this account. It does not deal with the relative deterioration of earnings of young males in many of the countries reviewed, nor with the relative increase in the cost of housing, each of which may have increased frustration at the opportunities forgone by parenthood in a context where images of material standards have become ever more affluent; nor does it deal with other events that may reflect on the legitimacy of an entire value system (the Vietnam War; educational and scientific advance that eroded the quasi-scientific basis of religious belief—a major cultural prop supporting earlier value systems); nor does it deal with changes in the assumption of state responsibility for childrearing, which some analysts argue may have undercut the social institution of marriage. While these factors and others would need discussion in a complete account, I believe that the three factors highlighted here were the principal actors during the period under review.

Japanese exceptions

In my earlier article I observed that the Japanese postwar fertility decline had a very different coloration from those of the English-speaking countries. It was earlier, more abrupt, and occurred at a much lower income level. The behavioral boundaries of marriage remained very important and perhaps even grew stronger. The predominant means of contraception remained inefficient and coitus-dependent. After an initial upsurge, abortion declined in frequency. By themselves, these differences point to the key role played by cultural and institutional factors in conditioning fertility change. A vivid reminder of the importance of cultural values in fertility was provided by the Year of the Fiery Horse; in 1966, Japanese fertility was more than 25 percent below its value for adjacent periods.

In view of the peculiarity of the Japanese case and its possible pertinence to other Asian countries, it is surprising how little attention it has received. Carl Mosk (1983) advances an economic explanation of Japanese fertility change. Rising costs of children and changing labor markets, he argues, eroded the merits of the patriarchal stem family as an organizational device. But he admits that such changes were very slow and could not account for the sudden postwar collapse of Japanese fertility.

It is likely that the rapid change in this period reflects a radically altered institutional and economic context resulting from the war and occupation, changes that abruptly altered the values attached to childbearing. Per capita income had fallen sharply from 1930s levels, creating a widespread perception that Japan was "overpopulated." Such indeed was the conclusion of a Population Planning Committee report of 1946 suggesting that the balance between population and carrying capacity had been destroyed and that unparalleled surplus population was an undeniable fact (Taeuber, 1958: 371). A Cabinet-commissioned Population Problem Council report of 1949 confirmed that "The solution of our problems demands suppression of population expansion through birth control but also emigration overseas" (1958: 372). Adding to this perception was a rapid postwar decline in mortality, fostered by the occupying forces, that produced the highest rate of natural increase in Japanese history (1958: 369; Davis, 1963). These reports were widely publicized, and the controversies that they both reflected and stimulated focused a great deal of public attention on the "population problem" (1958: 373). This issue re-emerged after the oil shocks of the 1970s. Shigemi Kono (1982) reports on a 1978 survey in which a majority of respondents considered that the population size of Japan was too large to support and that their economic situation had deteriorated owing to a scarcity of space and natural resources relative to population.

The earlier debates were important background for the National Eugenic Law of 1948, whose stated intent was to prevent the increase of inferior descendants and to protect women for whom pregnancy would involve severe health hazards (Taeuber, 1958: 269). Whatever the intent, the legalization of sterilization and abortion radically altered the context within which couples reproduced. During the years between the two World Wars, the Ministry of Home Affairs had outlawed the discussion of birth control methods in books, magazines, and public gatherings. Contraception was a "dangerous thought" covered by the Dangerous Thought Law (Mosk, 1983: 235).

A final change is more directly related to the occupation of Japan and the very different value premises that it imposed. The Supreme Commander of the Allied Powers invoked a series of legal changes that undercut the patriarchal stem family system. There was to be equality of inheritance, with no primogeniture for boys and no disinheritance for girls. There was to be equality of opportunity for all social classes, with education promoted as the principal equalizing force. Women were to be treated similarly to men both within and outside the family system (Taeuber, 1958: 371).

Clearly, the conditions of rapid postwar fertility decline in Japan bear at least surface resemblance to those that occurred a decade or two later in the English-speaking countries. In particular, the widespread perception of overpopulation and the greatly enhanced means for controlling fertility were present in both. The Japanese model remains very different in some basic respects, particularly the much greater importance of parent–grandparent relations (see, e.g., Morgan and Hirosima, 1983). The steeper age-profile of earnings, the higher relative cost of housing, and the very high premium attached to education would deserve emphasis in the account of why Japanese fertility remained so low. But the importance of value systems, and of exogenous shocks to those systems, would appear to deserve a central explanatory role in both Japan and the English-speaking countries.

Toward the future

If the analysis presented here is basically correct, then the future course of fertility in the English-speaking countries depends on whether and how values spring back. Among the important factors we identified in fostering recent changes in family-related values, economic growth is likely to continue to produce moderate downward pressure on fertility. The contraceptive advances of recent decades are largely irreversible, although similarly dramatic advances are not likely in the future. A sustained fertility upsurge seems likely only if the 1960s population/environmental consensus gets turned on its head. If children again become perceived as being in short supply, societies have formal and informal means at their disposal to enlarge the flow. One rationale for such action is the problems that a top-heavy age distribution pose for supporting the "old-age welfare state" that we have created (Binstock, 1985; Preston, 1984). How extreme this age distribution may become is indicated by Figure 1, which shows the age distribution that would result from indefinite continuation of Japanese female fertility and mortality of 1983. Under this scenario there are more 77-year-olds than infants.

After decades of calculations showing the huge net public cost of children due to their consumption of public resources long before they start yielding the (heavily discounted) stream of tax payments, the new age bias in public expenditures has reversed the charges. Ronald Lee (1985) estimates that the age pattern of interhousehold transfers in the United States is now such as to produce positive externalities to childbearing. Using comparative statistics, he reckons that a 1 percent increase in the population growth rate leads to a 4.4 percent increase in average lifetime consumption. The recognition that higher fertility and higher quality children are a boon to pay-as-you-go social security programs has been an important element in population and family policy in several European countries (McIntosh, 1983). In the United States, however,

FIGURE 1 Age composition of a stable population, assuming continuation of Japanese female fertility and mortality as of 1983

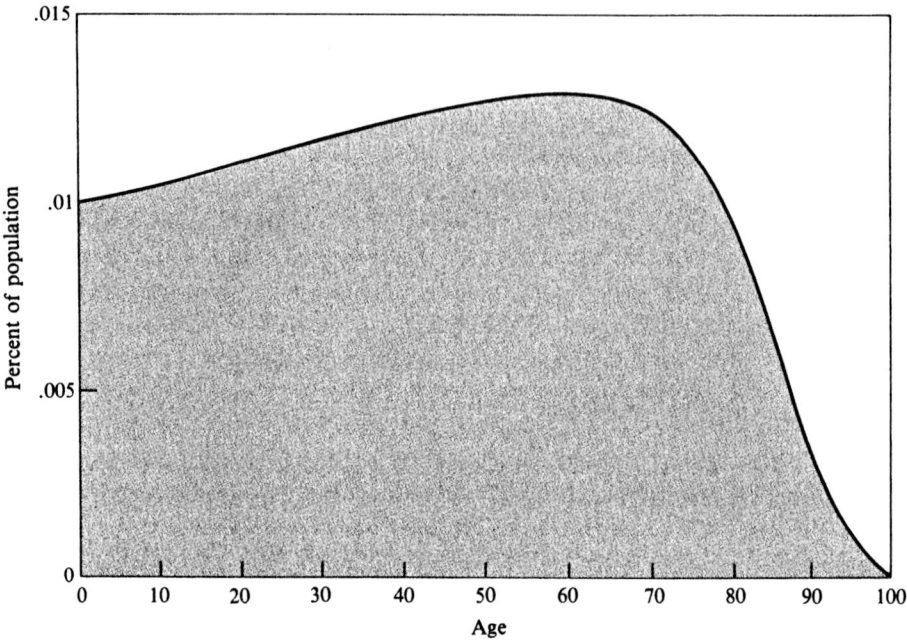

SOURCE: Computed from vital rates presented in Japan, Ministry of Health and Welfare, *Selected Demographic Indicators of Japan* (Tokyo: Institute of Population Problems, April 1985).

this recognition has yet to influence policy, and the depreciation of parenthood in the past several decades was clearly accompanied by a depreciation of childhood as well (Preston, 1984).

A second potential source of renewed parenthood values is the psychological cost associated with their erosion. The decline in social direction of adult lives has left a wake of introspection, soul-searching, and role confusion. According to Joseph Veroff et al. (1981), young adults in 1976 were much more anxious, uncertain, and pessimistic about the future than in 1957, the year in which the total fertility rate reached its postwar peak. These changes were accompanied by a sharply increased frequency of symptoms of psychological distress relative to 1957.

There are, in fact, signs of change in the United States, emergent value systems in which parenthood plays a more esteemed role. A fascinating finding of the 1982 National Fertility Survey is that fertility intentions have become strongly and positively affected by frequency of church attendance among Protestants, although not among Catholics. Protestant women who attend church at least once a month have a total fertility rate that is 0.6 children higher than those who do not, surely one of the largest current fertility differentials

(Mosher et al., 1985). Thornton et al. (1983) note a striking inegalitarian change in sex role attitudes among fundamentalist Protestants between 1962 and 1977, while the rest of the country was moving in the opposite direction. The extreme case of Mormon fertility and family practices is well known. Since elevation of the parental role is a central point on the agenda of family fundamentalists, it is not surprising that they have directed much of their political efforts toward restricting access to abortion. Do these groups represent a social reaction to excessive individualism, especially as it bears on the family, or simply a reactionary resistance to the march of modern ideas? The answer depends in part on their reception among social scientists, who have become principal agents of social change. The mild endorsement of fundamentalist lifestyles in *Habits of the Heart* (Bellah et al., 1985) thus itself becomes an important social datum, perhaps the harbinger of a revised social construction of parenthood and marriage.

Notes

The author is grateful to Caroline Bledsoe, Frank Furstenberg, Philip Morgan, and Susan Watkins for comments and advice, and to Katherine Condon for research assistance.

References

Atoh, Makoto. 1985. "Changes in fertility and fertility control behavior in Japan," in *Basic Readings on Population and Family Planning in Japan,* ed. Minoru Muramatsu and Tameyoshi Katagiri. Tokyo: Japanese Organization for International Cooperation in Family Planning (JOICFP), pp. 40–60.
Beaujot, Roderic P. 1978. "Canada's population: Growth and dualism," *Population Bulletin* 33, no. 2.
Becker, Gary S. 1981. *A Treatise on the Family.* Cambridge, Mass.: Harvard University Press.
Bellah, Robert N., Richard Madsen, William M. Sullivan, Ann Swidler, and Steven M. Tipton. 1985. *Habits of the Heart: Individualism and Commitment in American Life.* Berkeley: University of California Press.
Binstock, Robert H. 1985. "The oldest old: A fresh perspective or compassionate ageism revisited?," *Milbank Memorial Fund Quarterly/Health and Society* 63, no. 2: 420–451.
Blake, Judith. 1972. "Coercive pronatalism and American population policy," in *Aspects of Population Growth Policy,* Vol. VI, ed. Robert Parke, Jr. and Charles F. Westoff. Washington, D.C.: US Government Printing Office, pp. 85–114.
Caldwell, John C. 1981. "An explanation of the continued fertility decline in the West: Stages, succession and crisis." Canberra: Department of Demography, Australian National University.
Carmichael, Gordon. 1984. "The transition to marriage: Trends in age at first marriage and proportions marrying in Australia," in *Australian Family Research Conference Proceedings,* Vol. 1, *Family Formation, Structure, Values.* Melbourne: Institute of Family Studies, pp. 99–175.
Cherlin, Andrew J. 1981. *Marriage, Divorce, Remarriage.* Cambridge, Mass.: Harvard University Press.

Cleland, John. 1985. "Marital fertility decline in developing countries: Theories and the evidence," in *Reproductive Change in Developing Countries: Insights from the World Fertility Survey*, ed. John Cleland and John Hobcraft. London: Oxford University Press, pp. 223–252.

Cosford, Wendy, Margaret Neill, Jamie Grocott, Pat Caldwell, and John Caldwell. 1976. "Semi-structured interviews of individuals: The Canberra Survey and supplementary interviews," in *Towards an Understanding of Contemporary Demographic Change*, ed. John Caldwell. Australian Family Formation Project, Monograph No. 4. Canberra: Australian National University, pp. 55–116.

Davis, Kingsley. 1955. "Institutional patterns favoring high fertility in underdeveloped areas," *Eugenics Quarterly* 2, no. 1: 33–39.

———. 1963. "The theory of change and response in modern demographic history," *Population Index* 29: 345–366.

de Beauvoir, Simone. 1953. *The Second Sex*. New York: Knopf. (Originally published in France in 1949 as *Le deuxième sexe*.)

Easterlin, Richard A. 1980. *Birth and Fortune: The Impact of Numbers on Personal Welfare*. New York: Basic Books.

Ehrenreich, Barbara. 1984. *The Hearts of Men: American Dreams and the Flight from Commitment*. Garden City, N.Y.: Anchor Press.

Ehrlich, Paul R. 1968. *The Population Bomb*. New York: Ballantine Books Inc.

French, Marilyn. 1955. *The Women's Room*. New York: Summit Books.

Friedan, Betty. 1963. *The Feminine Mystique*. New York: Norton.

Glezer, Helen. 1984. "Changes in marriage and sex-role attitudes among young married women: 1971–1982," in *Australian Family Research Conference Proceedings*, Vol. 1, *Family Formation, Structure, Values*. Melbourne: Institute of Family Studies, pp. 201–255.

Jones, Elise F., and Charles F. Westoff. 1979. "The end of 'Catholic' fertility," *Demography* 16, no. 2: 209–218.

Kerouack, Jack. 1957. *On the Road*. New York: Viking Press.

Khoo, Siew-Ean. 1984. "Family formation and ethnicity," in *Australian Family Research Conference Proceedings*, Vol. 1, *Family Formation, Structure, Values*. Melbourne: Institute of Family Studies, pp. 409–450.

Kono, Shigemi. 1982. "Determinants and consequences of low fertility in low-fertility countries," in *Third Asian and Pacific Population Conference (Colombo, September 1982)*. United Nations, Economic and Social Commission for Asia and the Pacific, Asian Population Studies Series No. 58. New York.

Lee, Ronald. 1985. "Population growth and intergenerational transfers in a household setting." Berkeley: Department of Economics, University of California.

Lesthaeghe, Ron. 1983. "A century of demographic and cultural change in Western Europe: An exploration of underlying dimensions," *Population and Development Review* 9, no. 3 (September): 411–435.

McDonald, Peter. 1984. "The baby boom generation as reproducers: Fertility in Australia in the late 1970s and the 1980s," in *Australian Family Research Conference Proceedings*, Vol. 1, *Family Formation, Structure, Values*. Melbourne: Institute of Family Studies, pp. 13–52.

McIntosh, C. Alison. 1983. *Population Policy in Western Europe: Responses to Low Fertility in France, Sweden, and West Germany*. Armonk, N.Y.: M. E. Sharpe.

Meadows, D. H., D. L. Meadows, J. Randers, and W. W. Behrens. 1972. *The Limits to Growth*. New York: Universe Books.

Mincer, Jacob. 1984. "Inter-country comparisons of labor force trends and of related developments: An overview," *NBER Working Paper Series*, Working Paper No. 1438. Cambridge, Mass.: National Bureau of Economic Research.

Morgan, S. Philip, and Kiyosi Hirosima. 1983. "The persistence of extended family residence in Japan: Anachronism or alternative strategy?," *American Sociological Review* 48, no. 2: 269–281.

Mosher, W. D., D. P. Johnson, and M. C. Horn. 1985. *Religion and Fertility in the United States: The Importance of Marriage Patterns and Hispanic Origin.* Washington, D.C.: National Center for Health Statistics.

Mosk, Carl. 1983. *Patriarchy and Fertility: Japan and Sweden, 1880–1960.* New York: Academic Press.

Preston, Samuel H. 1984. "Children and the elderly: Divergent paths for America's dependents," *Demography* 21, no. 4: 435–457.

Rindfuss, Ronald. 1972. "Recent trends in population attitudes," in *Aspects of Population Growth Policy,* Vol. VI, ed. Robert Parke, Jr. and Charles F. Westoff. Washington, D.C.: US Government Printing Office, pp. 465–474.

———, and James A. Sweet. 1977. *Postwar Fertility Trends and Differentials in the United States.* New York: Academic Press.

Sloan, Wilson. 1955. *The Man in the Grey Flannel Suit.* Cambridge, Mass.: Bentley.

Summers, Robert, and Alan Heston. 1984. "Improved international comparisons of real product and its composition: 1950–1980." Philadelphia: Department of Economics, University of Pennsylvania.

Sweet, James A., and Ronald R. Rindfuss. 1983. "Those ubiquitous fertility trends: United States, 1945–1979," *Social Biology* 30, no. 2: 127–139.

Taeuber, Irene B. 1958. *The Population of Japan.* Princeton, N.J.: Princeton University Press.

Thornton, Arland. 1979. "Fertility and income, consumption aspirations, and child quality standards," *Demography* 16, no. 2: 157–176.

———, and Deborah Freedman. 1982. "Changing attitudes toward marriage and single life," *Family Planning Perspectives* 14, no. 6: 297–303.

———, Duane F. Alwin, and Donald Camburn. 1983. "Causes and consequences of sex-role attitudes and attitude change," *American Sociological Review* 48, no. 2: 211–227.

United States Bureau of the Census. 1975. *Historical Statistics of the United States: Colonial Times to 1970.* Washington, D.C.: US Government Printing Office.

Veroff, Joseph, Elizabeth Douvan, and Richard A. Kulka. 1981. *The Inner American: A Self-Portrait from 1957 to 1976.* New York: Basic Books.

Westoff, Charles F., and Norman B. Ryder. 1977. *The Contraceptive Revolution.* Princeton, N.J.: Princeton University Press.

Whyte, William Hollingsworth. 1956. *The Organization Man.* New York: Simon and Schuster.

Willis, Robert J. 1985. *Externalities and Population.* Stony Brook: State University of New York.

Comment: Harriet B. Presser

Why the convergence to low fertility in industrialized countries? I shall argue that an important missing explanatory link is the general trend toward postponement in age at first birth among women and the changing context of childrearing that this has generated. The significance of these neglected dimensions of fertility behavior will be elaborated upon after first considering the explanations offered by Samuel Preston.

In the opening section of this volume (Trends), Preston relates the fertility trends to changing marriage and divorce rates and documents the accompanying out-of-wedlock fertility rates. He also considers changes in contraception and abortion practice and in family size orientation. These are familiar demographic correlates of fertility change. Marriage is becoming less of a determinant of fertility, birth control methods are becoming more effective and more widely used, and expected as well as actual fertility is falling.

Preston then shifts in the immediately preceding article to a broader explanatory framework, identifying three principal sets of factors that influence fertility change: economic factors, contraceptive technology, and values. Social factors appear in this formulation to be subsumed under values, rather than vice-versa, which is a debatable issue. But Preston is right to say that we often neglect values as explanatory variables, and his discussion of them in the context of the recent fertility decline in industrialized countries poses some provocative questions, such as whether a changing commitment to "responsible parenthood" and the spread of "secular individualism" are relevant. It is a rare treat to hear a demographer talk about such factors as the constraints of parenthood and role identity at a macro level.

The two explanatory levels of analysis, however, leave a considerable gap. How do the proximate determinants of fertility link up with changing technology, changing economic conditions, and changing values to produce a fertility decline? The process of fertility decline needs further specification, and here is where the postponement of women's age at first birth and the changing context of childrearing become critical focal points.

Postponement in age at first birth

My central thesis is that our currently low levels of fertility in industrialized countries may be largely explained by social, economic, and technological changes that served to postpone women's age at first birth. This postponement, by providing more child-free time for women to participate as adults in activities outside the home, radically changed the context of childrearing—making motherhood more complex and costly, both in terms of time and money, and more inequitable in terms of sex differences in total workload. Women have responded by having fewer subsequent births.

When first births are postponed from the early to the mid-20s (or later), as is the case for the industrialized countries Preston is looking at, women increasingly are in the labor force when they are making decisions (often in conjunction with spouses) as to when to have their first child. Improved contraceptive technology and the legalization of abortion make the timing of births more truly a matter of choice than ever before. The longer women postpone childbearing, the more likely they are to be well educated and committed to long-term continuous participation in the labor force. The exception occurs when, as in Japan, the marketplace is organized so as to discourage married women from acquiring full-time salaried positions. But for the other industrialized countries, because of the postponement of childbearing the incompatibility between labor force participation and childrearing is keenly experienced. Why is this so?

Greater child care constraints

Good, dependable, inexpensive child care in industrialized societies is a major problem. The younger the child, the greater the problem. With the earlier return of mothers to the labor force after childbirth, the age of children placed in child care is becoming younger. In the United States in 1984, 46.7 percent of women with children under one year of age were in the labor force (US Bureau of the Census, 1985a). Institutional provision of child care for preschoolers, particularly young preschoolers, is limited in availability and frequently expensive relative to women's wages. The more common alternative is reliance on less stable and often multiple types of arrangements, frequently involving female neighbors and relatives (primarily the child's grandmother). The availability of such child care providers is declining, given their alternative employment opportunities. Many dual-earner spouses and unmarried mothers with preschool-age children work evenings and nights so as to share child care with their day-employed spouses and relatives at minimal or no cost. In 1980, one-third of full-time dual-earner couples in the United States with preschool-age children included a spouse who worked other than a day shift (Presser and Cain, 1983). Also, in 1982, one-fifth of full-time employed unmarried mothers with preschoolers worked evenings, nights, or miscellaneous shifts (Presser, 1986). The "latch key" phenomenon among somewhat older children also reflects this problem. It may be that women's real wages are rising, but it is not certain whether real wages minus the cost of child care have improved. Many industrialized countries have gone further than the United States in subsidizing child care. The United States provides government funds for the poor only, while other countries have provided subsidized child care for all employed mothers. For all of these countries, however, there is a large unmet need for satisfactory, affordable child care.

How does the availability of child care affect fertility? The Commission on Population Growth and the American Future (1972) argued that government provision of child care would have an antinatalist effect in the long run, since it would encourage female employment and thus lower family size. But W. B. Reddaway (1939) had argued, in response to the concern about declining fertility in England in the 1920s, that the provision of subsidized child care would be pronatalist, because it would reduce the burden of childrearing. (Implicitly, he meant for nonemployed women, since restrictions on women's employment were also proposed.) These positions are not as inconsistent as they may at first seem. To the extent that child care availability increases women's entry into the labor force, it may be antinatalist; and to the extent it reduces the burden of childrearing for those who are (and will remain) in the labor force, it may be pronatalist. In a society like the United States, where great numbers of mothers with young children are already in the labor force and where fertility desires exceed actual behavior, subsidizing child care for employed mothers would seem to be pronatalist. So would a reduction of the childrearing burden after women come home from work. Both aspects become increasingly problematic the older women are at the time of their first birth, because they are more likely to want to remain in the labor force with minimal interruption after their first child is born. They will be making subsequent childbearing decisions while they are employed and experiencing these difficulties. Thus, more women will decide against additional births after the first unless these difficulties are eased.

Greater time constraints and sex-role inequities

By relying heavily on neighbors and relatives in an ad hoc fashion, women in the labor force with young children reduce the economic cost of child care, but add considerably to constraints on their time, because the arrangements are often multiple, unstable, and provided outside the home. Moreover, when women come home from their outside jobs, a greater share of their home time is spent on general housework and caring for their child and spouse, if married, than would be the case if they were not employed. (Very few women have paid housekeepers who also care for their children.) This generates greater sex-role inequities. Despite particular cases in which men do their fair share at home, or have full custody of their children, men in general are not responding to the increased participation of women in the labor force by substantially increasing their participation in the home. A greater change may be the "industrialization of household labor" (Bergmann, in press)—the purchase of household services that were traditionally performed by the wife.

One of Preston's most significant points is that "long-term economic growth not only affected the quality/quantity tradeoff within the role of responsible parent; it also increased the incentives to abandon the role altogether"

(p. 179). He notes that for women, unlike men, this requires a "massive change in role identity" (p. 185). It is important to consider also whether these role changes occur for both men and women after as well as before the first birth. Later marriage, more nonmarriage, and more sexual partners represent greater freedom for both sexes, and clearly postpone age at first birth. However, if—after children have arrived—men are becoming less responsible fathers, it is hard for women to become less responsible mothers: Who is going to make up for lack of child support from fathers if children are to survive? The growing proportion of single-mother families—22.9 percent in the United States in 1984 (US Bureau of the Census, 1985b)—points to the seriousness of this problem, and to the potential for increasing, not decreasing, gender inequities regarding childrearing responsibilities.

Future expectations

A further postponement in age at first birth may promote marital stability and the sharing of childrearing and household tasks. The more time a woman and a man spend as a couple without children, the more power the woman will have relative to the man to negotiate child care and household responsibilities once they have children. And power is what is required. I agree with Margaret Polatnick's (1973–74) analysis that in all societies, childrearing is basically a woman's responsibility, not for biological reasons (which are limited to childbearing) but because men do not want to do it. Childrearing, while it has intrinsic rewards, is not a source of economic and social gain. It is an activity that ties one down as no other activity does, and women generally lack the power to get men more involved. A further postponement of childbearing would increase women's power, both because women would become economically more independent and thus able to negotiate with strength, and because their longer participation in adult roles in a child-free context would make them—and men—more aware of gender inequities. Women's greater economic independence also would make childrearing outside of marriage a more feasible option if they want to have children but have not found a desirable long-term partner.

No matter what the future trend in age at first birth, the great majority of both men and women will continue to want children. The desire to be a parent, to have an intimate link with the next generation, is in my view generally stronger than the desire to be legally married. Witness the high out-of-wedlock childbearing rates in Sweden, where such children have the same legal rights as those born in wedlock. However, it takes only one child to make one a parent, after which a person remains a parent indefinitely. With the postponement of childbearing, the desire for two or more children may linger on, but the marginal benefit of additional children relative to the increased workload they entail, especially for women, makes a second child increasingly unlikely. We may retain our generally negative view about the "only child" being spoiled, selfish, and lonely, but we may soon see attitudes change in this regard as well. Child care can provide sibling substitutes of the same age (a rarity in families), and of course more time and money can be spent on a single child. Let us not forget that the parents making these decisions in the future will themselves have been reared increasingly in alternative child care arrangements.

Will industrialized countries move toward even later ages at first birth, and will a growing proportion of people have one child, but desire two? Probably so. For one thing, the social and economic factors causing the postponement of first births over the past 15 to 20 years are still operative. There are some signs of change in the workplace toward more flexible hours, but employer-supported child care services are still minimal and likely to remain so as long as child care is defined as a woman's issue. The pressure will increase for men to participate more in childrearing and household tasks as women acquire greater family power. Whether men will do so and, if so, whether this participation will serve to decrease their family size desires, is an open question. Changes in men's behavior in the family may be the most interesting source of variation in fertility in the near future.

A final assessment: fertility decline in industrialized countries is good for women, just as it is in developing countries, even though the number of children at issue and the contexts are different. Having fewer children enhances women's status outside the home, increases their family power, and is certainly less tiring. If men want more children, and the society fears depopulation, perhaps serious efforts will be directed toward improving the context of childrearing—that is, improving the availability of satisfactory and inexpensive child care, making the workplace more compatible with childrearing, and reducing women's total workload as they continue to participate more fully in the labor force. However skeptical one may be about the likelihood of any of these changes occurring, the alternative response of declining female labor force participation seems far less likely.

References

Bergmann, B. In press. *The Economic Emergence of Women*. New York: Basic Books.
Commission on Population Growth and the American Future. 1972. *Population and the American Future*. Washington, D.C.: US Government Printing Office.
Polatnick, M. 1973–74. "Why men don't rear children: A power analysis," *Berkeley Journal of Sociology* 18: 45–86.
Presser, H. B. 1986. "Shift work among American women and child care," *Journal of Marriage and the Family* 48: 551–563.
———, and V. S. Cain. 1983. "Shift work among American couples with children," *Science* 219 (18 February): 876–879.
Reddaway, W. B. 1939. *The Economics of a Declining Population*. London: George Allen and Unwin Ltd.
United States Bureau of the Census. 1985a. *Current Population Reports*. "Fertility of American women, June 1984," Series P-20, No. 401, Table C. Washington, D.C.: US Government Printing Office.
———. 1985b. *Current Population Reports*. "Household and family characteristics, March 1984," Series P-20, No. 398, Table D. Washington, D.C.: US Government Printing Office.

CONSEQUENCES

Demographic Effects of Below-Replacement Fertility and Their Social Implications

Ansley J. Coale

Most of the social implications of sustained low fertility arise from how it affects the growth and the age composition of the population. In the absence of massive immigration, these effects are inevitable in any population in which low fertility continues for several generations. Fertility is the principal determinant of age composition; continued low fertility produces a population with relatively few young people and relatively many old people, whatever the mortality conditions. Continuous immigration modifies the effect of low fertility on the growth of the population but has less influence on the age composition deriving from low fertility.

The demographic effects of low fertility

I have chosen to illustrate the effects of continued low fertility by constructing projections of the US population from 1980 to 2100.[1] Alternative projections have been made with moderately low fertility (at a level that just reproduces each parental generation) and three levels of fertility successively lower than fertility that yields long-term replacement. I have assumed a constant regime of low mortality, with an expectation of life at birth for females of 80 years, a little greater than the current expectation of life in the United States. With this level of mortality, more than 99 percent of women survive to the mean age of childbearing, and 95 percent survive to age 60. With such high survival rates, an average of 2.07 births per woman leads to replacement of the mothers in each generation. They must bear an average of 1.01 daughters (to allow for the fact that about 1 percent of women die before reaching the mean age of childbearing) and 1.06 sons (since there are about 1.05 male births for every female birth). The total of 2.07 children thus guarantees that women on the average will produce just the number of daughters they must have to replace

FIGURE 1 Growth of the total projected population of the United States, 1980–2100, at alternative low levels of fertility, with and without net immigration

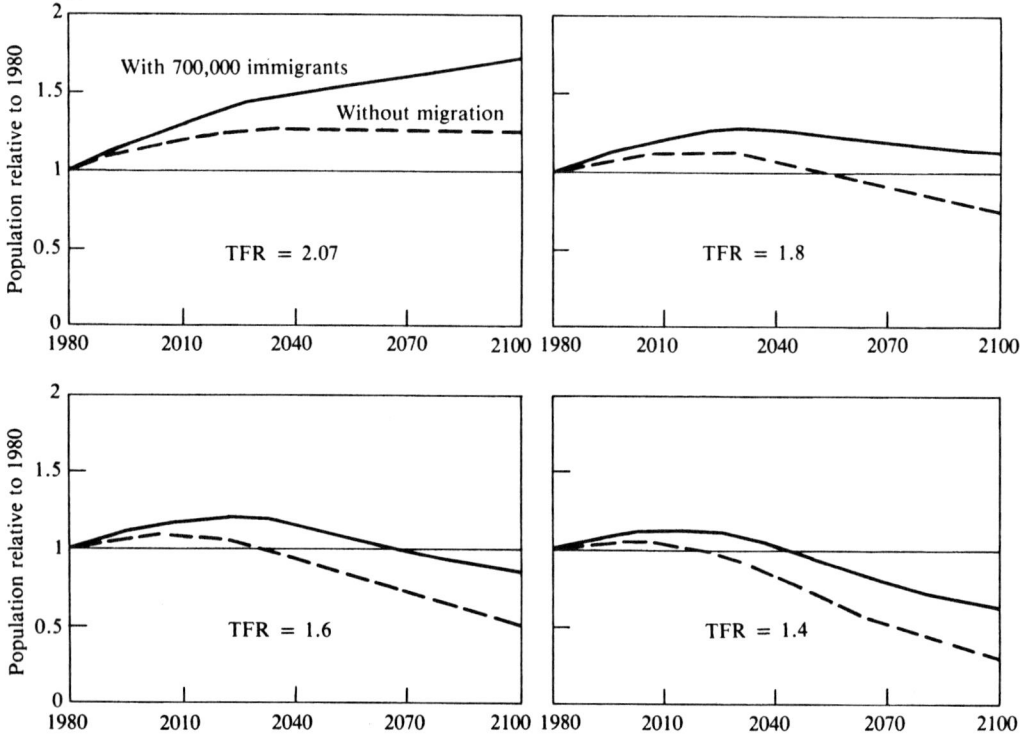

SOURCE: Calculations by the author.

themselves. The projection at this level of fertility yields a population that neither grows nor shrinks significantly after the year 2030. The population would grow for about 50 years even at the replacement level of fertility because the initial age distribution is favorable to producing more births than deaths. There will be many women in the principal ages of childbearing in the next few years because they were born during the baby boom. The death rate will only gradually rise to its ultimate level because the initially moderate fraction of the population at the higher ages will increase slowly.

In the alternative projections, fertility is assumed to remain lower than a total fertility rate of 2.07. The range of rates used in these projections corresponds to recently experienced levels of fertility in industrialized countries. (In the United States in 1985, the total fertility rate was 1.8.) Two sets of projections of the population of the United States have been made at each assumed level of fertility: one with an assumption of no immigration, and the other with an assumed net immigration of 700,000 persons per year.[2] This

TABLE 1 The effect of net immigration on the size of the projected population of the United States in 2100, at various low levels of fertility

Assumed total fertility rate	Population in 2100 relative to 1980		Population in 2100 with migration relative to population without migration	Required annual migration so that population in 2100 = population in 1980
	No immigration	700,000 annual immigration		
2.07	1.265	1.732	1.370	−396,000
1.80	0.748	1.130	1.511	464,000
1.60	0.492	0.824	1.675	1,017,000
1.40	0.336	0.627	1.870	1,594,000

SOURCE: Calculations by the author.

number is well in excess of the approximately 400,000 migrants (not including refugees) permitted under current immigration laws, but is less than some of the recent estimates of total immigration, including undocumented migrants.

Figure 1 shows the increase in the US population that would result from continued low fertility at various levels. In each panel of this figure the projected total population without migration is compared with the projected population with an annual net immigration of 700,000. The difference between the two projected totals is, of course, the contribution of the immigrants and their descendants to the total population of the United States. (The age composition of the annual immigrant stream is that assumed by Thomas Espenshade et al., 1982.) The postulated fertility and mortality rates of immigrants after arrival are the same as those experienced by the resident population.

Table 1 summarizes the cumulative change in population between 1980 and 2100 under the various assumptions. With replacement fertility (TFR = 2.07), the population would stabilize at a little more than 25 percent above its 1980 size before the middle of the next century. With net immigration of 700,000 per year, it would be nearly three-quarters again as large in 2100 as in 1980, and steadily increasing at about 4 million additional persons each year. The lowest fertility projection, with a total fertility rate of 1.4, would produce a population only one-third as large as in 1980 by the end of the next century in the absence of immigration, and a population about five-eighths as large as in 1980 if immigration occurred at the rate of 700,000 per year. The last column of Table 1 shows the net migration flow that would be required to produce a population at the end of the next century the same size as in 1980. Under replacement fertility, a net outflow would be needed to offset the temporary increase occasioned by the momentum inherent in the 1980 age distribution. If the total fertility rate were only 1.4, net immigration of 1.6 million per year would be required to produce a population in 2100 as large as in 1980.

The future age composition that would result from the continuation of low fertility is presented in Figures 2 and 3 and Table 2.

FIGURE 2 The percent age distribution of the projected population of the United States, selected dates from 1980 to 2100, with a total fertility rate of 2.07 and no immigration

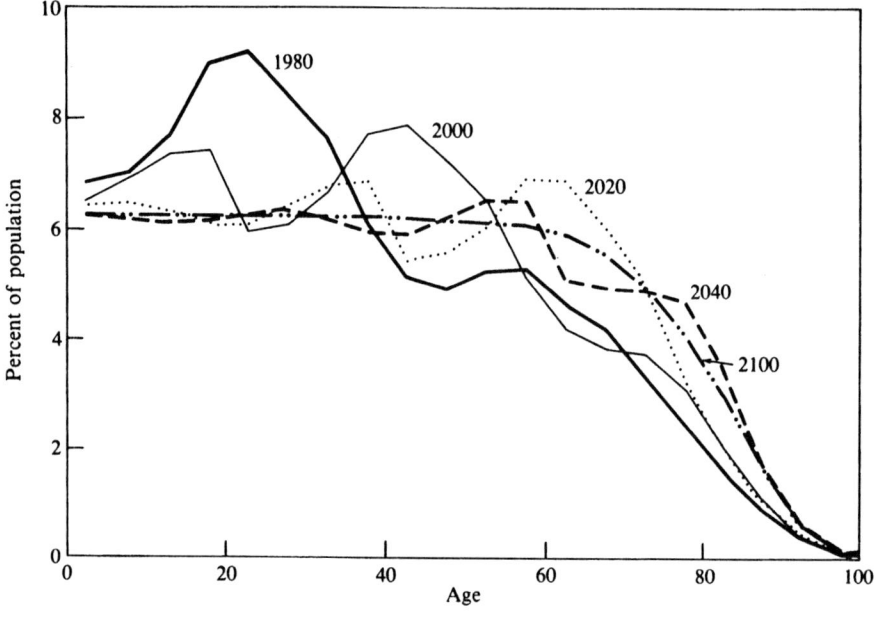

SOURCE: Calculations by the author.

Figure 2 shows how the age distribution would evolve until the end of the next century if fertility were at the replacement level and there were no migration. The approach to a stationary age distribution is clearly visible. The 1980 age distribution has a high point at ages 20–24, representing the peak in the number of births that occurred during the height of the baby boom in the late 1950s. The much lower proportion at ages 0–4 than at 20–24 in 1980 is the result of the much reduced fertility in the late 1970s. The hollow at ages 45–49 in 1980 is the product of the low fertility in the early 1930s. In the year 2000 the peak generated by the baby boom has moved to ages 40–44. The low fertility of the 1970s results in a low range at ages 20–29 in 2000. The high proportions at ages 10–14 and 15–19 in 2000 are a sort of echo of the baby boom because when women born in the boom years are themselves in the principal childbearing ages, the number of births is inflated, even with moderate fertility. These bumps and hollows move to older ages as time passes: by 2100 the age distribution is very close to the ultimate unchanging distribution produced in the long run by constant fertility and mortality.

Figure 3 illustrates the cumulative effect of various levels of low fertility on the age distribution by the end of the next century. Each of the panels shows the projected age distribution in 2100 for one of the four levels of fertility that we have considered. Two age distributions are shown in each panel: one under

FIGURE 3 The percent age distribution of the projected population of the United States in 2100 at various levels of fertility, with and without net immigration

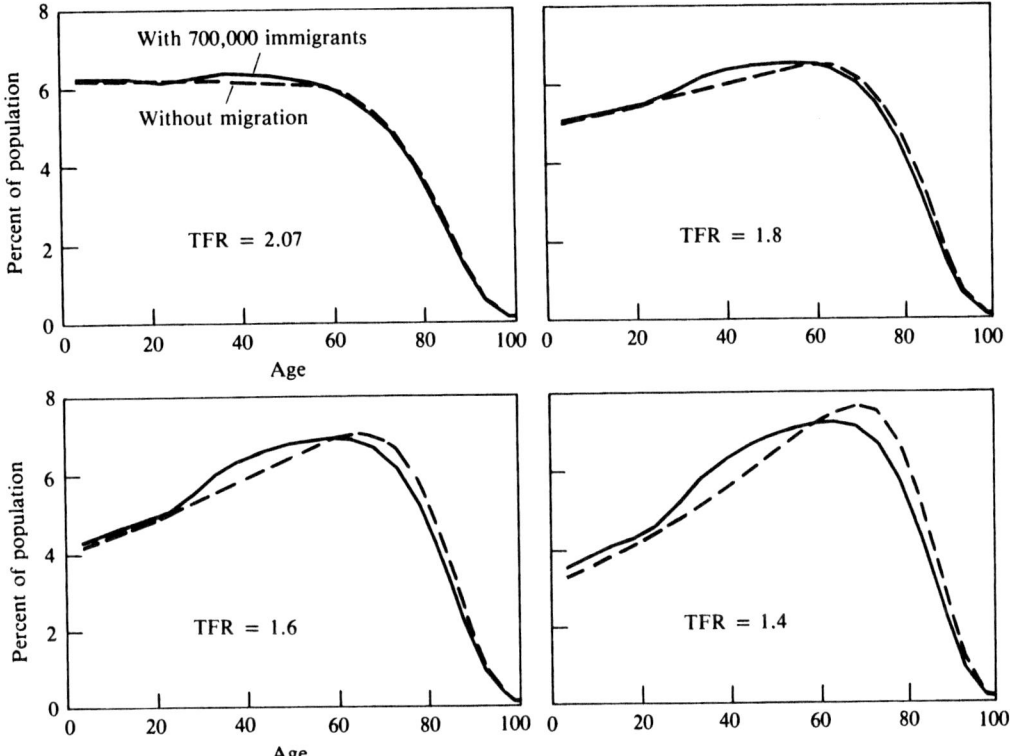

SOURCE: Calculations by the author.

the assumption of no migration, the other with an assumed net immigration of 700,000 persons per year.

Table 2 lists parameters of the projected populations in the year 2100 under the four assumed low-fertility regimes, with and without net migration. It also compares these parameters with the corresponding characteristics of the population in 1980. The increase in the proportion of the aged population and the decrease in the proportion under age 20 are the most conspicuous features when any of the projected populations at the end of the next century is compared with the population in 1980. As part of this shift of proportions, the median age (defined as the age below which 50 percent of the population is found) increases by about nine years between 1980 and 2100 even with replacement fertility. If fertility were as low as a total fertility rate of 1.4, the increase in the median age would be more than 20 years without migration, and 18 years even with 700,000 net immigrants each year. The fraction under age 20 is sharply reduced in any of the projections (by 50 percent with the lowest assumed

TABLE 2 Characteristics of age distributions in 2100, at various low levels of fertility

Assumed total fertility rate	Median age		Proportion in age intervals				P_{60-64}/P_{20-24}
	Whole population	Persons 20–64	0–19	20–64	65+	80+	
	No immigration						
2.07	37.7	39.7	0.249	0.551	0.200	0.054	.95
1.80	42.3	41.0	0.209	0.552	0.240	0.068	1.17
1.60	46.0	42.2	0.178	0.546	0.275	0.081	1.39
1.40	49.9	43.3	0.147	0.536	0.317	0.098	1.70
	Including net immigration at 700,000 per year						
2.07	37.5	39.7	0.248	0.558	0.193	0.051	0.95
1.80	41.5	40.9	0.210	0.565	0.226	0.062	1.16
1.60	44.3	41.7	0.182	0.567	0.251	0.070	1.35
1.40	46.9	42.5	0.156	0.569	0.275	0.079	1.59
1980 population	28.8	35.0	0.305	0.565	0.131	0.030	0.51

SOURCE: Calculations by the author.

fertility), whereas the proportion over age 65 changes in the opposite direction. As a result, the total proportion above and below the principal ages of labor force participation hardly changes at all, so that the fraction aged 20–64 is virtually unchanged in all of the projections. The proportion over 65 increases by anywhere from 50 percent to more than 100 percent, depending on the level of fertility assumed. The proportion of the very old (over 80) is multiplied by more than three in the projected population having the lowest fertility and no immigration.[3]

An important feature of the numbers given in Table 2 is the modest difference in the age distribution in 2100 between the projections that include net immigration and those that do not. (The same slight difference can be seen in Figure 3.) A substantial flow of net immigrants offsets to a marked extent the reduction in population growth occasioned by the continuation of very low fertility and leads to a steadily growing population if fertility is held at the replacement level. But if the immigrants and their descendants have the same low fertility as the resident population, their continuing arrival has only a modest effect on the drastic reordering of the age distribution caused by sustained low fertility.

Within the age span of heaviest participation in the labor force, the median age (in the age range 20–64) rises by nearly five years with a total fertility rate of 2.07 and by seven to eight years with a total fertility rate of 1.4. As shown in the last column of Table 2, the ratio of the number about to leave the labor force (at ages 60–64) to those just entering (ages 20–24) nearly doubles by 2100 with moderately low fertility and is multiplied by three or more with very low fertility.

The social implications of low fertility

A greatly altered age distribution is the most conspicuous result of continued low fertility. If there is popular and official concern about the prospect of shrinking numbers, the flow of migrants from parts of the world in which fertility has not yet declined to low levels can be encouraged. Our projections show, however, that if the migrant population and its descendants themselves have low fertility rates, the age distribution is altered only to a small degree by the net inflow. To avoid a large increase in proportions at older ages, a decrease in the proportions at young ages, and the attendant increase in mean age, high fertility would have to be imported with the immigrants.

Differences in the social environment persisting from early childhood to old age are implied by these gross differences in age composition. When low fertility has long continued, children grow up with fewer collateral relatives—fewer siblings, aunts and uncles, and cousins—but with many ancestral relatives as low mortality continues. Usually all four grandparents of young children are still alive and, at least in early childhood, several great-grandparents. In a low-fertility population, each of these ancestral relatives of course has few descendants.

In a cohort of women who bear only 1.4 children on the average, 45 percent of the total person-years lived would be spent without having borne a child, and 33 percent after the last child had reached age 20. Only about 22 percent of the cohort's aggregate lifetime experience would be spent with children under age 20.[4]

The difference between the 1980 population and the population in 2100—following upon sustained below-replacement fertility—would be highly visible in everyday life. The female population of Vienna in 1981, despite irregularities in age distribution caused by the great depression and the birth deficit during World War I, has an overall age structure typical of a population that has long had low fertility. In fact, the proportion under age 10 is lower, and the proportion over age 65 and the median age greater, than in the projected US population in 2100 with a total fertility rate of 1.8 (see Figure 4). The present-day difference in age composition between Vienna and any American city is visible to a casual observer. In an American city the streets, stores, and public conveyances are peopled largely by young adults born in the late 1950s and early 1960s. In Vienna the predominant impression is of gray-haired ladies prepared to intimidate with their walking sticks the rare unruly child who might sit near them on a tram.

The most conspicuous features of low-fertility age distributions are the very high proportions above 65 and above 80, proportions that will be still greater if major reductions in old-age mortality are achieved. The problem of providing material support for the aged is a major social implication of low fertility and is discussed elsewhere in this volume.

As noted earlier, continued low fertility changes the age composition of the labor force as well as the age structure of the whole population. In a lecture

FIGURE 4 The percent age distribution of the projected population of the United States in 2100 with total fertility rates of 1.4 and 1.8, compared with the US age distribution in 1980 and the age distribution of Vienna in 1981

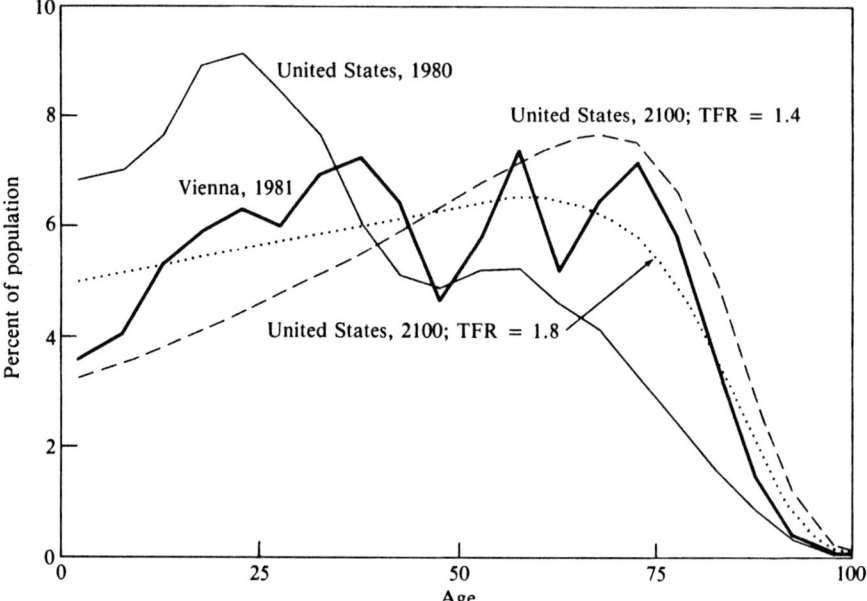

SOURCES: For the United States, calculations by the author; for Vienna, Census of Austria, 1981.

series entitled "Population, a problem for democracy" that Gunnar Myrdal gave at Harvard University in 1938, he noted that the pyramid of the number of persons at each age from 20 to 64 in a growing population is roughly congruent with the hierarchial pyramid of authority and responsibility in the labor force (Myrdal, 1940). Normally, persons enter the labor force in positions with low pay and little authority. With more experience and seniority they rise to positions where they may supervise a number of junior members of the labor force. There are necessarily fewer positions with higher status in this hierarchy. The congruence in a growing population between the age pyramid and the status and pay structure of the work force means that individual labor force participants have a reasonable expectation of promotion as the length of their service is extended. With the age distributions generated by continued low fertility—distributions in which numbers of persons increase with age—the normal expectation of advancement cannot be sustained. Length of stay in a given status is extended; promotion is slower (Keyfitz, 1973). At the same time, a small number of entrants relative to the number of older workers increases the demand for the qualities young workers offer, such as vigor and adaptability to new technology. When the population increases rather than diminishes with age from ages 20 to 64, the young enjoy a high demand for their services, but face the prospect of intense competition for the small number of advanced positions they might hope to occupy as they get older. They can expect a good starting wage, but very slow promotion.

Political effects of reduced numbers of children and increased numbers of the aged

In Samuel Preston's presidential address to the Population Association of America (Preston, 1984), he assembled US data for recent decades that showed very different changes in well-being of those under age 15 and those over age 65. The absolute number of children fell between 1960 and 1982 by 7 percent, while the number of persons aged 65 and over grew by 54 percent. The proportion of children living in households in poverty rose from 16 to 23 percent between 1970 and 1982, while the proportion of the elderly living in poverty declined from 24 to 15 percent. When adjustment is made for such noncash transfers as foodstamps and Medicare, the relative improvement in poverty status of the elderly compared with children is even greater. An age-neutral method for assessing changes in mortality rates reveals a larger reduction in mortality over age 65 than at ages 35 to 60, which reduction in turn was larger than the reduction at early adult ages and in childhood. Lowered mortality for the aged coincided with a very large expansion in public expenditures in support of health care for the elderly. Preston presents evidence that, in contrast, the quality of public schooling, the principal conduit for public transfers to the young, has deteriorated.

Conventional analysis of the 54 percent increase in the number of the aged and the 7 percent decrease in the number of children between 1960 and 1980 would lead to the expectation that these demographic changes would operate against the well-being of the elderly, and in favor of children. Smaller numbers of children should allow the use of more educational resources per child; and a substantial increase in the number of persons over 65 should increase the strain on government pension schemes and subsidized medical care. Preston argues to the contrary: the increase in the number of the elderly has contributed to their improved well-being, while the decrease in the number of children has served to worsen their relative position.

Political support for benefits given to the elderly is greater than support for benefits received by children. A high proportion of persons over 65 now participate in elections; a substantial increase in their numbers adds to their voting strength. Children do not vote. Adults aged 20–64 have more living parents than living children under age 20. The selfish interest of adults below the age of retirement leads them to support benefits for the retired, since they anticipate receiving such benefits themselves.

The relative decline in the well-being of children is associated with changes that contribute to the establishment and continuation of low fertility. A high proportion of the children living in poverty live in single-parent households headed by a woman, often deprived of support from the former husband in a dissolved marriage. The large increase in marital dissolution has helped both to reduce the number of children and to worsen their economic circumstances.

Preston notes that the increase in the number of older persons and the reduction in the number of children has strengthened the major industry supporting the elderly (medical care) and weakened the major industry supporting children (public education). Although expenditures per pupil have risen and the student/teacher ratio has fallen as the number of children has declined, the real income of teachers has diminished, and the quality of persons entering teaching, as measured by test scores, has deteriorated. In contrast, there has been a dramatic increase in funds supporting medical care, especially medical care for the elderly. It is not surprising that, increasingly, the ablest college graduates are choosing training for the expanding industry of medical care rather than entering the declining industry of public education.

The future of education

The potential trajectory of primary education with continued low fertility ranges from substantially downward with very low fertility to moderately upward if a large volume of immigration accompanies a return of fertility to replacement level. Unless fertility rises above replacement, primary education will not again become a high growth industry. The difficulty of attracting able young adults into public school teaching—a longstanding American dilemma—is not likely to be lightened by demographic factors. If the ratio of students to teachers remains constant, the demand for new teachers is proportional to the increase in enrollments. The number of children aged 5–14 rose rapidly when the children born during the baby boom succeeded the small cohorts born in the 1930s and 1940s. From 1950 to 1970 the number rose by 66 percent, then a decline began. The rapid rise in enrollment required the recruitment of many new teachers; the rate of retirement after such an expansion is low because of the large fraction of recently hired younger persons.

The shift from rapid growth to slower growth and then numerical shrinkage that earlier affected the primary schools is now occurring in college enrollments. From early in this century until about 1970 college enrollments increased at an average rate of 6 or 7 percent a year; thereafter, the rate of increase fell, and it will almost certainly be negative until about 1995. The rapid growth in enrollment was caused by two factors: the increase in the proportion enrolled among those of college age, and the increase in the number of persons at the usual ages for college attendance. The proportion of persons at these ages who were enrolled reached a peak around 1970 and has diminished slightly or not increased significantly since. The decline in fertility that began in the early 1960s is producing a shrinking number at the ages of college attendance in the 1980s. Enrollment has been projected as declining to a minimum in 1997, about 15 percent lower than in 1981 (Bowen, 1981).

The reduction in the rate of increase in the number of children attending elementary school, followed by the actual decline in numbers, has reduced the demand for public school teachers. The slowdown in growth and the prospective decline in college enrollment are now reducing the demand for new college faculty. According to the acceleration principle in economics, the demand for capital goods is proportional to the increase in the sale of consumer goods. An increase in the sale of flour calls for more milling equipment; without an increase, the demand is limited to the replacement of worn-out or obsolete equipment. Graduate schools are the capital goods industry for college education. A large proportion of graduate students working toward a Ph.D. expect to become instructors or assistant professors in colleges and universities. The rapid growth in college enrollments before 1970 created a large demand for newly trained faculty. With enrollments fixed, and even declining, the only demand for additional young faculty is to replace those who are retiring.

The number of retirements from college faculties in the United States is low in the 1980s because the recently ended rapid expansion in college enrollments created a faculty with a young age structure. The faculty now approaching retirement age entered college teaching 35 to 40 years ago when enrollments were much smaller. A recently enacted federal law overturning mandatory retirement before age 70 will further reduce the rate of retirement, especially in the next few years, but also in the long run. A proposed law to forbid the imposition of any mandatory age would reduce the rate still more. It is especially difficult to mandate retirement of faculty on any basis other than age, because senior members of college faculties have tenure. Contrary to popular opinion, the crucial importance of academic tenure is not to provide economic security to professors, but to sustain their academic freedom. When a professor has met the typically stringent requirements for appointment to tenure, he is safe from dismissal on the grounds that the departmental chairman and the college administration do not like him, or, in particular, do not like what he says. Tenure is necessary to protect the professor from removal because of the unpopularity of his views. In this context, a rule against age-related mandatory retirement implies that senior faculty may decide to remain employed well beyond age 70, further reducing the demand for new instructors and assistant professors.

The industrial structure of higher education has been shaped by a long period of rapidly increasing college enrollments. Graduate education in the arts and sciences expanded in response to the need for many teachers of undergraduates. William Bowen (1981) projected about 100,000 academic positions to be filled in the 15 years from 1980 to 1995, compared with 60,000 filled in just 5 years from 1971 to 1975. The number of Ph.D.s awarded was in the range of 30,000–35,000 per year in the 1970s, and about the same from 1980 to 1984. Degree recipients in some fields such as engineering, economics, and chemistry can find excellent professional positions other than teaching. In other fields the great majority who receive the Ph.D. look for academic employment. Graduate education programs designed to meet a large demand for new faculty, combined with stagnant or declining undergraduate enrollments, a young faculty, and no mandatory retirement before age 70, have produced a very serious lack of job opportunities for many of those completing their graduate training. The result is not merely frustrated job seekers. Shrinkage in public school enrollment has worsened job prospects for would-be school teachers and led able college students to plan careers in more promising fields. The stagnation and shrinkage of college enrollments has similar connotations for applicants to graduate schools in the arts and sciences.

Nathan Keyfitz (1978) warns that a reduction in graduate education and reduced entry of young faculty members into college and university employment threaten the quality of scholarship in the humanities and of research in the sciences. Both fields prosper when constantly replenished with an infusion of the best young minds. With reduced numbers of graduate students and young faculty, the volume of academic scholarship and scientific research will be hard to maintain; with reduced prospects, the best minds will increasingly go elsewhere.

Continued low fertility will dampen the increase in college enrollments that might otherwise begin in the late 1990s and perpetuate the difficulties graduate education and university scholarship now face.

Conclusion

Continued low fertility inevitably implies slower growth, even negative growth, of the total population. It also means a much lower proportion below, and a higher proportion above, every age than was ever experienced until now within any national population. If immigrants adopt the low fertility of the receiving country, importing migrants can offset to an important degree the tendency for a low-fertility population to shrink, but it will not greatly modify the aging of the population.

These demographic characteristics imply a social environment radically different from the environment that would be created if fertility were again to rise above the replacement level. In a low-fertility society children grow up with few collateral relatives; a small portion of a typical lifetime is spent in the role of parent of dependent children; the ease of getting a job and the chances of promotion are affected; transfer payments from the employed to the retired are enlarged; and so on.

Alfred Sauvy once said that a stationary population is a population of old people ruminating over old ideas in old houses. Such a depiction describes tendencies only, not inevitable characteristics. But such tendencies are even stronger in a population with sustained low fertility than in a stationary population.

Notes

1 Only the female population is projected. Increases in a projected male population and the changes in its age composition would closely parallel corresponding features of the female population. Male and female births are in a constant ratio. Had the male population been projected, male mortality would have been assumed constant at death rates slightly higher than female death rates, with an expectation of life at birth of 76.6 years, compared with 80 for females.

2 The effect of alternative levels of net immigration (from 0 to 2 million net migrants annually) on the population of the United States projected to 2080 at three fertility levels is analyzed in Bouvier, 1981. Espenshade et al., 1982, show that a constant immigrant stream, combined with fixed mortality and fertility below replacement, ultimately yields a stationary population, of size $Be_0/(1-NRR)$, where B is the fixed annual number of births to immigrant women, e_0 is the expectation of life at birth, and NRR is the net reproduction rate. Convergence to this stationary state is exceedingly slow. Convergence requires the disappearance of the calculated descendants of the original resident population; after three centuries with a total fertility rate of 1.8, the descendants of the original residents would still constitute 22 percent of the total population.

3 All of the projections were made with a life table in which the expectation of life at birth for females is 80 years. This is the "West" model life table that represents an estimate of the typical mortality experience at a very high expectation of life based on international data from many countries.

We made an experimental projection with even lower mortality rates at older ages (an expectation of life of 25.8 years instead of 21.8 years at age 60 and 11.5 years instead of 7.5 years at age 80). Lower old-age mortality increases the projected proportions at the upper ages in 2100 by a factor of 1.18 over age 65 and by a factor of 1.68 over age 80.

This model life table matches very closely (within one year) the sequence of remaining expectations of life at every age from zero to 100 in the two female populations with the highest recent life expectancy at birth (Japan, 1982–83, 79.7 years; Sweden, 1983, 79.6 years). Because of age overstatement at advanced ages, US life tables at ages above 75 or 80 seem to understate mortality. Thus, other projections that begin with the current US life table incorporate even more favorable old-age mortality than does our projection.

4 See Davis and van den Oever, 1982. This calculation was made on the assumption that 20 percent of the cohort have no children, 20 percent have one child, and 60 percent have two children. The first birth occurs at an average age of 25, and the second at an average age of 28.

References

Bowen, William G. 1981. *Graduate Education in the Arts and Sciences: Prospects for the Future*. Princeton University, Report of the President. Excerpted under the title "Market prospects for Ph.D.s in the United States," in *Population and Development Review* 7, no. 3 (September): 475–488.

Bouvier, Leon F. 1981. *The Impact of Immigration on U.S. Population Size*, Population Trends and Public Policy, No. 1 (Washington, D.C.: Population Reference Bureau).

Davis, Kingsley, and Pietronella van den Oever. 1982. "Demographic foundations of new sex roles," *Population and Development Review* 8, no. 3 (September): 495–516.

Espenshade, Thomas J., Leon F. Bouvier, and W. Brian Arthur. 1982. "Immigration and the stable population model," *Demography* 19, no. 1 (February): 125–133.

Keyfitz, Nathan. 1973. "Individual mobility in a stationary population," *Population Studies* 27, no. 2 (July): 335–352.

———. 1978. "The graduate schools lose their economic base," Harvard University, Center for Population Studies, Working Paper No. 104.

Myrdal, Gunnar. 1940. *Population. A Problem for Democracy*. Cambridge, Mass.: Harvard University Press.

Preston, Samuel H. 1984. "Children and the elderly: Divergent paths for America's dependents," *Demography* 21, no. 4 (November): 435–457.

Economic Growth with Below-Replacement Fertility

Geoffrey McNicoll

A demographic Laffer curve, discovered, let us imagine, sketched on a tablecloth in the Hoover Institution canteen, tells us that six-child families are bad for business and zero children bad for business, but somewhere in between is a fertility regime under which the economy can optimally thrive. Little more than a decade ago the US Commission on Population and the American Future explored the implications of the choice between three- and two-child families. In the economic arena the Commissioners' conclusion was unqualified: "we find no convincing economic argument for continued national population growth. On the contrary most of the pluses are on the side of slower growth" (US Commission, 1972: 40–41). A two-child average was to be welcomed. It soon came, and passed—with scant respect for the convention, embodied in most population projections, by which demographic transition ends comfortably on a floor of replacement-level fertility. A population commission set up in the late 1980s would have the task of examining two- versus one-child family averages—the latter, most would expect, likely to be found to lie clearly on the downward gradient of the Laffer curve.

In this article I take continuing below-replacement fertility as the premise and look to identify and weigh economic outcomes that plausibly follow. My interest is in the industrialized countries, principally the United States. As in a number of prior studies, the effects of low fertility on labor supply, technological change, and investment and consumption appear relatively slight.[1] I shall argue, however, that there *are* serious, potentially adverse, economic consequences of low fertility, chiefly found in the distributional changes that are generated or accentuated under these demographic circumstances and in the international setting in which low-fertility countries will find themselves.

Labor force implications of low fertility

The chief demographic effects of below-replacement fertility are familiar: eventual but often greatly delayed contraction in population numbers; a concentration of families around completed parities (number of children ever born by the end of childbearing years) of 0–3; substantial rises in the median age of the population and in the proportion of elderly; and a fall-off in the relative numbers of youth and in the ratio of labor force entrants to retirees under constant participation rates. Unlikely variants such as below-replacement fertility coinciding with increased rather than diminished variance in completed parity, or with massive levels of immigration, need not detain us.

For a developed country, total population size roughly sets the overall scale of the economy, but in view of the current plausible range of population growth rates, this attribute of a population is a given over the time horizon of most economic calculations. Of course, demographers can let their projections run on indefinitely, with even slight growth rate differences yielding arbitrarily large size disparities. It would be hard to claim that economic outcomes are neutral over differences in population size of a factor of two or more. Yet such variation is generated, for example, by fertility assumptions within what is deemed a realistic range over the 100-year horizon of the latest official US population projections—total fertility rates (TFR) of 2.3 (high), 1.9 (middle), and 1.6 (low). Combined with the middle mortality and migration assumptions (the latter being a net inflow of 450,000 per year), the US population is projected to grow as follows (in millions):

Assumption	1985	2000	2025	2050	2080
High fertility (TFR = 2.3)	239	273	330	380	453
Middle fertility (TFR = 1.9)	239	268	301	309	311
Low fertility (TFR = 1.6)	238	262	276	258	224

SOURCE: US Bureau of the Census (1984b: 111).

The 40 years or so that it takes for an absolute decline in the US population to occur even in the low-fertility case above is notable. That this is more a momentum phenomenon than an outcome of migration is seen by a corresponding low-fertility/*zero*-migration projection run, in which the peak population occurs around 2010, little more than a decade earlier. In Europe, as Hilde Wander (1978: 54) has pointed out, projected momentum effects are much smaller: by the end of the 1960s "the buffer effect of large fertile age groups had come to an end, so that a drop in fertility now tends to depress growth much more immediately than in the 1930s." Even so, radical fall-back in Europe's population numbers under current long-range projections is a feature of the second half rather than the first half of the twenty-first century (see Bourgeois-Pichat, 1981: 40).

The working-age population, say those aged 20–64 years, grows roughly in line with the total population. In the prime early labor force age groups, absolute declines set in sooner—in the 1990s for the age group 20–24 in most Western countries (see Table 1).

Changes in participation rates, unemployment, or hours worked per worker can potentially offset changes in aggregate labor force numbers, although these factors have other determinants and may not in fact do so. Indeed, the likelihood of substantial drops in labor demand emerging from current developments in technology makes an interest in complete offset for the future purely notional. In the important case of female labor force participation, part of the steady rise over recent decades can be attributed to a response to fertility decline or to (related) marital instability. Jacob Mincer (1985: S7) points out the causal complications, however: while "declines in family size and durations of marriage provide an increased scope and motivation for the greater labor market commitment of women," there is also an opposite connection, namely that "fertility and marriage patterns adjust to greater labor force commitments," and both may be jointly influenced by changes in wages, educational levels, urbanization, fiscal policies, and so on. James Smith and Michael Ward (1985: S60) find that more than half the post–World War II growth in the US female labor force measured in hours worked per year can be accounted for by rising wages (male and female), with half of this in turn being transmitted through fertility.

Gross female participation rates in Western countries still contain considerable slack potentially able to be taken up. In OECD countries (unweighted), the average female labor force of all ages as a proportion of the female population aged 15–64 is reported to have risen from 41 percent in 1950 to an estimated 51 percent now. The equivalent male proportions were above 95 percent in the 1950s, dropping to 85 percent in 1985. The Scandinavian countries show female labor force participation of around 70–75 percent, which even if close to an upper bound under low-fertility conditions suggests the scope for increases in other countries.[2] (See OECD, 1979: 110–111.)

Migration is in some ways a more straightforward offset to the labor force trends—in both size and age—implied by low fertility (and does not have a theoretical upper bound or the unclear welfare connotations of very high participation rates in the existing population), although here also labor demand is not alone in governing the process. Pure labor response is approximated in *gastarbeiter* programs and, in the US case, for those categories of

TABLE 1 Estimates and projections of population in the age group 20–24 in selected countries, 1960–2010 (indices, 1985 = 100)

Country	1960	1970	1980	1985	1990	2000	2010
France	67	96	99	100	97	86	87
West Germany	92	72	90	100	93	56	61
Italy	89	90	90	100	99	72	79
United Kingdom	75	94	90	100	97	73	78
United States	52	81	101	100	87	80	93

SOURCE: UN 1984 assessment, medium variant (United Nations, 1985).

migration for which Labor Department certification is needed. It is also reflected in much illegal migration into the United States and other Western countries, in that efforts to stem this flow are in part inversely proportional to labor demand in the industries most affected. Economic interests are not uniformly served by immigrant labor, however, even if the evidence on balance suggests a positive economy-wide impact (see Simon, 1984). An overall gain to the economy does not mean that no one suffers: some workers clearly are exposed to greater labor market competition and downward pressure on wages, the other side of the positive effect on returns to capital that accounts for the strength of domestic pro-migration interests. Political alignments respond accordingly. Perceptions that migrants usurp jobs otherwise available to native workers or hold down wage levels readily translate into populist political rhetoric. The perceived costs of cultural assimilation or of shifts in ethnic balance in plural societies also raise political opposition to large-scale migration.

The literal demographic replacement of work-hours lost in a contracting labor force–aged population covers only a subset of the possible supply-side responses that would tend to maintain economic growth. Technological adjustment through changing factor proportions or induced innovation, and other means by which labor productivity is raised, are probably more familiar kinds of response. These I will come back to shortly. Such further dimensions of flexibility would give additional grounds for discounting the labor-input effects of below-replacement fertility.

An exception sometimes made to such a conclusion is that fluctuations in fertility can indeed be economically disruptive and may be pronounced under long-run low-fertility conditions. Fairly sharp fluctuations have been an evident part of the empirical record in recent decades, although generally demographic transition is thought to have lowered vital rate variance over time. Some current theorizing posits links between fertility and the business cycle, or predicts generational waves in the birth rate. A perhaps equally likely possibility is that contemporary Western society is peculiarly subject to cultural fads, to switches in behavior in response to the tides of popular culture, and that fertility, notwithstanding economists' calculation of the heavy financial burden of children on parents, may not be sufficiently "serious" behavior to be insulated from such forces. A simple shift in the relative frequencies of one-, two-, and three-child families requires only modest behavioral change in a society, and the relevant indifference curves may be nearly flat over the change—and yet the aggregate outcome, channeled by "general currents of opinion" (Bourgeois-Pichat, 1976: 86), can be demographically substantial.

The economic effects of fertility fluctuations, sans policy response, are manifold. In postwar Britain, John Ermisch (1983: 309) writes, "fertility waves . . . have reverberated through the age distribution over time producing repercussions for education, labour force entry, unemployment, the relative earnings of different age groups, housing demand, social services provision and the state pension system." In most such cases, however, institutional adjustments could be envisaged that would have gone far to remedy the resulting problems. Where adjustments were neglected, it was not for want of lead time.

Technology and innovation

More people, goes a well-known argument, mean more geniuses. The link was suggested by Simon Kuznets (1960: 328) and is averred by Julian Simon (1981: 197, 210). Singapore's leaders have helpfully quantified it: one genius per five million people, though for them it unhappily translates to one-half a genius per generation. A parallel strand of argument posits population growth as a force inducing technological advance. Assertion of this possibility by Albert Hirschman (1958: 176–182), based in part on the elaborate marshaling of argument and evidence by Eugène Dupréel (1928), supplemented by some later practitioners of the new institutional economics, produces an eclectic amalgam of supporting material.

In only slightly caricatured form, this summary captures much of the writing on the connections between population size and growth and technological change. While the motivating interest has been chiefly the benefits and costs of moderating population growth in poor countries, the argument could readily extend to the present case. Below-replacement fertility, in other words, might on these grounds be expected to have adverse effects on innovation.

In looking to the sources of technological change in self-aware modern times, such relationships, whatever their historical validity, cannot be seriously entertained. Scale economies in research are not trivial, but the genius-in-numbers argument is dwarfed by selectivity effects and by the social organization of research and development. America's scientific prowess probably benefited as much from the numerically small migration of European refugee scientists in the 1930s and 1940s as from years of natural increase, and from the structure of its tertiary education system more than from either. Hong Kong and Taiwan gained crucial economic advantage from the entrepreneurial cream of China's pre-1949 private sector and created a business climate and infrastructure in which they could thrive. For many countries an obvious strategy to ensure the intellectual base for productivity growth is to tap the rest of the world for brains. (This is often a simpler matter than ensuring the best development and use of indigenous talent; in turn, improvements in the latter process are more obviously within a government's competence than engineering a higher rate of natural increase.) In a world in which multinational companies play a significant role in research and development and in which both states and corporations engage in the acquisition of foreign technological know-how, such selectivity need not even entail migration.

That there are technological effects of population growth, mediated through factor prices, is not in question: a labor shortage can elicit shifts to more capital-intensive production methods. The pace and direction of innovation generated by demographic change are harder to identify. In one sense, such is the capaciousness of the typical argument on the matter, low fertility could be as much a "challenge" to an economic system as high fertility, yielding a similarly positive productivity response, although the youthfulness, embodied skills, and receptivity to change that are invoked in the high-fertility case would be less significant. (Japan and West Germany, with total fertility rates of 1.7 and 1.3, are showing little evidence of technological decrepitude.) The theory of induced innovation provides more formal grounds for predicting a response. According to it, a higher wage–rent ratio resulting from low fertility should lead to labor-saving innovation. In its Hicksian variant, however, this theory has been criticized on the grounds that rising labor costs encourage entrepreneurs to search for any cost reductions, not necessarily labor-saving ones. More telling difficulties relate to what Nathan Rosenberg (1976: 111–112) terms the "compulsive sequences" of technological innovation. "Complex technologies," he writes, "create internal compulsions and pressures which, in turn, initiate exploratory activity in particular directions." The subject is elegantly developed by Brian Arthur (1985).

The emphasis on simple labor force numbers or other straightforward input indices gives rise to another kind of objection. In making for factor substitution or labor-saving technological change, these measures may have little direct bearing on effective labor costs. Much more important are likely to be skill levels and the less tangible aspects of labor quality: worker morale, nature of the instilled "work culture" (discipline, timeliness, flexibility, etc.), problems of recalcitrance and supervision—all the current issues in the debate on US productivity vis-à-vis Japan and the Asian newly industrializing countries.[3] Low fertility would not be a neutral factor here if it accentuated economic "sclerosis" in the sense of Mancur Olson (1982) or Alfred Sauvy (1978: 91); while this is not altogether implausible—see Dupréel (1928: 150–171) for ammunition for such a case—the contemporary evidence is I think slight, and the tendency to draw insights from this biological metaphor should probably be resisted.

In thinking about technology and productivity, one commonly has in mind machines—belts and cog wheels succeeded by computer chips, applied to produce more and better goods per man-hour. Yet as employment in services proliferates in mature economies, more and more of the workforce have jobs for which productivity is a social and accounting convention rather than a material fact. By no means all services are of this nature; on the other hand, there are numerous occupations in other industrial classifications where labor productivity is as arbitrarily measured (say, by remuneration or by the value of complementary inputs). An enlightening discussion of the fallacy of regarding the statistical aggregate of national product as a "production fund," notionally redistributable, is contained in Giffen (1979 [1885]: 338–340). Expensive services, for example much of the output of the professional occupations, are mostly exchanged among the better-off in a society: "such exchanges, counting very largely in the aggregate, go to swell the total [national income]; but to some extent the whole thing is merely nominal—it pleases those concerned to count them for so much, and that is all." The basis for the measurement of service productivity in any nonarbitrary sense is quite fragile, entailing an increasing amount of cantilevering from the well-grounded image of a factory-based economy equipped with capital, K.

Investment and consumer demand

A good deal of attention to economic consequences of declining population in the 1920s and 1930s was focused on demand effects. Keynes's 1937 Galton lecture, W. B. Reddaway's *Economics of a Declining Population* (1939), and Alvin Hansen's 1941 book on fiscal policies each stressed the problem of deficient investment. (See Serow, 1975, for a brief survey of the pre–World War II literature.) This concern is almost totally absent in more recent writings on economic consequences. After decades of relatively fast economic growth, capital deepening rather than capital widening is seen as the major process of accumulation in developed countries, with investment demand thus little dependent on demographic change. Moreover, the massive expansion of trade in the postwar world has lifted many restrictions based on the size of the domestic market. It can even be argued that income growth and hence increase in aggregate demand will be faster under lower fertility (this was the position of the US Commission on Population), making the dependency an inverse one. For the United States, Larry Neal (1978: 103–104) allows a negative effect of fertility decline on investment but one without major net consequences: "Neither in the short run of the next 2 or 3 years nor in the long run of 20 to 30 years . . . is it likely that the adverse effects of declining population growth upon investment demand will also lower the rate of growth of per capita income."

There are, of course, changes in the composition of consumer demand tied to population aging. The most often noted are substitutions among consumption goods—inane illustrations abound, of the sort: fewer prams, more bath chairs—that are likely to be trivial above the level of the firm.[4] But there are nontrivial consumption changes also. The most important is probably the increase in demand for health services. The demographic link here is both direct (the private demand of the increased numbers of elderly in the population) and indirect (through the public demand for health services as amplified by the growing political power of the elderly). Services directed at the young—schooling and child welfare services, for example—correspondingly suffer, perhaps disproportionately so. (See Preston, 1984 on the distributional issues in this area. Some of them I refer to below.)

A more general prospective shift in consumer demand, but one in which income growth and demographic change are tightly intertwined, is a gradual rise in demand for services at the expense of commodities in the consumption basket. Engel's Law–type satiation has not proven much of a limit on the demand for goods, given their pace of qualitative change and the offsetting process in which some services are replaced by goods (for instance, cinemas by video cassette players). Even Herman Kahn (1979: 142), however, was prepared to concede that one of the "main limits on economic growth will be caused by decreasing marginal utility for more production per capita."

The general conclusion that I believe comes from this cursory review is that, insofar as these factors are concerned, low fertility, even somewhat below replacement level, presents no great difficulty for a modern economy. Its effects are likely small compared with business-cycle fluctuations in economic performance, and reasonable flexibility in adjustments to complementary factor inputs and technology and in fiscal management should enable continuation of a satisfactory pace of economic growth, both aggregate and, a fortiori, per capita. Radical diminution of population, like radical growth in population, would presumably raise a host of problems that would alter this complacency, but that scenario is not under scrutiny here. (The West German case may nearly qualify for this exception: see, for example, Chesnais, 1981.) The counterfactual against which such a comparison is made—what would have happened to the economy had fertility not declined?—is necessarily hazy, in that fertility is in some measure a response to the same forces that influence economic performance and in some measure too a response to that performance. Nevertheless, for the range of factors considered the conclusion seems fairly robust.

Those factors, however, are only part of the picture. In particular, I have paid little attention to the likelihood that a low-fertility trajectory will have marked effect on the distribution of income and assets (including human capital) in a population and may alter the pattern of relationships between the society experiencing it and the rest of the world. Both of these classes of effect are important in reaching a fuller judgment on economic consequences.

Distributional implications

Even in elementary demographic terms a population is not a simple concept. It is in some respects a collection of atomistic individuals, in others a grouping of family units; for some purposes, a succession of cross-sectional snapshots of age and family distributions, for others an intricate mesh of overlapping individual and family life cycles played out over time. These possibilities (one could add many others) in combination yield several different ways of apprehending the same reality, each giving a distinct picture and interpretation of the distributional effects of low fertility. A bent toward the individual or toward the family as the basic unit of society, a choice on which the US tax code, for example, is perennially ambivalent, and a particular stance on entitlements tied to birth or life cycle attributes may make one or other of these facets salient. Two are of particular interest for the present topic: the atomistic/cross-sectional and the family/life cycle.

In an atomistic, cross-sectional view of population, low fertility shows up as an age-structure characteristic—the fact, for example, that a stable

("West" model, 75-year life expectancy) population has the following sequence of age patterns under successively lower fertility levels (in percent):

	0–14	15–44	45–64	65+	Total
TFR = 2.1	20	38	25	17	100
TFR = 1.9	18	37	26	19	100
TFR = 1.6	14	34	28	24	100

A population declining by one percent per year, as in the last of these cases, and as projected for West Germany and Switzerland by 2025 in the current United Nations low-variant projections, has no greater total dependency burden by the conventional definition in comparison to replacement fertility, but a 50 percent greater proportion at old ages.

Seen in this way, the main distributional problem is that of ensuring transfers from producers to consumers at each point in time; the simplest device to solve it in this family-less society is by direct transfers for the old—an unfunded (pay-as-you-go) pension scheme—and by tacitly assuming that children are in effect consumption items for their parents and thus need not appear in their own right in the calculation. (Familiar consumption values of children to their parents include contributions to parental self-esteem, fulfillment of the ideal of family continuity, and parental expectations of emotional support in old age.) As fertility declines, the drop in child dependency is thus no public gain, but the rise in old-age dependency puts a growing burden on the pension program. US Social Security is an obvious case in point. President Carter's Budget Message for 1980 contained the calculation that maintenance of the ratio of retirement benefits to average wages (assuming that budgeted expenditures for other purposes remained a constant share of gross national product) implied that the total US tax burden would rise from 33 percent of GNP in 1980 to almost 50 percent by 2030. (See "Long-range effects," 1979.)

Other prospective shifts in transfers would go in the opposite direction—benefiting younger age groups. In the United States, the chief among these, emphasized by Laurence Kotlikoff (1985), is the trend toward increased reliance on consumption taxes instead of income taxes in the future—giving potentially large benefits to net savers (working-age adults) at the cost of net dissavers (the old). But there are many other mechanisms of redistribution also in play.[5] "Considering the impact of Social Security holding all other redistributive policies constant is instructive for understanding the consequences of net changes in government intergenerational redistribution, but it is surely a rather implausible counterfactual exercise" (ibid., p. 490). More plausible would be to assume that the polity on balance favors a more or less unequal distribution of consumption and can employ a variety of means to bring it about.

A different distributional problem generated by low fertility in this population model is the slowing of upward mobility, a point discussed by Nathan Keyfitz (1982: 65) and Brian Arthur (1983). But while a population pyramid with a contracting base may describe the aggregate societal age distribution, there is no a priori reason for organizational groupings within the population to mimic this pyramid. Moreover, countervailing Easterlinian effects—benefits accruing to small age groups by virtue of their size—may also be present.

Retaining an atomistic view of population but giving its members a life cycle draws attention to the lifetime profiles of earnings and consumption, and to the disposal of private assets at or before the death of the owner. The formal life-cycle analysis of the relationships between population and economic growth mostly fits here—in particular, studies of intergenerational transfers (e.g., Arthur and McNicoll, 1978). Solow-type neoclassical models, however, are ill-suited to tracing effects of below-replacement fertility. Reduced ad absurdum, an economy could have a population that is exponentially vanishing while enjoying surging consumption per capita down to the last caput. Without more institutional meat, the important distributional issues elude us.

Introducing a family structure to the population, even ignoring its life-cycle dimension, is a major advance toward institutional realism. Cross-sectional data on family arrangements can be highly misleading, however, because of the radical shifts in such arrangements that families experience over their existence. An apparent stability of income distribution across families can disguise a rapid turnover in the individual families falling in any particular economic category. This indeed has been one of the principal findings of the elaborate Michigan Panel Study of Income Dynamics (see Duncan, 1984: 10). The high rates of marital instability and illegitimate births, the proliferation of unconventional living arrangements, and the increase in single-person households all but defeat simple summary descriptions of family organization in postindustrial societies. (See Le Bras, 1979, for heroic grapplings with OECD family statistics.)

Some progress can be made toward identifying fertility-related distributional effects among families by classifying women by completed parity, disregarding other demographic details of family life. A fertility decline can be characterized by its particular pattern of change in the distribution of women by completed parity. (For fertility declines among younger women, this pattern cannot be conclusively read for another 15–20 years.) Some relevant data from the US Current Population Survey are set out in Table 2. Fertility in the United States has been changing predominantly through a drop in completed parities of 3 or above and concentration at parity 2.

A long-run total fertility rate of 1.6, as in the low variant of the official US projections cited earlier, would imply some breakthrough in this pattern toward greater prevalence of one-child families and childlessness. That this is not unprecedented in the United States is seen by the fertility experience of the cohort of women born in 1910–14, whose peak childbearing coincided with the Depression years. More women of this cohort had zero or one child than had more than two children. The 19 percent projected proportion childless in the 1951–55 birth cohort, shown in the last line of Table 2, suggests a return to Depression-era levels, but with fertility likely to be further diminished by the more truncated parity distributions of today.

TABLE 2 Distribution of women aged 35–39 by number of children ever born, selected years 1950–84, and estimated proportion of women aged 25–29 in 1980 who will remain childless: United States (in percent)

Year of survey	Year of birth	Number of children					Total
		0	1	2	3	4+	
		Women aged 35–39 by children ever born					
1950[a]	1910–14	26	19	23	14	18	100
1960[a]	1920–25	16	14	25	20	25	100
1972[a]	1932–36	12	8	23	24	33	100
1984	1944–48	15	16	35	21	13	100
		Women aged 25–29 by projected lifetime births[b]					
1980	1951–55	19		81			100

[a] Assuming respondents declaring themselves "never-married" to be childless.
[b] Estimated from Coale–McNeil marriage model fitted to CPS data.
SOURCES: Current Population Reports, Series P-20, No. 147 (Table 1), No. 248 (Table 12), No. 401 (Table 1); and (last row) Bloom and Trussell (1984: Table 1).

Instances of possible futures for parity distributions under differing levels of childlessness are the two given below. The first is the 1925–30 West German birth cohort with total fertility 1.9 (Le Bras, 1979: 44), the second a hypothetical distribution with total fertility 1.4 posited by Hervé Le Bras and Georges Tapinos (1979) based on more recent German experience (in percent):

	0	1	2	3	4+	Total
TFR = 1.9	13	28	30	16	13	100
TFR = 1.4	26	31	23	11	9	100

I am not concerned with the factors that might bring about the fertility collapse shown in the second of these situations—with a majority of women having at most one child—but with the economic effects of such patterns. These effects depend on the distributions of families by average socioeconomic status within parity groups, which determine the degree of disjunction between the welfare of families selected by adult members and the welfare of families selected by child members. Arbitrarily, suppose women are divided into those with completed parity 2 or above and those with completed parity 0 or 1—crudely denotable as "breeders" and "nonbreeders." Most children, of course, are born to breeders—some 80 percent of children in the TFR = 1.4 case above. Yet 57 percent of women in that population are nonbreeders. If there are significant differences between the two categories of women in family socioeconomic status over the years of childrearing, as indeed there are likely to be, the fertility pattern may have an important distributional impact.[6]

Family income is one aspect of such status differences, education another. In the United States, Current Population Survey data for 1982 on children ever born to ever-married women aged 35–44 show averages of 2.3 children for those with family income above $25,000, 3.0 for incomes below $15,000. Childlessness among women aged 35–44 of all marital statuses was 18.6

percent for those (about one-third) who had one or more years of college, 9.7 percent for those with high school education or less (US Bureau of the Census, 1984a.) Other relevant contrasts—for example, births to teenagers—could similarly be drawn. The differences are only moderate at present, but the prospect of their becoming larger as low fertility persists is clear.

Cross-sectional data throw only a dim light on this topic, however. To probe further into intergenerational distributional changes calls for a full-blown family/life-cycle view of a population—at the cost of highly intricate data (witness the Occupational Change in a Generation surveys or the Michigan Panel Study) and probably limited scope for formal modeling.[7]

A connection between size of a man's family of origin and his later occupational status was shown for the United States by Peter Blau and Otis Dudley Duncan (1967: 328–330). The idea, of course, has a long prehistory. Education appears as the critical intermediate variable. A large family dilutes the resources available for the education of each child, and thereby, and in interaction with other conditions in the family, limits educational attainments and subsequent occupational success. A two-earner family concentrating its resources on the upbringing of one or two children, the increasingly prevalent modern pattern, has fairly strong assurance of at least perpetuating family status in the next generation. Even in poor family economic circumstances, lower fertility seems associated with better prospects for upward intergenerational mobility. A recent reanalysis of Occupational Change in a Generation data by Judith Blake (1985: 93) concludes: "At least with regard to education, the 'system' appears to have been remarkably open for those coming from small families [1–2 children] and relatively rigid for those coming from large ones."

The broader problems of selectively disadvantaged upbringing add to those of formal education. As Thomas Sowell (1983: 255) writes, "many— perhaps most—of the more fortunate people are recipients of windfall gains that derive from the accident of their being born where they were, if not to immediate affluence, then into families, communities, or nations where the values and patterns of life were a human capital that made economic success more readily attainable." The problems of the reproduction of human capital in this broad but wholly legitimate sense of that term are some of the most important (and sensitive) issues connected with likely patterns of low fertility in modern societies.

Sowell's concern in this regard is with the striking observed differences in economic mobility among certain ethnic and immigrant groups, principally in the United States, and with the tendencies for economic incentives to push fertility below replacement in the most upwardly mobile of them. Reproduction of human capital (in his sense) in the population as a whole thereby suffers. Since divisions according to such groups are often long-lasting and show up in how societies organize themselves socially and economically, between-group fertility differentials may be significant even when within-group fertility variance is considerable.[8]

The picture of the US income distribution by families over time given by the Michigan Panel Study—of families moving into and out of poverty, especially as their composition changes, with few of them remaining long in that state—at first sight looks very different from the "culture of poverty" notion that sees an existing or emerging semipermanent underclass. If the circulation in fact mostly takes place within layers in a society, the contradiction vanishes. The possibility that current patterns of low fertility directly or indirectly accentuate such layering, expanding the absolute or relative numbers of those with little prospect themselves of economic improvement and at the same time damping currents of intergenerational economic mobility, deserves careful scrutiny. Quite aside from the value judgments that may be assigned to particular distributional and mobility outcomes, there are broader implications in that opportunities for economic mobility plausibly contribute to the overall vigor of the economic system.

In Western Europe, where economic mobility is less a proclaimed value than in the United States but economic equality somewhat more of one, the streams of immigrants from now-halted guest-worker programs, (once) relatively free migration from former colonies, and continuing family reunion have created a seemingly permanent ethnic minority—and one in which the variegated economic achievement of immigrants in the US case is replaced by a more uniform picture of disadvantage. Convergence of immigrant fertility toward dominant European patterns is fairly rapid, with greatly narrowed differences in the second generation. Convergence in economic status distribution and in patterns of mobility, where cultural factors and discrimination both play a role, may be much slower.[9]

There is nothing intrinsic about low fertility that would compel these distributional effects. It is conceivable that fertility variance will diminish much further, or that differentials by socioeconomic status will be reversed, or that the institutional means and political will can be found to counter the intergenerational transmission of economic disadvantage. On this last score, however, efforts to remedy the consequences as they stand—to enhance human capital in Sowell's sense—have had a generally poor success record. It matters greatly in judging the economic consequences of low fertility whose fertility (and whose migration) is left.

International contexts of low-fertility societies

An overwhelming reality that confronts and will continue to confront the rich low-fertility countries as a whole is their demographic marginalization. The ratio of the population in the more developed countries (by the UN's definition) to that in the less developed is currently 1:3. Forty years hence, in the medium-variant UN projection (keeping group boundaries fixed), it will be 1:5. For young adult age groups (say, ages 20–40), the equivalent ratios are 1:4 and

1:6 (United Nations, 1985). This matters for the present subject both because demographic trends influence factor price differences among nations and because population weight conveys power or voice in world affairs, or claims of entitlement to such. The implications of low fertility thus need to be assessed against this global backdrop.

The factor price changes that declining fertility may generate over time in a single country exist already and in extreme form across countries. Trade flows, transfers of capital and know-how, and (to some extent) migration are the main resulting processes that make for equalization of returns to factors. International trade in accord with standard criteria of comparative advantage brings downward pressure on wage levels in high-wage participating countries, just like migration. Joseph Grunwald and Kenneth Flamm (1985) examine the effects on a subset of US industries—electrical equipment and electronics, motor vehicles, and apparel—that employ substantial numbers of unskilled workers. For industries such as these they see a steady process of plant relocation overseas. "[T]he continued displacement of the unskilled [in manufacturing] will mean the end of their relatively high income in Western industrial societies" (p. 224). Grunwald and Flamm conclude, however, in the conventional antiprotectionist vein: that there are nevertheless compelling reasons in favor of the process. "Apart from the clear advantages of a prosperous and stable world system, US consumers benefit from lower costs of a growing volume of traded goods, US producers benefit from broader markets for their products, and US workers benefit from reduced foreign immigration" (pp. 237–238).[10]

A problem with this reasoning is its assumption that rich economies can progressively move up a technological gradient toward ever more sophisticated and capital-intensive products, as lower-productivity lines are taken over by newcomers. With such a progression, low fertility would indeed seem little hindrance to a nation in maintaining rank among its trading partners and its place in the international income hierarchy. But nearly all economies have a wide range of technological levels and labor skills, and limited scope for concentrating merely on the upper end. Productivity levels at that upper end may be so high as to make it contribute little directly to employment under realistic size constraints on the market. Elsewhere in the economy, the "natural" protection thought to be enjoyed by many labor-intensive activities, principally in the service categories, may be in significant part illusory. Moreover, efforts to adjust to a continually shifting international division of labor are politically costly—as Paul Demeny (1983: 35–36) remarks: "The compelling global economic logic supporting free trade and free capital movements notwithstanding, there is no reason to expect the exercise of national sovereignty in deciding about the desirable speed of structural transformation to be abdicated by countries of the North in deference to the aggregate reproductive decisions of couples in countries of the South." Protectionist pressures in US industry will not vanish with devaluation of the dollar.[11]

The populist appeal of opposition to low-wage competition from the labor-surplus South is clear. Other things equal, it would probably dominate developed-country debate on international economic relations and lead to further restraint on manufactured imports from less developed countries—especially as the populous low-wage nations (India and China, most notably) seek a footing on the trade and technology ladder previously ascended by the newly industrialized countries. Technological changes under way or in prospect may undercut this debate, however, though not to the advantage of low-wage countries. These changes are the progressive introduction of computer-aided manufacturing and its various analogues in the white-collar occupations.[12] Job losses ascribable to this process could come to rival those of "deindustrialization," although to some degree offset by relocation of manufacturing back to the rich countries. (Low-wage nations may find it difficult to resist the same labor-displacing technological trends, even, for many of them for several decades more, in the face of growing rather than diminishing cohorts of labor force entrants.)

Sheer demographic weight is the second area where possible international ramifications exist. While the pace of Third World fertility decline will have the dominant influence on the developed countries' share of world population, especially when international migration is taken into account, the effect of fertility levels in the developed countries themselves on this share is by no means negligible. Whether population weights will gain in significance—whether the populous, so to speak, will inherit the earth—depends heavily, however, on whether the current technological (and related military) dominance of today's developed countries persists.

The likelihood in most cases that it can seems fairly high. The advantages the rich nations enjoy in terms of educational institutions and traditions, research facilities, and amenities of life will make competition exceedingly difficult. Immigration of technological and entrepreneurial talent will continue—countering the increasing entropy of international wage-leveling (to draw an analogy from thermodynamics) by something akin to Maxwell's Demon. The United States and to a lesser degree Japan also benefit from the positive externalities generated by the sheer scale of their expenditures on research and development—gains that are motivating the hesitant but evolving technological collaboration of the EEC nations. It is possible for poorer countries to promote high-technology enclaves within which privileged workers are insulated from less fortunate compatriots—take, for example, nuclear physics in India or China, or perhaps the entire defense industry and its associated research establishment in the Soviet Union—but this option hardly makes for economy-wide strength. While second-tier technological success through skillful adaptation of existing knowledge—licensed or not—combined with high-quality engineering can continue, leading to affluence for some nations, the present easy access to this route may well be eroded by the new production technologies mentioned above. Japan's own rapid and largely unforeseen movement to the technological frontier over 1950–70 should, however, give pause to any cavalier dismissal of such possibilities elsewhere, remote as they might presently seem.

One major caveat should be entered in this guarded projection of the technological status quo. The present international system is one in which demographic weights play little part. As more large nations acquire the technological level (civilian and military) to be regarded as "modern" in at least a significant enclave of their economy, it is hard to imagine there not being substantial adjustments in that system. The rules of the game now governing international trade and finance cannot be projected forward as givens. A "new international economic order" is of course not likely to resemble the models popular in UN forums in the 1970s, but it may equally differ from today's order. If demographic marginalization is accompanied by diminished political and cultural influence in world affairs, as could readily be imagined, technological prominence may count for less. Analogies of such circumstances that might be culled from high-technology but demographically dwarfed nations or ruling minorities in the contemporary world are not happy ones.

I have discussed the international context of low-fertility societies from the standpoint of those societies qua nations. There are of course other standpoints. Take, for example, that of the utopian liberal in one of the rich nations who does not see liberalism halting at national boundaries. Unfortunately, it is not easy to envisage alternative institutional arrangements to national governments in ordering a global economy. One reason that efforts to do so seem highly unreal is the difficulty with the demographic dimension—the inherent anarchy of reproductive decisions and hence the potential role for a territorially defined entity, the functional equivalent of a national government, in attempting to reconcile individual and social demographic interests when these appear to diverge.[13]

The standpoint of a more distanced observer of global developments in this century could also be imagined. Such an observer might well express regret (if not stronger distaste) at the needless multiplication of humanity at the expense of the natural world and its nonhuman inhabitants and perhaps at the expense also of more considered design of social organization. And he might, with William McNeill (1984), see resonances in the present of the experience of Europe's high civilization of the Middle Ages—a period that witnessed "a swarming of population": massive sporadic flows from the steppe hinterlands that could be seen both as successive nomadic conquests and as the recruitment needed "to sustain human skills and numbers." "Die-off at the center (or at least a rate of reproduction inadequate to fill all available jobs) and recruitment from ethnically diverse peripheries again prevail in post-1950 Europe and America. Consequently, polyethnic lamination—clustering different groups in particular occupations and arranging them in a more or less formal hierarchy of dignity and wealth—is again asserting itself . . ." (pp. 17–18).

No essay of this length can do much more than touch on selected issues in a subject as complex and elusive as this. Moreover, judgments on what are major and what minor effects of low fertility depend on one's time horizon, on where and how far a society is thought to be able to adjust, whether through natural resiliency or by deliberate policy, and on what length of collective memory and stability of values is needed for continuity of a society's identity. In my comments above I set out by agreeing with what I judge to be a loose consensus among economists writing on the subject in recent years that adjustments to an older labor force, altered factor prices, and shifts in consumer demand need not be economically damaging. Social security problems generated by population aging are indeed widely recognized to be highly important; but they are properly seen as an aspect of an intricate mesh of distributional relationships—some involving age categories, others family units, still others socioeconomic and ethnic groups—that are part of the fabric societies must weave in attempting to reconcile their often-conflicting goals of solidarity and economic growth, and their conceptions of entitlement and equity. I have also stressed the likely changes in international economic relationships in a world in which the group of industrialized low-fertility countries is fast becoming demographically insignificant, but in which the technological and human capital differentials that might make this fact of little importance cannot be presumed permanent.[14]

The broad themes I have used are those of distribution and selectivity: distribution across time, across social strata and other groupings, and across states; selectivity in recruitment to national elites, to middle class well-being, to citizenship in the affluent, low-fertility world. The social processes thus defined are modified by new patterns of fertility both directly and through the responses of government. The resulting economic effects of low fertility depend in large measure on the combinations in which and the degree to which those processes are changed. While I have not sought to make a case for government intervention to raise fertility, certainly not in situations (as in the United States) where completed parity has barely dipped below replacement, I see no reason to doubt that the fertility-related issues discussed in this essay will increasingly require deliberation and policy attention.

Notes

Comments on an earlier draft of this paper by W. Brian Arthur, Jean-Claude Chesnais, Thomas J. Espenshade, Allen C. Kelley, Georges Tapinos, and Michael P. Todaro are acknowledged.

1 Notable sources of such studies are the proceedings of five conferences held during the past decade: the Council of Europe's 1976 Strasbourg conference on the Implications of a Stationary or Declining Population in Europe (Council of Europe, 1978); the joint US National Institutes of Health–World Health Organization 1977 conference on Social, Economic and Health Aspects of Low Fertility (Campbell, 1980); a second NIH-sponsored meeting in 1977 titled The Economic Consequences of Slowing Population Growth (Espenshade and Serow, 1978); the Third European Population Seminar in Belgrade in 1978 (Macura, 1979); and the Conference on Population Economics held in Paderborn, West Germany in 1983 (Steinmann, 1984). For surveys of recent scholarship bearing on the subject see Espenshade (1978b) and relevant sections of Clark, Kreps, and Spengler (1978). The research reports of the 1972 US Population Commission touched on consequences issues

but did not delve into the then quite unexpected situation of below-replacement fertility (see Morss and Reed, 1972).

2 Cf. Davis and van den Oever (1981: 8): "There must be a level of childbearing below which people will not go, and this point may be high enough to give women a childbearing and child-rearing role sufficient to keep them from ever equaling male labor force participation in middle adult ages. Also, the same forces that are pushing men out of the labor force are likely soon to affect women as well."

3 In a different comparison, Morawetz (1980) emphasizes many such factors in accounting for why Colombia cannot compete with Hong Kong in clothing manufacture despite Colombia's significant wage cost advantages.

4 And hard to pin down empirically, even using detailed categories of household consumption expenditure, given the confounding and offsetting effects of higher per capita income and changing household size. "The goods and services which an older society would acquire relatively more of are largely those of which a wealthier society would purchase relatively less, and vice versa"—Espenshade (1978a: 158). See also Serow (1984: 175–176).

5 Inflation is one such mechanism, resolving competing claims of wage earners, pensioners, and rentiers to national product by eroding the value of claims that are expressed in nominal terms or less than fully indexed. Colin Clark (1977: 257) quotes Alfred Sauvy's description of inflation as "a revolt of the younger and more active elements in the population against having too large a part of their product taken away from them. . . ."

6 For an illuminating quantitative study of this issue in the United States, see Preston (1976). For a group of women with completed childbearing whose distribution by children ever born, x, is $f(x)$, and ignoring mortality, Preston derives the relationship between the average number of children ever born, $\bar{x}$, and the average completed family size (in terms of number of children) in which a child finds itself, $\bar{c}$: $\bar{c} = \bar{x} + \text{var}(x)/\bar{x}$. The two parity distributions given in the text yield the following rough estimates:

	$\bar{x}$	var$(x)/\bar{x}$	$\bar{c}$
TFR = 1.9	1.9	1.1	3.0
TFR = 1.4	1.4	1.4	2.8

In the latter case, for example, a woman on average has 1.4 children, while a child on average comes from a family with 2.8 children.

7 Among the few instances of formal modeling I am aware of is a study by Straub and Wenig (1984) that explores analytically one aspect of the problem posed here.

8 The magnitude of effects of between-group fertility differentials can be illustrated by black–white projections in the United States. In 1980, 14 percent of the population but 20 percent of births were "nonwhite" (predominantly black); under the Census Bureau's middle-fertility/middle-migration assumption, by 2030 these proportions will have risen to 20 and 25 percent (US Bureau of the Census, 1984b).

9 In Western Europe some 7–10 percent of the population in most countries (over 4 million each in France, West Germany, and the United Kingdom) live in households with a foreign-nationality head (Castles and Kosack, 1985: 490). Evidence for a European melting pot is thus far scant: Castles and Kosack (1985: 505) comment: "Liberal views on assimilation and individual integration, current in the sixties and early seventies, have not stood the test of time. As the migrant workers have become settlers, and established new communities, the division between them and the rest of the population has not grown less. Racism and discrimination have prevented this, but so have the wishes of the minorities for cultural and ethnic identity."

10 The same interlinked trends can of course be described in very different ways: for Butz et al. (1982), low US fertility yields a tight labor market and increased immigration, the latter including low-skill labor that "may be all that is keeping some industries from going out of business or moving overseas" (p. 26).

11 See also Demeny (1985). The demographic case against free trade is put strongly, indeed stridently, by Culbertson (1984, 1985). He argues that defenders of free trade ignore

the prospect of a deteriorating trade balance for the North in North–South trade and thus promote a policy that in effect tends to make the world a "population commune"—as much as if they were advocating free migration. Economic integration through free trade "brings into play an evolutionary structure in which no region can effectively defend its standard of living by limiting its own population" (1985: 35). (In the blandly apolitical world of many trade theorists, the rich could of course become rentiers, living off Third World investments.)

12 On the prospects for retrenchment in management and services as well as among production workers as expert systems and other computer applications become more widespread, see the review article by Draper (1985).

13 A somewhat bizarre libertarian utopia, peopled by telecommuters living where they please, is that sketched out by *The Economist*'s Deputy Editor, Norman Macrae (1984). In it the withering of national governments is as complete as Marx could ever have hoped. The social limits to growth of the sort depicted by Hirsch (1976)—the constraints inherent in the hierarchies that emerge in virtually all societies in the course of competition for truly limited resources such as power and prestige—are notably absent in the description, although perhaps they are implicit in Macrae's faith that the amenities he values (such as an unspoiled Tahiti) will be preserved in 2024.

14 On one topic that is often found in writings on fertility decline, especially in the French literature, I have said little: the possible negative effects of low fertility on "optimism," on "ethos," on the cultural milieu that may make the difference between dynamic and lackluster economic performance. Adam Smith and Keynes both gave credence to such a connection. Dupréel (1928) wrote subtly and at length on it. Sauvy (1978) accords it importance. The distributional issues that I have discussed are probably implicated in any such association. For example, the "British disease"—Britain's long, steady course of relative economic decline—is often traced to class rigidities and a class-based value system. Might not some different array of rigidities give rise to a "Japanese disease" in the future? The United States, still relatively open to migration from all sides but willing more than most to struggle against social barriers, would seem to be as well positioned as any nation to elude such an outcome.

References

Arthur, W. Brian. 1983. "Age and earnings in the labour market: Implications of the 1980s labour bulge," in Paul Streeten and Harry Maier (eds.), *Human Resources, Employment and Development*, vol. 2. London: Macmillan.
———. 1985. "Competing technologies and lock-in by historical small events: The dynamics of allocation under increasing returns," CEPR Publication No. 43, Center for Economic Policy Research, Stanford University.
———, and Geoffrey McNicoll. 1978. "Samuelson, population and intergenerational transfers," *International Economic Review* 19: 241–246.
Blake, Judith. 1985. "Number of siblings and educational mobility," *American Sociological Review* 50: 84–94.
Blau, Peter M., and Otis Dudley Duncan. 1967. *The American Occupational Structure*. New York: Wiley.
Bloom, David E., and James Trussell. 1984. "What are the determinants of delayed childbearing and permanent childlessness in the United States?" *Demography* 21: 591–611.
Bourgeois-Pichat, Jean. 1976. "The economic and social implications of demographic trends in Europe up to and beyond 2000," *Population Bulletin of the United Nations*, No. 8, pp. 34–88.
———. 1981. "Recent demographic change in Western Europe: An assessment," *Population and Development Review* 7: 19–42.
Butz, William P., et al. 1982. *Demographic Challenges in America's Future*. Santa Monica, Calif.: Rand Corporation (Rand report R-2911).

Campbell, Arthur A. (ed.). 1980. *Social, Economic and Health Aspects of Low Fertility*. Washington, D.C.: National Institutes of Health. (NIH Publication No. 80-100).

Castles, Stephen, and Godula Kosack. 1985. *Immigrant Workers and Class Structure in Western Europe*. Oxford: Oxford University Press, 2nd edition.

Chesnais, Jean-Claude. 1981. "Le modèle économique de l'Allemagne fédérale est-il compatible avec son modèle démographique?" *Revue d'Economie Politique* 91, no. 2: 163–177.

Clark, Colin. 1977. *Population Growth and Land Use*. London: Macmillan, 2nd edition.

Clark, Robert, Juanita Kreps, and Joseph Spengler. 1978. "Economics of aging: A survey," *Journal of Economic Literature* 16: 919–962.

Council of Europe. 1978. *Population Decline in Europe: Implications of a Declining or Stationary Population*. London: Arnold.

Culbertson, John M. 1984. *International Trade and the Future of the West*. Madison, Wis.: 21st Century Press.

———. 1985. *The Dangers of "Free Trade."* Madison, Wis.: 21st Century Press.

Davis, Kingsley, and Pietronella van den Oever. 1981. "Age relations and public policy in advanced industrial societies," *Population and Development Review* 7: 1–18.

Demeny, Paul. 1983. "International development and population policy," paper presented at the Harvard-Draeger Conference on Population Interactions between Poor and Rich Countries, Cambridge, Mass.

———. 1985. "A note on world population growth and protectionism in international trade," *Zeitschrift für Bevölkerungswissenschaft* 11, no. 2: 141–146.

Draper, Roger. 1985. "The golden arm," *New York Review of Books*, 24 October.

Duncan, Greg J. 1984. *Years of Poverty, Years of Plenty: The Changing Economic Fortunes of American Workers and Families*. Ann Arbor, Mich.: Institute for Social Research, University of Michigan.

Dupréel, Eugène Gustave. 1928. "Population et progrès: essai sur les conséquences des variation démographiques," in his *Deux Essais sur le Progrès*. Brussells: Maurice Lamertin.

Ermisch, John. 1983. *The Political Economy of Demographic Change: Causes and Implications of Population Trends in Great Britain*. London: Heinemann.

Espenshade, Thomas J. 1978a. "How a trend towards a stationary population affects consumer demand," *Population Studies* 32: 147–158.

———. 1978b. "Zero population growth and the economies of developed nations," *Population and Development Review* 4: 645–680.

———, and William J. Serow (eds.). 1978. *The Economic Consequences of Slowing Population Growth*. New York: Academic Press.

Giffen, Robert. 1979 [1885]. "Some general uses of statistical knowledge," reprinted in *Population and Development Review* 5: 319–346.

Grunwald, Joseph, and Kenneth Flamm. 1985. *The Global Factory: Foreign Assembly in International Trade*. Washington, D.C.: The Brookings Institution.

Hansen, Alvin H. 1941. *Fiscal Policy and Business Cycles*. New York: Norton.

Hirsch, Fred. 1976. *Social Limits to Growth*. Cambridge, Mass.: Harvard University Press.

Hirschman, Albert. 1958. *The Strategy of Economic Development*. New Haven: Yale University Press.

Kahn, Herman. 1979. *World Economic Development: 1979 and Beyond*. New York: Morrow.

Keyfitz, Nathan. 1982. *Population Change and Social Policy*. Boston: Abt.

Keynes, John Maynard. 1937. "Some economic consequences of a declining population," *Eugenics Review* 29: 13–17. (Reprinted in *Population and Development Review* 4: 517–523.)

Kotlikoff, Laurence J. 1985. "The distributional impact of social security: A framework for analysis," *International Population Conference, Florence 1985*. Liège: IUSSP. Volume 3.

Kuznets, Simon. 1960. "Population change and aggregate output," in *Demographic and Economic Change in Developed Countries*, a report of the National Bureau of Economic Research. Princeton: Princeton University Press.

Le Bras, Hervé. 1979. *Child and Family: Demographic Developments in the OECD Countries*. Paris: Organization for Economic Co-operation and Development.

———, and Georges Tapinos. 1979. "Perspectives à long terme de la population française et leurs implications économiques," *Population* 34: 1391–1452.

"Long-range effects of population change on the US budget." 1979. *Population and Development Review* 5: 373–377.

Macrae, Norman. 1984. *The 2024 Report: A Concise History of the Future 1974–2024*. London: Sidgwick and Jackson.

Macura, Miloš (ed.). 1979. *The Effect of Current Demographic Change in Europe on Social Structure*, Proceedings of the Third European Population Seminar, Beograd, 1978. Belgrade: Ekonomski Institut.

McNeill, William H. 1984. "Human migration in historical perspective," *Population and Development Review* 10: 1–18.

Mincer, Jacob. 1985. "Intercountry comparisons of labor force trends and of related developments: An overview," *Journal of Labor Economics* 3 (Supplement): S1–S32.

Morawetz, David. 1980. *Why the Emperor's New Clothes Are Not Made in Colombia*. Washington, D.C.: The World Bank (Staff Working Paper No. 368).

Morss, Elliot R., and Ritchie H. Reed (eds.). 1972. *Economic Aspects of Population Change*. Washington, D.C.: US Government Printing Office. (US Commission on Population Growth and the American Future, Research Reports, Vol. 2.)

Neal, Larry. 1978. "Is secular stagnation just around the corner? A survey of the influences of slowing population growth upon investment demand," in Espenshade and Serow (1978), pp. 101–125.

Olson, Mancur. 1982. *The Rise and Decline of Nations: Economic Growth, Stagflation and Social Rigidities*. New Haven: Yale University Press.

Organization for Economic Co-operation and Development. 1979. *Demographic Trends, 1950–1990*. Paris.

Preston, Samuel H. 1976. "Family sizes of children and family sizes of women," *Demography* 13: 105–114.

———. 1984. "Children and the elderly: Divergent paths for America's dependents," *Demography* 21: 435–457.

Reddaway, W. B. 1939. *The Economics of a Declining Population*. London: Allen and Unwin.

Rosenberg, Nathan. 1976. *Perspectives on Technology*. Cambridge: Cambridge University Press.

Sauvy, Alfred. 1978. "De la baisse de la fécondité en Europe occidentale," in Macura (1978), pp. 81–92.

Serow, William J. 1975. "The economics of stationary and declining population: Some views from the first-half of the twentieth century," in Joseph J. Spengler (ed.), *Zero Population Growth: Implications*. Chapel Hill: Carolina Population Center.

———. 1984. "The impact of population changes on consumption," in Steinmann (1984), pp. 168–178.

Simon, Julian L. 1981. *The Ultimate Resource*. Princeton: Princeton University Press.

———. 1984. "Immigrants, taxes, and welfare in the United States," *Population and Development Review* 10: 55–69.

Smith, James P., and Michael P. Ward. 1985. "Time-series growth in the female labor force," *Journal of Labor Economics* 3 (Supplement): S59–S90.

Sowell, Thomas. 1983. *The Economics and Politics of Race: An International Perspective*. New York: Morrow.

Steinmann, Gunter (ed.). 1984. *Economic Consequences of Population Change in Industrialized Countries,* Proceedings of the Conference on Population Economics, Paderborn, West Germany, June 1983. Berlin: Springer-Verlag.

Straub, Martin, and Alois Wenig. 1984. "Human fertility and the distribution of wealth," in Steinmann (1984), pp. 68–86.

United Nations. 1985. "World population prospects: Estimates and projections as assessed in 1984." New York. (Computer tape.)

United States Bureau of the Census. 1984a. *Fertility of American Women: June 1982.* Washington, D.C. (Current Population Reports, Series P-20, No. 387).

———. 1984b. *Projections of the Population of the United States, by Age, Sex, and Race: 1983 to 2080.* Washington, D.C. (Current Population Reports, Series P-25, No. 952.)

United States Commission on Population Growth and the American Future. 1972. *Population and the American Future.* Washington, D.C.: US Government Printing Office.

Wander, Hilde. 1978. "The working population," in Council of Europe (1978), pp. 53–71.

Comment: Ester Boserup

Persistent below-replacement fertility results in diminishing ability to finance infrastructure investment and leads to other disadvantages due to loss of advantages of scale. But these consequences are only significant in the long run or in the case of extremely rapid decline of fertility. Other unfavorable effects of changes in the age composition are felt more rapidly. The changing age composition poses two problems: on the one hand, the declining share of persons below working age and the increasing share of the elderly; on the other hand, the aging of the labor force. Both Geoffrey McNicoll's article in this volume and general public discussion of the problem focus mainly on the first of these problems, but the second one is by no means less serious.

The economic effects of below-replacement fertility vary with the institutional setting. Large variations exist among industrialized countries in the extent to which expenditures in kind and in cash for the young generation, as well as for the old one, are financed by families, by employers, or by general taxation. Some European countries not only provide liberal support of the elderly and all their health care costs but also impose high taxation in support of persons below working age. High-quality education is free for all age groups, with loans and grants for the maintenance of adult students. Subsidies are granted for high-quality daycare institutions for infants and small children, and tax deductions or direct subsidies are provided for all children. In other industrialized countries both child services and free education are of poor quality, so that ambitious parents incur heavy costs in paying for private care and education, and old-age benefits are so low that those who can afford to do so must supplement them by private savings.

If per capita investment in the young generation remains unchanged when fertility descends below replacement level, the shift in age composition will reduce productive investment in the young. But, according to my reading of his article, McNicoll expects that productive investment per child will increase as a result of below-replacement fertility. The improved quality of the labor force will compensate for declining numbers, since in the industrialized countries the quality of the labor force is more important than the quantity. The expectation of increasing the quality of education as a result of below-replacement fertility derives from the theory that the parental burden of educational costs is a main cause of the very low fertility in industrialized countries. It is assumed that to reduce the number of children is a means of improving their quality. This theory does not agree well with the fact that the countries in which parents pay least for the education of their children are the ones with the lowest levels of fertility. Moreover, research on educational levels in one- and two-child families in the United States reveals only marginal differences. Only in large families are educational levels significantly lower (Blake, 1981).

The main cause of the decline in fertility levels below replacement is probably the change in female lifestyle. This in turn has resulted from the decline of household work and greater control over fertility as a result of improved technology. The disadvantages for women of the old lifestyle can be avoided by increasing levels of education and of labor market participation. The extremely low incomes and low status of divorced women who have given priority to childrearing in a traditional family setting are strong inducements for the new generation of women to give lower priority to stable marriages and to rearing of children. These female lifestyle changes are recent, and the ways in which various societies adapt to them will influence future fertility levels, determining whether below-replacement fertility is to be a temporary or a more permanent feature.

Increasing per capita family income by reducing the number of children is more likely to stimulate parental consumption, especially female consumption, than to increase educational expenditure per child or to expand private savings. Historically, economic and social development in the industrialized countries has strongly reduced the motivation for private savings. In Europe, the large majority are wage and salary earners with extensive access to public security schemes, and in the countries with the most comprehensive systems nearly all motivation for private savings has disappeared. Today, establishment of new homes for young people leaving the parental family is not being financed by savings by either the young or their parents, but rather in some countries by credits for building and furnishing homes. New consumer credits are being added in step with the payment of earlier debts. Fewer and fewer members of the young generation are making any attempt to replace payments on debt with private savings.

In contrast to private savings, the relationship between fertility levels and public savings or dissavings is important. Public budgets are already burdened by increasing expenditure due to the longer lifespans of the elderly and the high cost of life-prolonging health expenditure for old people. The decline to below-replacement fertility causes a further acceleration of this trend. In addition to the increase in relative numbers of the elderly, the mounting political pressure from voters who benefit from these public services or who anticipate such benefits in the near future has brought an increase in pension benefits, a reduction in the pensionable age, and easier access to public services for more and more groups of the population. The result is a growing imbalance between rapidly increasing expenditures and declining or less rapidly increasing numbers of people to finance them. In the United States expected future deficits in these services are viewed with alarm, but in parts of Europe with earlier and larger declines of fertility some systems are already in grave financial crisis. Not only demographic experts, but ordinary people are beginning to realize that they have no hope of getting back the money that they are paying in contributions or taxes to finance public services for the elderly.

Indications exist that insecurity regarding the future extent and quality of public services for the elderly is inducing people to attempt to solve their own problems of satisfactory income and health care in old age. They are doing so by increasing rates of private personal savings and insurance. This trend is likely to become stronger, leading to widespread attempts to replace payments to the public system with private insurance, at higher cost but with better and more reliable services. As a result, the political pressure for a high level of public services is weakened, and the shift in public resources in favor of the elderly may be somewhat reduced. On the other hand, it seems less likely that a similar shift toward deterioration of public services and "privatization" of expenditures will take place with respect to the young generation, due partly to official fear of deterioration in the quality of the candidates for high-level education and jobs, and partly to the fear of further fertility decline.

With persistent below-replacement fertility, the problems posed by the aging of the labor force are no less serious than those posed by the age shift in the nonworking population. In some European countries, the increasing share in the labor force of older, less mobile and flexible workers has given rise to retraining schemes for older personnel, thus shifting a share of the training expenditures from younger to older persons, probably with significant loss of productivity gain per person trained. Moreover, an attempt is made to retard the shift in age composition from young to old by offering attractive retirement schemes to persons below pensionable age, which of course further exacerbates the problem of financing payments to the elderly.

In spite of concern for the effects on productivity of an aging labor force, many of the industrialized countries with high unemployment have a heavy concentration of unemployment among the young. As is well known, persons over 40 years of age have difficulty in obtaining new jobs similar in status and pay to the ones they have left. Therefore, employed workers, salaried staff, and trade unions insist on the use of the principle "first-in, last-out" and on avoidance of dismissals by regrouping and retraining of existing staff. The result of this recruitment and dismissal policy is to accelerate the aging of the *employed* labor force even more rapidly than the aging of the labor force in general.

In consequence, more mature workers have considerable job security, but only as long as the enterprise or company survives. The real risk for older workers is that their employer will become uncompetitive and close down. This risk can be reduced or eliminated by protection of the industry against foreign competition, by government subsidization, or by government takeover. Older workers therefore constitute a strong pressure group for government support to outmoded and sluggish enterprises and industries. The older the labor force in an industry or service becomes, the stronger the political pressure for government support. Protection and other subsidization of uncompetitive enterprises already places a large burden on government budgets in industrialized countries, and fertility decline to below-replacement levels will inevitably cause additional distortion of the investment pattern in favor of traditional and old industries. Labor and capital accumulate in these industries, and the financial burden of their subsidization and the distortion of the price structure act as a brake on technological progress and the development of newer, more efficient industries. Labor strikes to prevent the introduction of new technology are more likely the older the labor force and the industry.

The large increases in population size and in the ranks of the young labor force in the developing countries are already creating pressures for adaptation by the international economy, and the decline of fertility to below-replacement level in industrialized countries augments these pressures. There are two means by which the world economy can adapt to large regional differences in fertility and incomes: by movements of labor and of labor-intensive products from the countries with high fertility and low incomes to those with low fertility and high incomes, and by movements of capital and of labor-intensive industries in the opposite direction.

In recent decades the movements of labor and of labor-intensive products from developing to industrialized countries have been large, and the resistance to them in the receiving countries has been growing. With below-replacement fertility in industrialized countries, and continued rapid growth of entrants to the labor market in developing countries, both demand for and resistance to legal and illegal migration of the young working-age groups from the developing countries becomes sharper. The same is the case with demand for and resistance to imports of labor-intensive products.

Where these movements of products and labor from developing to industrialized countries are curtailed, the pressure for adaptation through movements of capital and of labor-intensive industries from the industrialized to the developing countries increases. Already in the nineteenth century, at the early stage of the European demographic transition, capital flows from the countries with the lowest rates of population growth to those with the highest rates played an important role in the national and international economy, with France, Russia, and the United States as spectacular examples. Similarly, the early stages of the demographic transition in the Third World have been accompanied by large capital flows from the industrialized countries with low population growth to a large number of developing countries, which thereby could accelerate their rate of economic growth to very high levels. But increased propensity to consume and mounting government deficits have, in many industrialized countries, pushed up interest rates and curtailed the supply of capital exports. Less capital has become available for rescheduling of debts and new loans.

Today, the increasing difficulty in obtaining international loans provides developing countries with a strong motive to attract direct investments by transfer of enterprises from industrialized countries, with all the means at their disposal. Less and less is being heard of objections to such investments, once voiced out of fear of resulting economic and political dependency. Also, many owners of enterprises in industrialized countries have strong motivation for moving production elsewhere in step with the need for reinvestments, because wage differentials between industrialized and developing countries are larger than productivity differences, where such exist. Intensive competition for shares in the world market leads businesses to set up production where costs are lowest. The tendency, mentioned by Ansley Coale in this volume, for persistent below-replacement fertility to tip wage differentials in industrialized countries in favor of young labor can only reinforce the desire of managers in these countries to locate increasing parts of their production in low-wage countries. Moreover, governments of developed countries are less able to prevent reinvestment in other countries than to curtail immigration and imports.

If below-replacement fertility leads to restrictions on trade and migration, it accelerates the trend toward concentration of production in large multinational companies. These enterprises, less dependent upon national governments, are in a much stronger bargaining position vis-à-vis governments both at home and abroad than are local industries. By legal and illegal means, large multinational companies are better able to circumvent government restrictions, and the increasing importance of multinational companies reduces the ability of governments to yield to national pressure groups that attempt to obtain protection.

Research is a labor-intensive industry, heavily dependent upon the availability of young and flexible labor. McNicoll asserts that the United States has hitherto been able to attract highly qualified researchers from other countries, by building up the quality of its educational system and by the beggar-your-neighbor policies of offering high wages and favorable work conditions. A large share of industrial research as well as related training and basic research is conducted not in universities and other public institutions, but in the large multinational companies. If an increasing scarcity of qualified youth and steeply rising wages for such labor accompany the decline of fertility, multinational companies may be induced to move research departments and training centers to other countries, instead of attracting nationals from these countries to the industrialized countries with the offer of high wages. They may contribute to a gradual geographical decentralization of research capabilities and a reduction in differences in levels of technology.

Reference

Blake, Judith. 1981. "The only child in America: Prejudice versus performance," *Population and Development Review* 7, no. 1 (March): 43–54.

Comment: Thomas Gale Moore

On the whole, I have no real criticism of Geoffrey McNicoll's article, but perhaps a slightly different approach might bring to light some interesting facts. For instance, there are two main effects of below-replacement fertility: the effect of age distribution and the effect of changes in the size of the population. Below-replacement fertility implies a population with a higher median age and an older work force, and also, without migration, a declining population size.

Changes in the age distribution have certain social effects. For example, fewer people in the 12–20 age bracket means fewer movies will be produced, though it is possible that the home use of video cassette recorders may stabilize this trend. An older population will decrease the popularity of what is called "pop" music and will increase the market for classical music. An older society will experience less crime and consequently decrease the need for police and for prisons.

Moreover, an older population has some distinct economic implications. The savings rate will be higher, while unemployment will be reduced. An older work force will bring with it more expertise through on-the-job training and will be a more stable work force with less job turnover. This implies a higher level of productivity. Homes can be smaller and multi-family units will be more common, resulting in lower housing and energy costs.

An older population will mean a less innovative society, demanding more services and fewer goods. Medical costs will be increased, while costs for education will be reduced. On balance, the cost increases for medical care may outweigh the savings in education. Overall, an older population probably means a slightly higher growth rate and gross national product.

A decline in the size of the population has other implications. Fewer people may mean fewer geniuses and less diversity, although this point is controversial and depends on whether geniuses are born or made. From an economic standpoint there undoubtedly will be reduced economies of scale.

On balance, declining population size probably reduces growth and gross national product. Therefore, given the offsetting effects of the age distribution and size of population, it is to be expected that below-replacement fertility would have a negligible effect on growth. In any case, it should be noted that the negative impact of a decline in population size due to low fertility can be offset by immigration.

Comment: Carmel U. Chiswick

The quantity/quality model of reproduction motivation (Schultz, in this volume) assumes that adults receive utility from "child services," a term intended to convey the joys of parenthood. While more children would increase parental utility, it is possible to some extent to compensate for fewer children by enjoying each child more intensively (i.e., raising child "quality" as a source of parental pleasure). It follows that the cost to parents of additional "child services" depends on whether they are going to have an additional child or to improve the quality of their existing children. Their decision in this matter is influenced by the relative costs of these two possibilities.

In keeping with this model, an observed decline in fertility may be the aggregate result of parental decisions to substitute child quality for quantity. But the consequent decline in the size of the labor force, which must eventually result from below-replacement fertility, need not imply a reduction in labor inputs into the production of goods and services. If parental expenditures that serve to raise child quality also effectively increase human capital attributes, the labor inputs provided by the younger generation may even exceed those provided by their parents. At worst, the per-worker quality increase will partially offset the reduction in cohort size, so that per-worker production will necessarily rise.

Perhaps the most interesting question raised by the quantity/quality model as an explanation of low fertility is whether below-replacement growth rates can persist as a long-run equilibrium. In other words, if parents have few children because it is relatively more expensive to increase family size than to enjoy a small family more intensively, is it possible that market forces may reduce the cost of additional children and raise the relative price of quality per child? If so, would this reverse the trend within, say, a generation or two? Several possibilities come to mind from reading the articles in this volume.

First, having another child has become increasingly expensive in the industrialized countries because children require much parental time and that time is becoming very expensive. This is true in general as worker productivity rises; it is especially true of maternal time, which has become even more expensive as women's opportunities for market work increase at a faster rate than men's. But, as parental time becomes more expensive, the return to time-saving innovation increases. Changes in childrearing techniques, in institutional arrangements, and in social values are already taking place (Preston, in this volume), and we shall probably continue to see more evolution in this direction for some time to come.

A second source of adjustment is a declining time-intensity of additional quantity relative to additional quality, implying a reduction in the relative cost of having more children. "Experts" increasingly support the view that the quality of parental time is more important for the child's emotional well-being than the actual number of hours spent together, and today's childrearing wisdom places great emphasis on spending "quality time" with one's child. At the same time, raising an additional child today in a middle-class American family probably requires fewer hours of maternal time, *ceteris paribus,* than it did a generation ago because of increased market services, both private and public (e.g., after-school care, evening hours at the pediatrician's office), and because of increased social acceptance of the corners that working mothers are inclined to cut in order to save time (e.g., reductions in housekeeping and meal preparation time).

Third, it is possible that recent fertility decisions were based on an incorrect assessment of costs, an error that market forces will eventually correct, though not for many years, if not decades. A possible example is the benefit derived from "grandchild services"—the obvious pleasure gained by having grandchildren, a pleasure that requires having had children beforehand. Following through on McNicoll's example (from Preston, 1976) of a fertility rate of 1.4 children per woman, suppose 26 percent of adult women have no children and 31 percent have only one child. This means that fully 42 percent of the mothers have only one child. If only-children tend toward mutual self-selection as marriage partners, the one-grandchild family results. (This phenomenon is increasingly being discussed in the context of China's one-child population policy.) Sharing one's only grandchild with three other grandparents, each more eager than the other to enjoy his or her relationship with the child, can create strains for all seven family members. This is a future cost related to economies of scale in family size. If there has been no prior experience with small extended families, or if there is no historical memory on the part of decisionmakers, the realized cost of low fertility may be higher than anticipated. If so, a future generation of decisionmakers can be expected to be better informed and therefore to have fewer one-child families.

Another set of questions is raised by the notion that an aging population implies a "dependency burden." In the example of a 1.4 total fertility rate just used, fully 57 percent of the adult women have no children or one child. People in this category are generally viewed as being in a good position to spend their money on other things, including (or perhaps especially) saving for their own retirement years. In fact, the quantity/quality model of low fertility suggests that the smaller cohort of workers in the next generation will embody more human capital than their parents while the elderly will have greater private savings to finance their own retirement.

There is a benefit to having the elderly around in an improved state of health. Adult children derive utility if their own parents (and, of course, their children's grandparents) are independent, active participants in family life. Just as the joys of parenthood must be netted out of the costs of children (Becker and Barro, in this volume), so the benefits to working-age adults derived from "parent services" and/or "grandparent services" must be netted out of the cost of the elderly. Insofar as the over-65 generation has an increasing number of members who are dependents in name only, the benefits for family social and economic life may well outweigh the costs.

The costs of supporting the elderly, especially costs related to health care, are frequently described as rising dramatically as the elderly population grows larger. It is probably the case, however, that many of the observed recent cost increases are transitory and will be offset in the long run as the market adjusts to the aging population. The sheltered position of the health care industry from market forces is being eroded, and costs will continue to fall in this industry as competition is increasingly permitted.

Finally, McNicoll spends some time in his article on the distributional aspects of fertility decline. In short, if low-fertility families are making large human capital investments in each child while high-fertility families are not, a large proportion of the children (some 80 percent in the TFR = 1.4 example) will enter adulthood with relatively low investments in human capital. If high-human-capital couples tend to have fewer children, the possibility arises of an ever-increasing gap between the high-quality "nonbreeders" and the low-quality "breeders." It should be emphasized that this outcome depends crucially on low intergroup mobility, either because of self-selection among marriage partners or because of social barriers. The very attributes of child quality that low-fertility parents desire may even serve as the basis of self-selection, social barriers, or both. While the historical evidence (some of which is quite contemporary) suggests that high-human-capital groups can be very successful at holding their own even when vastly outnumbered, it would seem prudent (if nothing else) to direct our intellectual energies toward reducing social barriers to mobility and encouraging the creation of human capital among children of families who are not inclined to invest privately. Such an approach, for which there is both historical precedent and contemporary social support, can go far toward forestalling the adverse distributional effects of below-replacement fertility.

Reference

Preston, Samuel H. 1976. "Family sizes of children and family sizes of women," *Demography* 13: 105–114.

Population Dynamics with Immigration and Low Fertility

Thomas J. Espenshade

Since 1965 fertility rates in many industrial countries have fallen substantially below the level needed to replace their populations in the long run. While fertility levels have been falling, international migration to these countries—much of it from Third World countries—has been accelerating, both in absolute numbers and as a proportion of total population growth. Though not recognized as such until recently, these international movements have become one of the most important demographic changes of the period (Teitelbaum and Winter, 1985). Immigration to Great Britain, France, and the Netherlands was spurred by decolonization, to Sweden and West Germany by various guest worker programs designed to alleviate labor shortages in the 1950s and 1960s, and to the United States and Canada by immigration reforms in the 1960s that ended discrimination against entrants from non-European countries. Recent estimates suggest that the United States is now accepting nearly twice as many immigrants and refugees as all other nations combined (Lamm and Imhoff, 1985), and that legal and illegal immigration together account for about one-third of annual US population growth. In 1970 the foreign-born population in the United States comprised 4.8 percent of the total population, but low birth rates coupled with growing levels of immigration in the following decade boosted this figure to 6.2 percent by 1980 (*Economic Report of the President*, 1986).

When immigration is predominantly from Third World countries, it contributes to population growth in two ways: through the addition of the immigrants themselves and from the fact that immigrant fertility is often higher than native fertility. West Germany registered a natural increase of 366,300 in 1965 when the excess of births over deaths among the native German population was 334,000, and among immigrant workers, 32,300. But by 1975, natural increase had turned negative. Births among the native population lagged deaths by 235,600, whereas the surplus among immigrants rose to 99,000. Thus immigration and natural increase among immigrants accounted for all of West Germany's population increase. Similarly in France, of the total population growth between 1950 and 1975 of 11 million, 7 million was due to immigration and 4 million to natural increase. And since 1975, nearly all of the growth in the French population has been due to high birth rates among immigrant North Africans (Carlson, 1985). Michael Teitelbaum and Jay Winter (1985) have called attention to the demographic significance of low fertility in the presence of immigration:

> The convergence of the baby bust with the growth of international migration has led to a new demographic phenomenon of great relevance to debates about population decline. Put simply, the combination of record-low fertility and high immigration (especially from countries of higher fertility than the receiving countries) means that immigration must account for a large and increasing proportion of Western population growth. (pp. 91–92)

In the absence of immigration, populations with below-replacement fertility are in incipient decline, but if immigration fills the gap changes may be expected in the ethnic, racial, cultural, and linguistic composition of the population—changes that some people believe are matters of national concern. In those Western European countries where these compositional changes are occurring more quickly than in the United States, concern is sometimes magnified to a high level. For this reason, Teitelbaum and Winter (1985) comment: "Recent developments in France and Germany once more highlight the extent to which the matters raised [here] go far deeper than the administrative and technical, touching sensitive and important political issues likely to cloud and complicate present and future policy debates" (p. 120).

Before policymakers can deal intelligently with these issues, it is important to understand the demographic implications of continued low fertility combined with immigration. Most discussions of long-term population dynamics are couched in terms of stable population theory, a theory of the growth and structure of human populations that was developed for populations assumed to be closed to immigration and emigration. When migration is recognized, it is often to note that migration rates can be incorporated into survival rates so that no substantial modifications of the stable model are required (Lopez, 1960; Hyrenius, 1959; Sivamurthy, 1982). Only in the last decade or so have demographers turned their attention to the formal properties of so-called open populations, and they have generally proceeded by focusing on long-run equilibrium solutions. Important gaps in our knowledge remain, however, with respect both to the paths followed by these open populations on the way to a long-term equilibrium and to the time it takes to achieve an equilibrium outcome.

Previous related studies

Mathematical models have treated migration both as rates of migration and as numbers of migrants. We begin our review with those models that have taken the first approach. Nathan Keyfitz (1977) has studied the long-run properties of populations subjected to repeated outmigration. Suppose, for example, that a population that is closed to immigration and emigration has an intrinsic growth rate of r and that the objective is to lower that rate to r^*. When $r^* = 0$ so that a stationary population is the ultimate aim, Keyfitz produces a simple formula for the fraction of the population at age x that must emigrate each year. Because examples of emigration at just one age are difficult to find in practice, it is worthwhile to generalize these results to incorporate emigration at several ages simultaneously. Hannes Hyrenius (1959) and I (1984) have made a start by adding emigration rates to age-specific death rates.

Approaches to inmigration and outmigration have been combined in work by Andrei Rogers (1975), who extended the classical mathematical demography of single regions to multiregional population systems. Rogers considers a closed multiregional system that experiences internal migration but no emigration or immigration. Long-run equilibrium conditions are then explored under the assumption that multiregional age-specific rates of fertility, mortality, and internal migration remain constant. With these postulates, the entire multiregional system and each region separately eventually grow at the same constant rate. Each region has a stable age distribution, though not necessarily the same as the age distributions in other regions.

M. Sivamurthy (1982) has studied the effects of migration on the growth of a population and on its age-sex structure when migration is specified by an overall net migration rate and an age-sex composition of the net migrants at the time of migration. These impacts are compared with those that occur when there is no migration and when migration is specified by age-sex-specific net migration rates. He concludes that the continuation of a fixed set of fertility, mortality, and migration rates leads eventually to an equilibrium-state population with an unchanging age-sex structure and a constant growth rate. Sivamurthy also examines the time required for convergence to such an equilibrium-state population. If there is net immigration at all ages, then convergence occurs more quickly than in the absence of migration; if there is net emigration at all ages, convergence takes longer than if migration were zero.

For many purposes it is more appropriate to characterize immigration by the number of migrants than by the rate of migration, not only because most countries have policies to limit the absolute size of the annual immigration flow but also because the population at risk of immigrating is not the population in the host country but the population in the rest of the world.

In a paper prepared for the US Commission on Population Growth and the American Future, Ansley Coale (1972) asked how much of a reduction in fertility below the replacement level would be needed in an initially stationary population to maintain a stationary population with the same annual number of births if a steady stream of immigrants were permitted to enter the population. Coale also considered the effect on long-term population growth of adding immigrants to a stationary population in which everyone maintained replacement-level fertility. In the latter case, growth would occur at a constant arithmetic rate; each year the addition to the population would be the same as in the previous year.

John Pollard (1973) has shown that any fixed below-replacement fertility schedule, when coupled with a constant number and age composition of immigrants, leads to a stationary population. Somewhat more general than Coale's, Pollard's analysis shows that the level of below-replacement fertility that leads to a stationary population is not unique. On the other hand, Coale preserves the distinction between immigrant and native fertility, whereas Pollard assumes the same reproductive behavior for all women.

Espenshade, Leon Bouvier, and Brian Arthur (1982) have shown that if, starting at some arbitrary point, the age-specific birth and death rates of a population are fixed, if fertility is below replacement, and if the yearly number of immigrants to the population as well as their age-sex composition is constant, then that population will evolve in the long run to a stationary state with a constant size and an unchanging age-sex distribution. Such characteristics of the long-run stationary population as its size and age composition do not depend on the size or the age-sex structure of the starting population, but only on the underlying assumptions regarding future fertility, mortality, and immigration. Moreover, the conclusion that a stationary population eventually results under these circumstances is unaffected by how far below replacement fertility declines or by the precise level of immigration. For this conclusion to hold, it is not necessary for immigrant women to adopt the fertility patterns of native women. Immigrant women may have fertility rates substantially above replacement, and so may their descendants in the first, second, and later generations. All that is required for an equilibrium stationary population to materialize in the long run is that, at some point in the generational chain— whether beginning with the first generation, the tenth, or the fiftieth—one generation of immigrant descendants must adopt, and subsequent generations must maintain, below-replacement fertility.

Finally, S. Mitra (1983) has examined the asymptotic properties of populations with a constant annual influx of immigrants and with fertility rates below, at, and above replacement. He reproduces the result that a long-run stationary population is the outcome when fertility rates are constant and below replacement. Like Coale, he finds that a population experiences arithmetic growth if fertility is at replacement; and if fertility rates are above replacement, Mitra shows that the long-run population approaches the same intrinsic growth rate it would have in the absence of immigration.

In sum, the current literature focuses on proving the existence of long-run equilibrium solutions when fertility, mortality, and migration are assumed to be constant, and on deducing the characteristics of the equilibrium population (e.g., its size, growth rate, and age composition) from underlying assumptions about vital rates. Much less is known about population dynamics in the years separating the start of a projection from the attainment of an eventual equilibrium and about the number of years required to reach an equilibrium-state population. We turn next to a consideration of these two issues in the context of below-replacement fertility.

Concepts

To study the dynamic path toward a long-run equilibrium stationary population when fertility is constant and below replacement and when there is a constant annual influx of immigrants, we find it useful to imagine that the host country is divided into a "western" half and an "eastern" half. Let us assume that the population that is alive at time $t = 0$, the time when underlying fertility, mortality, and immigration conditions become constant, lives entirely in the western half, that there is no migration into or out of this region for values of $t > 0$, and that there is no intermarriage with future residents of the other region. The eastern region, which is assumed to be empty at $t = 0$, is reserved for subsequent foreign-born immigrants and their future descendants.

Under these conditions, the population in the west eventually disappears. Closed to immigration and emigration and with fertility below replacement, the western population has a negative intrinsic growth rate, and therefore its size will eventually approach zero. The long-run path taken by the western population depends on the size of the stable equivalent population, Q_0, and on the intrinsic growth rate, r. As time increases beyond $t = 0$, $Q_t = Q_0 e^{rt}$ traces out a declining exponential population trajectory to which the size of the western population converges.[1]

The population-building process in the eastern half of the country is more complex. The first point to recognize is that a constant annual flow of immigrants after $t = 0$ leads to a resident population of foreign-born persons whose size and age composition are eventually constant. This stationary population of immigrants is built up in much the same way that an ordinary life-table stationary population is generated except that, in the former case, people can enter the population at any age and not just age zero. After immigrants have been arriving for t years, the foreign-born population will be stationary at all ages less than or equal to t. For example, after about 45 or 50 years, the number of foreign-born women will be constant through the end of the child-bearing ages. The total foreign-born population will be stationary after about 100 years. Because immigrants enter the population at all ages and not just at age zero, however, the age distribution of the foreign-born population will not follow the shape of the life-table survival curve, even when the number of foreign-born persons is stationary at all ages.

Next, assume that the native-born children of immigrant women and all of their subsequent descendants also live in the eastern portion of the country. If we designate the foreign-born population as the "zeroth" generation, their native-born children as the "first" generation, their grandchildren as the "second" generation, and so on, we can see how each of these generations evolves from the preceding one. The annual number of first-generation births to immigrant women at time t, $B_1(t)$, starts off at zero for $t = 0$ and then rises steadily as the number of immigrant women in the childbearing ages increases. Once the value of t surpasses the oldest age of childbearing, β, the number of foreign-born women of childbearing age becomes stationary and $B_1(t)$ levels off at a fixed annual ceiling of B_1.

The number of second-generation births at time t, $B_2(t)$, depends on the number of first-generation women in the childbearing ages. If the age at which childbearing begins is denoted by α, births in the second generation do not appear until after $t = \alpha$, the point at which women in the first generation reach the childbearing ages. Thereafter, because of the monotonic behavior of $B_1(t)$, $B_2(t)$ increases continuously until it, too, reaches a fixed annual ceiling. This ceiling is attained when $B_1(t)$ has been constant for β years, that is, when $t = 2\beta$. At that point, $B_2(t)$ can be written as

$$B_2(t) = B_2 = B_1 \cdot \mathrm{NRR}_1 ,$$

where NRR_1 is the value of the net reproduction rate for first-generation women.

In general, the number of births at time t in the ith generation is $B_i(t)$. Reasoning as before, $B_i(t)$ is zero until women in the parent or $(i-1)$th generation enter their childbearing years. $B_i(t)$ then increases continuously until it reaches a maximum of $B_i = B_{i-1} \cdot \mathrm{NRR}_{i-1}$. The times at which the successive generational birth sequences, $B_i(t)$, first acquire nonzero values and when they finally reach their maximum values are shown in Table 1.[2]

Up to this point, in describing the evolution of the population in the eastern half of the country, we have not made use of the assumption that fertility is below replacement. The discussion has been sufficiently general so as to apply to any level of generation-specific fertility. But only if fertility is

TABLE 1 Time paths followed by successive generational birth sequences, $B_i(t)$

Generation (1)	Births begin at $t =$ (2)	Births become stationary at $t =$ (3)	Duration of convergence (4) = (3) − (2)
$B_1(t)$	0	β	β
$B_2(t)$	α	2β	$2\beta - \alpha$
$B_3(t)$	2α	3β	$3\beta - 2\alpha$
⋮	⋮	⋮	⋮
$B_i(t)$	$(i-1)\alpha$	$i\beta$	$i\beta - [(i-1)\alpha]$ $= (\beta - \alpha)i + \alpha$
⋮	⋮	⋮	

below replacement will the equilibrium-state population in the east be a stationary population. As t progresses to larger and larger values, the annual birth flow in the eastern population, $B(t)$, is the sum of births in all generations, or

$$B(t) = B_1 + B_2 + \ldots + B_i + \ldots .$$

If all generations exhibit the same below-replacement fertility, so that $NRR_i = NRR < 1$ for every generation, then

$$B(t) = B_1 (1 + NRR + NRR^2 + \ldots) \text{ and, in the limit,}$$

$$B(t) = B = B_1 / (1 - NRR) .$$

The total stationary population that arises in the east is made up therefore of many smaller stationary populations. There are H foreign-born persons, and if life expectancy at birth is represented by e_0, there are in addition $B_1 e_0$ first-generation persons, $B_2 e_0$ second-generation persons, and so on. The relative size of successive generations of native-born persons is governed by the value of the net reproduction rate in the parent generation. Lastly, the ages of people in each native-born generation are distributed as the life-table survival curve.

To summarize, if a population with an arbitrarily chosen size and age-sex composition is projected assuming fixed below-replacement fertility and a constant annual number of immigrants whose age-sex composition is held constant, the equilibrium-state outcome is a stationary population. The initial population and its descendants eventually die out because fertility rates are inadequate to replace this population. While that is happening, a new population of recent immigrants and immigrant descendants is forming. This new population consists of a succession of smaller stationary populations—one of immigrants themselves, one of first-generation native-born persons, one of second-generation native-born persons, and so on. The stationary population of foreign-born persons is formed first, followed by the population of first-generation descendants, and so on down the generational chain. Total population size is the sum of the number of people in each generation, and this sum converges to a fixed total provided the number of people in successive generations becomes progressively smaller, that is, provided fertility rates are below replacement.

Application

To illustrate these conclusions we have projected the 1980 US population by age and sex assuming that fertility and mortality rates remain constant at their 1980 levels and net migration is constant in absolute numbers and in age and sex distribution at the level for 1983 legal immigration. In 1983 559,800 lawful permanent residents were admitted to the United States.[3] The projection parameters for the initial period, 1980–85, are given in the first column of Table 2.

TABLE 2 Summary demographic measures of the US population, 1980–85, and eventual stationary population achieved with constant levels of fertility, mortality, and annual net immigration

Item	1980–85	Eventual stationary population
Total fertility rate (per woman)	1.835	1.835
Net reproduction rate (NRR)	0.874	0.874
Male births per 100 female births	105.3	105.3
Female life expectancy at birth (years)	77.5	77.5
Male life expectancy at birth (years)	70.0	70.0
Population size (millions)	232	170
Yearly births (millions)	3.67	1.94
Yearly deaths (millions)	2.14	2.50
Yearly net immigrants (millions)	0.56	0.56
Annual rates per 1,000 population		
Births	15.8	11.4
Deaths	9.2	14.7
Natural increase	6.6	−3.3
Net migration	2.4	3.3
Population increase	9.0	0.0

SOURCE: Author's projections. For sources of data for the 1980 baseline population, see note 4.

The results of this projection are shown in Figure 1 (the line labeled "total") and the right-hand column of Table 2. There were 226.5 million persons enumerated in the 1980 US census. Under the assumptions described above, total population size increases to a maximum of 280.8 million in the year 2025 and then begins a long and gradual decline toward an eventual 169.7 million. In the eventual stationary population, the sum of the annual number of births (1.94 million) and the annual number of immigrants (0.56 million) is just enough to offset the annual number of deaths (2.50 million). In addition to being smaller, the stationary population is also older than the 1980 population. The median age for females is 42.3 years in the stationary population, compared with 31.3 years in 1980. For males the corresponding ages are 38.8 and 28.8 years, respectively.

Figure 1 also shows the individual projections for our hypothetical western and eastern portions of the total population. The closed population in the west continues to increase for a time after 1980 due to the effects of population momentum, reaching a maximum of 252 million in 2015 before beginning a decline toward zero. Soon after the population in the west begins to shrink, its "growth" rate settles down to a constant rate of −0.0052 per annum. The "West" line in Figure 1 may be interpreted as a projection of US population size in the absence of immigration and emigration after 1980.

The population in the east rises from zero in 1980 to an eventual total of 169.7 million. It is appropriate to think of the eastern population as a

FIGURE 1 Projections of the total US population and the hypothetical eastern and western populations

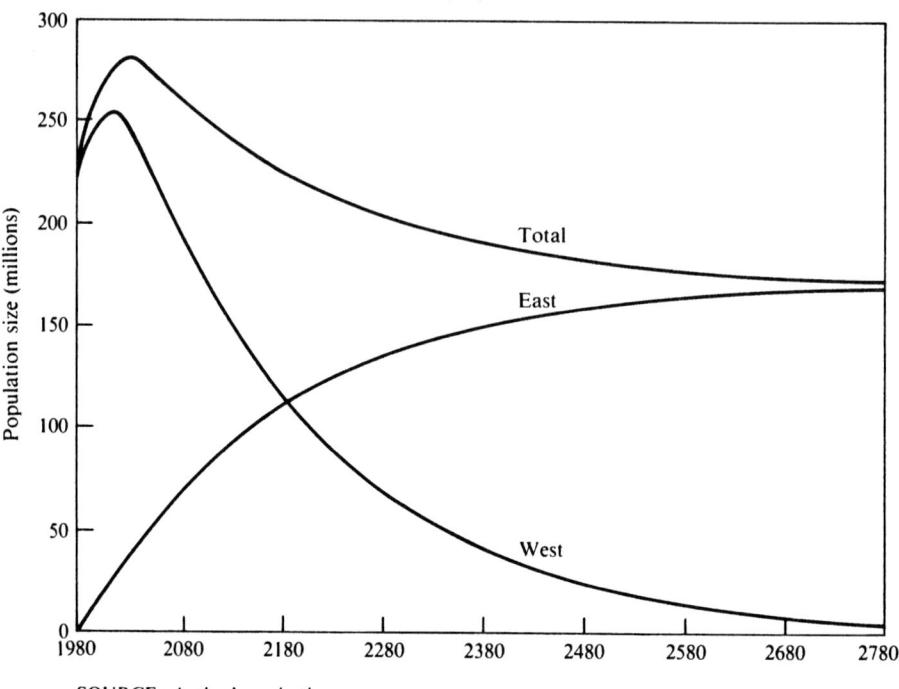

SOURCE: Author's projections.

"layered" population, much like sedimentary rock, with the successive generations of immigrants and their descendants constituting the layers. The bottom stratum would be the immigrant generation. First-generation native-born persons constitute the layer above that, and so on. The reason that the rate of growth in the eastern population decreases over time is that progressively smaller generations are being added to the total because the underlying net reproduction rate is less than one.

It is clear from Figure 1 that the eastern population comprises a rising share of the total population. These fractions are tabulated in terms of the western population's share of the total US population in Table 3. The western population falls to three-fourths of the total within 100 years of the start of the projection and to one-half in just over 200 years.

The concepts developed earlier paid special attention to the generational components of population growth. The behavior of the eastern population's generational birth flows, $B_i(t)$, is shown in Figure 2. Only births in the first six generations are included. Births in subsequent generations would appear lower and to the right in the diagram. Each generation's birth path is characterized by the same general pattern; it begins at zero, increases to a fixed annual ceiling, and then remains constant. As the order of the generation

TABLE 3 Projected size of the hypothetical west population and the total US population, selected dates

Year	West population (millions)	Total US population (millions)	West population as percent of total
1980	226.5	226.5	100
2000	248.2	261.1	95
2020	251.9	279.3	90
2080	192.2	257.7	75
2190	108.9	219.5	50
2350	47.6	191.5	25
2540	17.8	177.9	10
2680	8.6	173.7	5

SOURCE: Author's projections.

increases, it takes longer for births to appear and longer for births to attain their maximum value. Once births have become constant at an upper ceiling, the number of births in each generation is equal to the number of births in the previous generation multiplied by the value of the net reproduction rate—in this case 0.874.

Figure 1 indicates the time frame of the convergence process. It takes many centuries for an equilibrium-state stationary population to materialize with immigration and below-replacement fertility. We may with reason admit to little policy interest in this distant prospect. Substantial compositional changes in the population come much earlier, however.

In the particular hypothetical example used in this article, based on US parameters, the western population falls to about 75 percent of the total population after 100 years. In other words, in just 100 years, 25 percent of the total population consists of post-1980 immigrants to the eastern region and their descendants. Had we been more realistic and assumed higher fertility among immigrants and their near-term descendants than among the "native" population in the western region, these compositional changes would have occurred sooner. In addition, it is important to recognize that significant changes in the ethnic and racial balances of the US population are already under way and that these changes were evident well before 1980. The same is true for Western Europe. Indeed, in the short run at least, the potential for change in the ethnic, racial, linguistic, religious, and other compositional aspects of national populations is perhaps greater in Europe than in the United States because Europe did not experience a fertility upswing following World War II comparable either in magnitude or duration to the US baby boom. As a result, European populations do not have age distributions with the same degree of built-in momentum for future growth as the age distribution of the US population, and therefore they lack a "protective mantle of natural increase"[5] that softens and to some extent obscures immigration-related compositional trends.

FIGURE 2 Projected annual births by generational status in the hypothetical eastern population

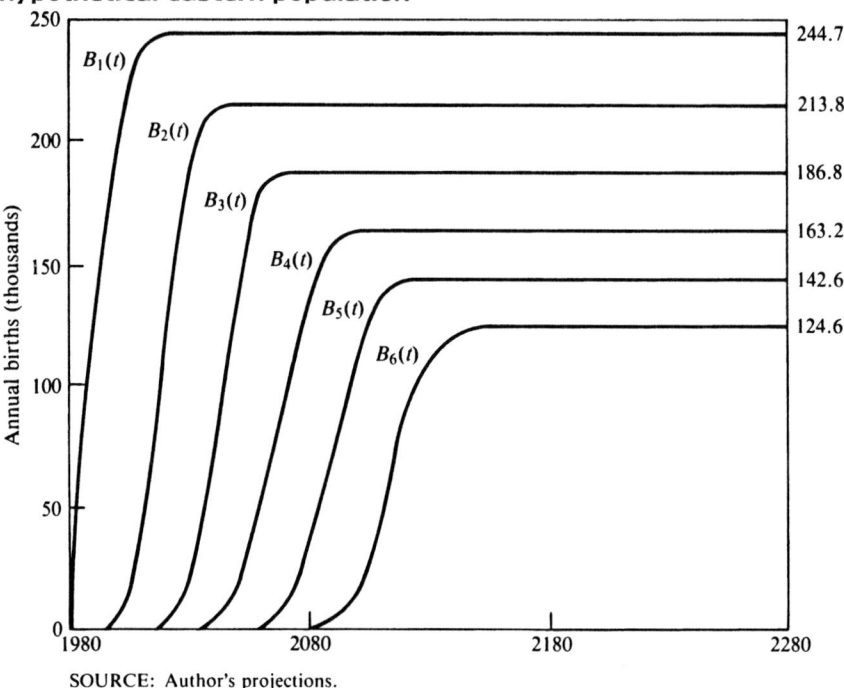

SOURCE: Author's projections.

Concluding remarks

When a population experiences both immigration and low fertility, we have seen that a kind of demographic transfusion occurs as it proceeds to a long-run stationary state. The initial population and its descendants diminish under the pressures of below-replacement fertility, to be replaced by a new population of immigrants and their descendants. Whether these findings trigger policy concerns depends on the particular context in which immigration arises and on the degree of similarity over time between the original population and the immigrants and their descendants.

The dilemma facing policymakers in developed countries with respect to immigration and low fertility is clear. Because fertility rates are now at levels that are insufficient to replace these populations in the long run and because there is little hope that they will rise above replacement any time soon, immigrants are needed for their contribution to demographic stability. At the same time, the public's dissatisfaction over the presence of a large and growing immigrant community swells as the proportion of the total population growth attributable to immigration rises. It is for this reason that many writers doubt that an "immigration solution" to allay fears of population decline will prove to be politically acceptable. Teitelbaum and Winter (1985), for example, conclude: "It seems doubtful, therefore, whether large-scale immigration can ever serve as a politically viable response to declining population over a considerable period of years, unless the immigrant streams are considered similar in character to the indigenous population" (p. 150).

If industrial democracies of the West want a migration solution to the demographic dilemma they face, then more attention must be paid to the character and tempo of immigrant adaptation and adjustment processes. It cannot be acceptable for minority immigrant populations to comprise an underclass existing "at the margins of white tolerance" (Markham, 1986). Barriers to immigrant adjustment must be removed and additional facilitators to immigrant adaptation must be found to speed the process of incorporating immigrants and their children into the mainstream of society.

The United States has an immigration policy, but it lacks an immigrant policy. US immigration policy consists in large measure of a simple gatekeeping function of determining who is and who is not eligible for entry. Once immigrants have been admitted, the federal government acts as though its responsibility to them has ended. Policies and programs to ease the adjustment of immigrants to their new surroundings are a missing component in the 1986 round of US immigration reforms.

Notes

This paper draws on research supported by the Center for Population Research, NICHD, US Department of Health and Human Services, under grant number 1 R01-HD18240-01 and by the Weingart Foundation. The author thanks Terri Murray, Tracy Ann Goodis, and Francesca Moghari for their capable technical assistance.

1 The interested reader may consult Espenshade and Campbell (1977) for details of the stable equivalent population and its relevance to population momentum.

2 Another instance in which the succession of generations arises has been discussed by Keyfitz (1968, pp. 117–126). Keyfitz uses the term "generation" in the context of projections of closed female populations. It refers to how many generations separate the children from the population alive at time zero. Specifically, the zeroth generation denotes births, $G(t)$, to women alive at time zero. The first generation, $B_1(t)$, denotes births to $G(t)$ women. In this situation there are only a finite number of births in each generation. In contrast to the immigration model developed in this article—in which the number of births in each generation is infinite (though the annual number is finite) because the population is continually replenished by immigrants—in the case Keyfitz considers, the limiting value of $B_i(t)$ as t tends to infinity is zero.

3 Although these projections ignore emigration and undocumented immigration, these two components are roughly offsetting. According to Warren and Kraly (1985), ". . . the estimated number of non-US citizens emigrating and undocumented migrants counted in the census were roughly of the same magnitude during the 1970s, 1.2 and 1.5 million respectively" (p. 7). Making a small adjustment for the emigration of US citizens boosts current total emigration to more than 150,000 people each year (p. 2). Beginning in January 1986, the US Bureau of the Census's postcensal estimates and Current Population Survey controls included an annual allowance of 200,000 for undocumented immigration and 160,000 for legal emigration for each year since 1980.

4 Sources of data for the 1980 baseline population of the United States, as they appear in Table 2, are as follows: US Bureau of the

Census, *1980 Census of Population,* Vol. I: Characteristics of the Population, Chapter B: General Population Characteristics, Part I: United States Summary, PC80-1-B1, Table 44, May 1983. Fertility rates for 1980 are from National Center for Health Statistics, Advance Report of Final Natality Statistics, 1982, *Monthly Vital Statistics Report* 33, no. 6, Supp., DHHS Pub. No. (PHS) 84-1120 (Hyattsville, Maryland: Public Health Service, Table 4, September 1984). Death rates for 1980 are from National Center for Health Statistics, *Vital Statistics of the United States, 1980,* Vol. II, Sec. 6, Life Tables, DHHS Pub. No. (PHS) 84-1104 (Public Health Service, Washington, D.C.: US Government Printing Office, Table 6-1, 1984). Immigration numbers for fiscal year 1983 are derived from Immigration and Naturalization Service, *1983 Statistical Yearbook of the Immigration and Naturalization Service,* Table IMM4.1.

5 To my knowledge, Peter Morrison (1978) was the first to use this metaphor.

References

Carlson, Allan C. 1985. "The 'population' question returns," *Persuasion at Work* 8, no. 12 (December): 1–10.
Coale, Ansley J. 1972. "Alternative paths to a stationary population," in US Commission on Population Growth and the American Future, *Demographic and Social Aspects of Population Growth,* ed. Charles F. Westoff and Robert Parke, Jr. Vol. I of Commission Research Reports, pp. 589–603. Washington, D.C.: US Government Printing Office.
Economic Report of the President. 1986. Washington, D.C.: US Government Printing Office.
Espenshade, Thomas J. 1984. "Comment on Mitra's generalization," *Demography* 21: 431–432.
———, and Gregory Campbell. 1977. "The stable equivalent population, age composition, and Fisher's reproductive value function," *Demography* 14: 77–86.
———, Leon F. Bouvier, and W. Brian Arthur. 1982. "Immigration and the stable population model," *Demography* 19: 125–133.
Hyrenius, Hannes. 1959. "Population growth and replacement," in *The Study of Population: An Inventory and Appraisal,* ed. Philip M. Hauser and Otis Dudley Duncan. Chicago: The University of Chicago Press, pp. 472–485.
Keyfitz, Nathan. 1968. *Introduction to the Mathematics of Population.* Reading, Mass.: Addison-Wesley Publishing Company.
———. 1977. *Applied Mathematical Demography.* New York: John Wiley.
Lamm, Richard D., and Gary Imhoff. 1985. *The Immigration Time Bomb: The Fragmenting of America.* New York: Truman Talley Books—E. P. Dutton.
Lopez, Alvaro. 1960. *Problems in Stable Population Theory,* unpublished Ph.D. dissertation, Department of Mathematics, Princeton University.
Markham, James M. 1986. "Minorities in Western Europe: Hearing 'not welcome' in several languages," *The New York Times* (5 August), p. A6.
Mitra, S. 1983. "Generalizations of the immigration and the stable population model," *Demography* 20: 111–115.
Morrison, Peter A. 1978. "Emerging public concerns over U.S. population movements in an era of slowing growth," in *The Economic Consequences of Slowing Population Growth,* ed. Thomas J. Espenshade and William J. Serow. New York: Academic Press, pp. 225–246.
Pollard, John H. 1973. *Mathematical Models for the Growth of Human Populations.* New York: Cambridge University Press.
Rogers, Andrei. 1975. *Introduction to Multiregional Mathematical Demography.* New York: John Wiley.
Sivamurthy, M. 1982. *Growth and Structure of Human Population in the Presence of Migration.* London: Academic Press.

Teitelbaum, Michael S., and Jay M. Winter. 1985. *The Fear of Population Decline*. Orlando, Florida: Academic Press.

Warren, Robert, and Ellen Percy Kraly. 1985. "The elusive exodus: Emigration from the United States," in *Population Trends and Public Policy*, no. 8 (March). Washington, D.C.: Population Reference Bureau.

Immigration as a Counter to Below-Replacement Fertility in the United States

David M. Heer

Let us make the assumption that the United States, without change in fertility policies, will sustain its current net reproduction rate, which has been below replacement level since 1972, 100 years into the future. Under what circumstances will immigration keep the given population from declining? Obviously, immigration will prevent declining population if enough persons enter the United States.

Leon Bouvier (1981) showed that if annual net immigration to the United States were 750,000, if life expectancy at birth were to continue at its current level of 72.8 years, and if the total fertility rate were to continue at its current rate of 1.8 births per woman, population growth in the United States would still be occurring in 2080. In that year, the population would have increased to 301 million (from an estimated 222 million in 1980) and would still be growing at a rate of 0.5 per thousand. On the other hand, if annual net immigration were only 500,000, eventual population decline could not be avoided. In that case the population of the United States in the year 2080 would be only 268 million and would be declining at a rate of 0.6 per thousand. More recently, Thomas Espenshade et al. (1982) demonstrated that a stationary population (i.e., one that never increases or decreases) will be formed at some population level by any constant flow of net immigration regardless of how low the net reproduction rate is. They also showed that under the fertility and mortality conditions of 1977, an annual net immigration of 840,000 would preserve the US population indefinitely at its 1980 level of 226 million (after a temporary rise to almost 300 million). Conversely, under the same fertility and mortality assumptions, a level of net immigration of only 400,000 per year would result in an eventual stationary population of only 108 million.

Neither Bouvier nor Espenshade et al. consider what the time pattern for annual net immigration would have to be to ensure that the US population would remain indefinitely invariant at its 1980 level. However, Bouvier's finding that without any net immigration the population would grow to 245 million by 2030 implies that the best way to ensure zero population growth over the long term would be to have net *emigration* for at least the next 40 years and thereafter a rapid rise in net *immigration* so that, by around 2080, it would be about 840,000 per year.

Is it reasonable to believe that the United States could achieve by 2080, if it wanted, a net immigration of 840,000 per year, that is, a level sufficient to prevent the population from ever declining below its size in that year? There can be no doubt that the answer is yes. According to the US Bureau of the Census, net immigration averaged 431,000 per year during the 1970–80 decade, despite a restrictive immigration law (Passel and Robinson, 1984). This amount was made up of an annual net flow of 279,000 legal immigrants (437,000 immigrants minus 158,000 emigrants) and an annual net flow of 152,000 undocumented, or illegal, immigrants. It seems certain that net immigration could be doubled if the government were to change the current law, which restricts quota immigration to 270,000 persons per year.

Even assuming no change in immigration law—this article omits consideration of the recent Immigration Control and Reform Act of 1986—the annual net flow of immigrants could hardly be expected to remain at the 1970–80 level. Refugee and nonquota immigration, which in recent years has comprised almost half of all legal immigration, will probably continue to increase at least as fast as world population growth. Unless preventive legislation is enacted, undocumented immigration, which now represents a substantial proportion of total net immigration, is also likely to increase at least as fast as the rate of world population growth. Accordingly, even if there is no change in immigration policy, the US population will probably not decline, in the long run, below its 1980 level.

After outlining current US policy with respect to fertility and immigration, I shall discuss options for a more pronatalist fertility policy and a less restrictive immigration policy. I then conclude by evaluating the consequences of such policy alternatives according to five criteria that I consider the most important bases for evaluating such alternatives. These criteria can be stated in the form of the following questions. First, what is the effect of the fertility or immigration policy on per capita income in both the near term and the long term? Second, what is the effect of the policy on the distribution of income? Third, what is its effect on the "quality" of the population, defined to include desirable characteristics in the population gene pool as well as a high level of education and health for each individual? I shall assume that the higher the quality of the population, the higher the level of per capita income in the long term. Fourth, what is the effect on the degree of conflict between ethnic groups within the United States? Finally, what is its effect on the influence of the United States in international affairs? Clearly, a policy that is best by one of these criteria may not be so by others. However, before making any judgments concerning the consequences and desirability of policy alternatives, let us briefly describe current policy on fertility and immigration.

Current policy on fertility and immigration

Relative to other industrial countries, the fertility policy of the United States tends toward antinatalism. Since the Supreme Court in 1973 declared state restrictions to be unconstitutional, abortion has been permitted throughout the country. Moreover, the United States is one of the very few industrial countries that do not provide child allowances to all families with a minimum number of children. The only subgroup in the United States provided with a liberal monetary subsidy for childrearing is unmarried mothers. The $9.2 billion spent on the program of Aid to Families with Dependent Children (AFDC) in the United States in 1975 was equal to 0.8 percent of the national income (Heer, 1980). Under the Reagan presidency, the $12.9 billion spent for this program in 1982 was only 0.5 percent of the national income (US Bureau of the Census, 1985). It should be noted, however, that the AFDC program is administered separately in each state and that payments per family vary substantially among states. Finally, mention should be made of the foodstamp program, which in 1982 provided some $10.8 billion in benefits to poor families, defined on the basis of income and number of members but without regard to marital status (US Bureau of the Census, 1985).

Let us now turn to current US immigration policy. With respect to legal immigrants, current law distinguishes between quota immigrants, nonquota immigrants, and refugees.

With the exception of some numerically unimportant groups, the only persons who can enter the United States without restriction are the immediate relatives of US citizens, including spouses, unmarried children under 21 years of age, and parents of US citizens who are themselves aged 21 or older.

The Refugee Act of 1980 established a uniform procedure for admission of refugees from all countries without numerical quota based on a United Nations definition of a refugee. However, this act also gives very broad power to the President of the United States. Under President Reagan's administration, persons seeking refugee status from communist-dominated countries have been freely admitted, but very few persons from either El Salvador or Guatemala have been granted refugee status.

Other legal immigrants to the United States are admitted within the worldwide annual quota of 270,000. Within this quota, no more than 20,000 immigrants can be admitted from any one country.

Immigration policy includes guidelines for the treatment of undocumented immigrants. Currently, no legislation bars employers from hiring such individuals. Undocumented immigrants are ineligible for benefits from entitlement programs; moreover, their employers can always threaten them with deportation. Accordingly, many employers prefer undocumented immigrant employees to employees who are either US citizens or legal immigrants.

Another important point to be made about current legal guidelines is that the children of undocumented immigrants who are born in the United States are, according to the provisions of the Fourteenth Amendment to the Constitution, automatically US citizens. Hence, although undocumented immigrants are not themselves eligible for benefits from such programs as AFDC, foodstamps, and Medicaid, their US-born children are. Moreover, even those children of undocumented immigrants who were themselves undocumented have recently been bestowed rights. The US Supreme Court ruled in 1982 that the State of Texas must provide free education to undocumented children. A California State court decided in 1985 that undocumented persons who were in fact residents of California have the right to attend the University of California and the California State University under the same status as other Californians.

Options for a more pronatalist policy

Let us now consider alternative fertility policies. One legislative change to consider is a reversal of the current legalization of abortion. Of course, strong support for such a step already exists among conservative groups. In 1983, the latest year for which data are available, the ratio of induced abortions per thousand live births in the 13 states reporting abortion data was 361 (Powell-Griner, 1986). The experience of Romania, which in 1966 abolished a previously liberal abortion law, indicates that restrictive abortion laws can have, at least temporarily, a very substantial effect on fertility (Teitelbaum, 1972).

Additional options with respect to a more pronatalist policy involve various financial inducements. These can be classified according to four major types: (1) child allowances, (2) aid to children of poor families, (3) increased income tax exemption for children, and (4) maternity-leave subsidies for working women.

Almost every European country now provides child allowances to all families with a specified minimum number of children, regardless of the parents' income. France has perhaps the most liberal program of child allowances: in 1974 the child allowance payments in that country constituted 2.6 percent of the national income (Heer, 1980).

Aid to children of poor families is exemplified by a program instituted in the Soviet Union in 1974. Under that program families with a total per capita income from all sources of less than 50 rubles a month receive a payment of 12 rubles per month for each child under age eight. In 1974, the program provided benefits for families with as few as two children if the husband and wife did not each earn much above the minimum legal wage of 70 rubles. As of the same year, for families in which both husband and wife earned the average wage, the new program provided benefits only to those with more than four children (Heer, 1977).

In direct contrast to programs that aid solely children of poor families are those that provide an income tax exemption for each child. Since the income tax is progressive in the United States, a flat exemption per child tends to favor families with greater income in terms of the absolute subsidy received.

A subsidy for working mothers is exemplified by 1981 legislation in the Soviet Union that provides working women a partially paid leave for one year following each birth of 35 rubles a month in most parts of the Soviet Union but 50 rubles a month in Siberia, the Far East, and the far northern regions (*Current Digest of the Soviet Press*, 1981).

Consequences of alternative fertility and immigration policies

Let us assume that the foregoing pronatalist fertility policies are successful. By the standard of per capita income in the short term, any policy of subsidizing fertility is bound to be less desirable than either current policy or a policy to encourage greater immigration. This is so because a pronatalist policy in the short term adds only to the dependent population of the country, whereas a generous immigration policy adds immediately to the population of economically active young adults (Simon, 1984). Moreover, a pronatalist policy might also reduce per capita income by reducing the proportion of females in the labor force. Compared with current policy, a more generous immigration policy might in the short term either increase or decrease per capita income depending on the quality and age composition of the immigrants and on the number of children they eventually have.

By the standard of per capita income in the long term, a pronatalist policy may also be relatively disadvantageous. First, the enactment of such a policy carries the risk that fertility will become excessive, unduly stimulating the growth of population, with the familiar disadvantages of that situation. An important point in this connection is that a pronatalist policy, once enacted, may prove difficult to repeal because of the vested interests it would create. If enacted in the near future, a more generous immigration policy might also, and for the same reasons, result in a long-term reduction in per capita income. However, the likelihood of this is less, if only because it is probably easier to secure legislative repeal of a generous immigration policy than of a pronatalist policy.

What would be the effect of the policy alternatives on the distribution of income? Let us first consider pronatalist policies. It is likely that a more restrictive policy with respect to abortion would result in a less equalitarian distribution of income. For instance, for the 11 states reporting such data, women with 16 or more years of schooling have a ratio of abortions per thousand live births (250) that is smaller than that for all women (364) (Powell-Griner, 1986). It is probable that specific financial aid to poor families would not only stimulate fertility but also favor a more equitable distribution of income. The latter effect is not certain since such a policy would increase family income by virtue of the subsidy while simultaneously reducing per capita income to the extent that it increased the number of children within such families. On the other hand, depending on the index of inequality being used, an increase in the exemption for dependents on the federal income tax might result in a less equitable distribution of income since the financial subsidies from such a policy would be greater for upper income groups.

Whether a more generous immigration policy would increase or decrease the inequality of income distribution would be largely dependent on the educational attainment of the immigrants. According to results from the 1980 census, the educational attainment of immigrants varies substantially depending on country of origin. Immigrants from most sending nations have a high level of educational attainment; however, immigrants from Mexico, about half of whom are undocumented, have a low level of education (US Bureau of the Census, 1984). Moreover, my own data show that undocumented Mexican immigrants have a lower level of educational attainment than legal immigrants (Heer and Falasco, 1982).

What would be the consequences of the various policy alternatives on the quality of the population? This is a more difficult question to answer because quality has no well-defined meaning. If we assume that quality is associated with the educational attainment of the mother, both restrictive abortion legislation and aid to children of poor families, other things equal, would lower population quality. Changes in immigration policy that increased the proportion of immigrants with low educational attainment would also tend to reduce the quality of the population, at least in the short run.

What effect would the policy alternatives have on ethnic conflict within the United States? Again the answer is highly speculative. Let us consider first the effect of pronatalist policies. Let us assume, following the viewpoint of H. M. Blalock (1967), that the white population's fear of blacks is a positive function of the proportion of the total population that is black, and further that the pronatalist policies adopted either restrict abortion or give financial aid to children of poor families. Such policies will increase the proportion of the total population that is black and, under the given assumption, would thus enhance the potential for ethnic conflict. In substantiation of this chain of reasoning, we may note that in 1983 for 13 reporting states, the ratio of abortions per thousand live births was 304 for whites and 644 for blacks (Powell-Griner, 1986). Furthermore, in 1982 35.6 percent of the black population was below the poverty level, compared with only 12 percent of whites (US Bureau of the Census, 1985).

A more generous immigration policy might also enhance the potential for increased ethnic conflict, if one may judge from the past history of such conflict in the United States whenever new immigrant groups have grown rapidly in comparison with the growth of more established ethnic groups.

Finally, what would be the effect of the various policy alternatives on the strength of the United States in the international arena? Obviously, to the extent that the power of the United States is a positive function of sheer numbers of persons, a pronatalist policy, if successful, could increase the power of the country relative to present policy. On the other hand, if the number of taxpayers or males of military age is the important criterion of strength, a more generous immigration policy would provide a faster increase in the ratio of such persons to total population than would a pronatalist policy that had the same effect on population numbers, and hence might be more desirable. Nevertheless, it is not certain that an increase in population size would increase US influence in international affairs.

Moreover, it should be recognized that immigrants of certain nationalities may weaken the influence of the United States in international affairs because they preclude effective alliances with countries that might otherwise wish to be allies of the United States. For example, the antipathy of Greeks and Armenians in the United States to Turkey makes it difficult for the United States to have an effective alliance with Turkey. Conversely, certain changes in the direction of a more generous immigration policy might increase the influence of the United States in international affairs. For example, a friendly government in Mexico is important to the United States because of the common land border and because of Mexico's valuable petroleum resources. It might be advantageous for the United States to enact some type of legalization of status (not necessarily granting the full privileges bestowed on permanent legal residents) not only for the large number of undocumented Mexican immigrants currently in the United States but also for many of those who will wish to enter the country in the future.

Conclusion

Assuming the continuation of a total fertility rate of about 1.8 and a goal of eventually maintaining a stationary population at the level of the 1980 population, some change in either fertility policy or immigration policy may be necessary, although not until the second half of the twenty-first century. For the reasons outlined above, a generous immigration policy is likely to be economically more advantageous than a pronatalist policy. On the other hand, the United States may not want a larger flow of net immigration than takes place under current legislation. Both fertility and immigration policies in the future, as in the past, seem more likely to be adopted for political or equity reasons than for demographic purposes.

References

Blalock, H. M., Jr. 1967. *Toward a Theory of Minority-Group Relations*. New York: John Wiley.
Bouvier, Leon F. 1981. "The impact of immigration on U.S. population size," *Population Trends and Public Policy*, No. 1. Washington, D.C.: Population Reference Bureau.
Current Digest of the Soviet Press. 1981. "More benefits for families, pensioners," 33, no. 13 (29 April): 9–10 and 23.
Espenshade, Thomas J., Leon F. Bouvier, and W. Brian Arthur. 1982. "Immigration and the stable population model," *Demography* 19, no. 1 (February): 125–133.

Heer, David M. 1977. "Three issues in Soviet population policy," *Population and Development Review* 3, no. 3 (September): 229–252.

———. 1980. "Population policy," in *Contemporary Soviet Society,* ed. Jerry G. Pankhurst and Michael Paul Sacks. New York: Praeger, pp. 63–87.

———, and Dee Falasco. 1982. "The socioeconomic status of recent mothers of Mexican origin in Los Angeles County: A comparison of undocumented migrants, legal migrants, and native citizens," unpublished paper presented at the Annual Meeting of the Pacific Sociological Association, San Diego, California.

Hirschman, Charles. 1978. "Prior U.S. residence among Mexican immigrants," *Social Forces* 6, no. 4 (June): 1179–1201.

Passel, Jeffrey S., and Gregory Robinson. 1984. "Revised estimates of the coverage of the population in the 1980 Census based on demographic analysis: A report on work in progress," unpublished paper presented at the Annual Meeting of the American Statistical Association, Philadelphia, Pennsylvania.

Powell-Griner, Eve. 1986. "Induced terminations of pregnancy: Reporting states, 1982 and 1983," *Monthly Vital Statistics Report* 35, no. 3 (Supplement).

Simon, Julian L. 1984. "Immigrants, taxes, and welfare in the United States," *Population and Development Review* 10, no. 1 (March): 55–69.

Teitelbaum, Michael S. 1972. "Fertility effects of the abolition of legal abortion in Romania," *Population Studies* 26, no. 3 (November): 405–417.

United States Bureau of the Census. 1984. *1980 Census of Population,* Volume I, Chapter D, Part 1, Section A. Washington, D.C.: US Government Printing Office.

———. 1985. *Statistical Abstract of the United States 1985*. Washington, D.C.: US Government Printing Office.

United States National Center for Health Statistics. 1984. *Vital Statistics of the United States, 1980,* Volume I, *Natality*. Washington, D.C.: US Government Printing Office.

United States National Office of Vital Statistics. 1950. *Vital Statistics, Special Reports,* Selected Studies 33, no. 4: 68.

Comment: Barry R. Chiswick

Citing the work of Leon Bouvier and Thomas Espenshade, David Heer asserts that in a mechanical sense the net flow of immigrants to the United States can be adjusted to attain nearly any desired rate of growth of the total population, regardless of the native fertility rate. In addition, native fertility rates can, in principle, be influenced by public policy. Thus, target levels of the rate of growth of the native and total populations can be achieved by policies that affect native fertility and net immigration.

The appropriate public policy depends on the "social welfare function." In Heer's view five arguments enter the social welfare function. Two refer to levels of well-being—a higher per capita income and a higher "quality" of the population. Lower income inequality, reduced tensions among ethnic groups, and greater harmony in international affairs are his other three objectives. It is important to recognize that there may be tradeoffs at the margin among these objectives. For example, an immigration policy that favors highly skilled workers may have positive effects on four of the five objectives, but if some sending countries (e.g., India, the Philippines, Korea) object to the "brain drain," and others (e.g., Mexico) object to a closing of their "safety valve" for low-skilled workers, international harmony may decrease. We have no guidance as to how much of a shortfall in achieving one policy objective can be offset by advancing the other policy objectives.

Part of the difficulty in considering the implications of alternative pronatalist and pro-immigration policies for increasing the population is the heterogeneity among the instruments that may be used. Some pronatalist policies, such as increases in benefits to low-income families and restrictions on legal abortions, are likely to increase fertility rates and may lower average child quality. On the other hand, consider raising the income tax deduction for the children of taxpaying parents, expanding private-sector daycare programs in high-income communities, and providing greater subsidies for higher education and private schooling. These policies may raise fertility and child quality simultaneously.

Immigration policy could raise the average quality of the labor force and per capita income by limiting immigration to highly skilled workers with readily transferable skills. Or, it could lower labor force quality and income by admitting only unskilled workers.

For these reasons, Heer's conclusion that "a generous immigration policy is likely to be economically more advantageous than a pronatalist policy" (p. 268) is unfounded. Policymakers need to be cognizant of the mix of pronatalist and pro-immigration policies. The task is not merely to view fertility and migration policies as alternative mechanisms for achieving population targets, but also to consider the implications of the wide range of instruments that can be used to implement each of these policies.

POLICIES

Social Security in Aging Societies

Carolyn L. Weaver

For social security and other retirement income systems, there may be no more important consequence of low fertility than the aging of the population. Since 1950, the proportion of people aged 65 and older has increased by a third or more in the United States and the United Kingdom, and by half or more in West Germany, and has doubled in Japan (United Nations, 1985). Further aging of the population is projected for all industrial nations in the decades ahead. For some countries, the United States included, the transition to a considerably older population will be abrupt, with a major shift after the year 2000 as the baby boom cohorts move into retirement.[1]

Neither public mechanisms (such as social insurance) for transferring income across generations nor private mechanisms (such as private pensions and family support systems) are immune to these developments. Everywhere the challenge is the same—how to respond to and plan for a potentially dramatic escalation in the per capita cost of the aged in the face of a deteriorating ratio of workers to retirees, or, within the context of the family, a deteriorating ratio of young adults to elderly parents and grandparents. This challenge is heightened by the prospect for continued improvements in health and medicine that increase the number of years people spend in retirement, all the while drawing on the resources of public and private institutions.

In the United States, as elsewhere, the effects of population aging on social security have been masked by the effects of social security aging, or at least this was the case roughly through the 1970s. With pay-as-you-go financing, characteristic of social insurance systems around the world, there is a start-up period of several decades during which the relation between benefits received and taxes paid is extremely favorable. These are the golden years for social security programs. Taxes can be kept deceptively low relative to the implicit debt being piled up. As these systems mature, however, the economic and demographic constraints on long-term performance begin to be felt.

Just at the time social security systems were facing this difficult adjustment to maturity, economic growth slumped while fertility rates were falling, setting into place the elements of a worldwide crisis. Whereas economies have generally rebounded, fertility rates have not. If sustained, low fertility and the consequent aging of populations will strike at the heart of social insurance systems as we know them today. This concern was voiced clearly in 1979 by Stanford Ross, then US Commissioner of Social Security, when he said, "We are confronting a worldwide issue which goes to the very viability of the institution" (1979: 9).

The aging of populations and of social security

The populations of the world's industrial nations are relatively old and are growing slowly, if at all. Europe, the slowest growing region, has an average annual population growth rate of 0.33 percent, about half the rate that prevailed 20 years ago.[2] The growth rate in northern and western Europe now stands very close to zero. Among the slowest growing countries are the United Kingdom and Sweden, which are barely replacing their populations, and Austria, Belgium, and West Germany, which have actually begun to shrink in size.[3]

TABLE 1 Population age in selected countries and regions of the world, 1985[a]

	Median age	Percent aged 65 and older
Europe	33.9	12.4
Western Europe	35.6	13.3
Austria	35.5	14.2
Belgium	35.3	13.3
France	33.7	12.4
West Germany	37.8	14.0
Italy	35.4	13.4
Netherlands	33.5	11.9
Sweden	37.6	17.0
Switzerland	39.8	15.7
United Kingdom	35.1	14.7
North America	31.2	11.3
Canada	30.5	9.6
United States	31.3	11.5
Asia	22.0	4.4
Japan	35.1	9.9
Africa	17.2	3.0
Latin America	20.7	4.4

[a] Projected for 1985 on the basis of intermediate assumptions for fertility, mortality, and net migration.
SOURCE: United Nations (1985).

(Certain Arab and African countries, by contrast, have populations that grow by 4, 5, almost 6 percent a year—fast enough to double in 15 years or so.)

In turn, the industrial nations have the greatest relative numbers of aged persons.[4] Looking simply at the proportion of the population aged 65 and older, the 20 "oldest" populations include the United States, ranked number 20 with 11.5 percent of the population aged 65 and older; Sweden, ranked number 1 with 17 percent of the population aged 65 and older; and 18 European countries in between. (The proportion of the population aged 65 and older runs as low as 1–2 percent in some regions of the world.) Europe has a median age of 34 years, some 50 percent higher than in Asia and nearly twice that in Africa (see Table 1).

Although influenced by mortality and migration, population aging is "traceable mainly and essentially to a decline in fertility or gross reproduction"; it is "a concomitant of the approach of a population to stationarity" (Clark and Spengler, 1980: 5–6).[5] All of the industrial nations that now rank among the world's "oldest" have below-replacement fertility rates. This includes the United States, the United Kingdom, and France, with total fertility rates averaging 1.7–1.8 births per woman (1983 data); Austria, Sweden, Italy, Switzerland, Belgium, and the Netherlands, with total fertility rates averaging 1.5–1.6; and West Germany, with a total fertility rate as low as 1.3 (Bourgeois-Pichat, in this volume, p. 5). The link between low fertility, slow population growth, and an aging population is thus a strong one.

Table 2 presents, for 12 industrial countries, the proportion of the population aged 65 and older for the period 1900–1980, and as projected by the United Nations (intermediate assumptions) to 2025. As illustrated, population aging became apparent in the various countries at quite different times—by

TABLE 2 Proportion of the total population aged 65 and older, selected countries, 1900–2025 (projected)[a]

	1900	1930	1950	1980	1985	1990	2000	2010	2020	2025
Austria	5.0	6.8	10.4	15.5	14.2	14.8	15.2	16.9	18.5	19.8
Belgium	6.2	7.6	11.1	14.3	13.3	14.3	15.9	16.1	18.8	20.3
Canada	5.1	5.6	7.7	8.9	9.6	10.6	11.8	12.7	16.1	18.1
France	8.2	9.4	11.4	13.7	12.4	13.2	14.8	14.9	18.1	19.4
West Germany	4.9	7.4	9.4	15.0	14.0	14.8	16.5	20.2	21.2	22.1
Italy	6.2	7.4	8.3	13.5	13.4	14.3	16.2	17.3	18.8	19.6
Japan	—	4.8	4.9	9.0	9.9	11.2	14.9	18.0	21.0	20.6
Netherlands	6.0	6.2	7.7	11.5	11.9	12.8	14.1	16.1	20.8	22.7
Sweden	8.4	9.2	10.3	16.2	17.0	17.7	17.2	18.8	21.9	22.3
Switzerland	5.8	6.9	9.6	14.8	15.7	17.3	20.6	23.9	26.8	27.1
United Kingdom[b]	4.7	7.4	10.7	14.8	14.7	15.1	14.9	15.3	17.4	18.3
United States	4.1	5.4	8.1	11.3	11.5	11.9	11.7	12.2	15.4	17.2

[a] Proportions for the years 1985–2025 are projected on the basis of intermediate assumptions for fertility, mortality, and net migration.
[b] Data for 1900 and 1930 are for Great Britain.
SOURCES: United Nations (1956, 1985); Clark and Spengler (1980).

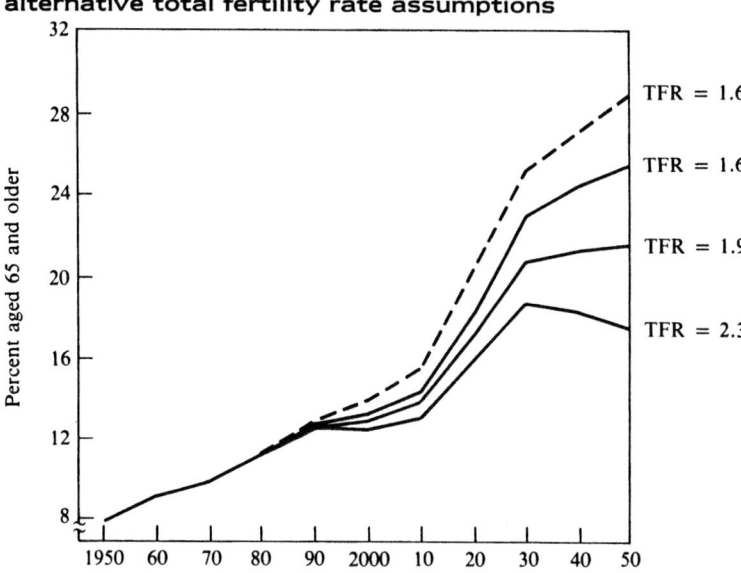

FIGURE 1 Proportion of the US population aged 65 and older, 1950–2050, projected according to alternative total fertility rate assumptions

NOTES: Projection indicated by dashed line is based on high assumptions for mortality improvements and migration; all others based on intermediate mortality and migration assumptions.
SOURCE: US Bureau of the Census (1984, pp. 5, 10, 18).

the turn of the century in France and Sweden, and more than a half-century later in Japan—but the trend is the same everywhere. In each country, persistent and in some cases dramatic aging has accompanied the general decline in fertility during this century. Four countries (the United States, United Kingdom, West Germany, and Austria) experienced a doubling of the proportion elderly between 1900 and 1950; almost all of the countries have experienced an increase on the order of 40–60 percent in the past three decades.

For the future, the United Nations projects that after a brief respite in the 1990s, there will be another surge in the relative size of elderly populations.[6] Over the period 2000–2025, the proportion of the population aged 65 and older is projected to increase by one-third in West Germany and Austria and by as much as one-half in the United States, Canada, and the Netherlands. The elderly would comprise about one in five persons in the United States by the year 2025—about twice the proportion of elderly residing in that country today. In Switzerland, the number would exceed one in four. The median age by then would be over 40 in most industrial countries.

It is worth bearing in mind that the conditions we expect to prevail in the year 2025 are of great importance for the retirement policy decisions we make today. After all, everyone who will be elderly in that year (and even in the year 2050) is already alive today.

A closer look at aging trends in the United States helps highlight the range of possible futures and the relatively dramatic role played by fertility. Figure 1 illustrates the proportion of the population aged 65 and older projected through 2050 based on "low," "intermediate," and "high" fertility assumptions.[7] As illustrated, the proportion aged 65 and over is projected to grow rapidly—by 40–60 percent or more between 1980 and 2020—under any of the fertility rates assumed. Low fertility, however, generates a considerably older population, with fertility alone accounting for a difference of almost 50 percent in the proportion that is elderly in 2050—the year the 1985 birth cohort turns 65. If low fertility is combined with a significant further reduction in mortality (shown by the dashed line), nearly 30 percent of the population in the United States is projected to be 65 or older in the year 2050.

Aged dependency ratios

In any society, the elderly possess a set of claims—contractual or otherwise—on the current output and income of an economy. Population aging thus assumes economic importance for many reasons, but especially because of its implications for the changing mix of "producers" and "consumers" and the demands placed on public and private institutions fulfilling those claims. The aged dependency ratio (the number of persons 65 and older per 100 people aged 15–64) bears directly on the burden of social security and other income support systems. Historical data and future projections of aged dependency ratios are illustrated for several countries in Figure 2. There are presently about 17 elderly people per 100 working-age people in the United States. This ratio is projected to remain in the range of 17–18 percent through 2010, when the first wave of baby boom cohorts reaches age 65, and then jump by a third in 10 years and by half in 15 years, reaching 27.4 percent by 2025. In West Germany, the aged dependency ratio peaked once, at 22.7 percent in 1980, and is expected to soar again after the turn of the century—exceeding 30 percent by 2010, and reaching 35.8 percent in 2025. Japan, now noticeably younger than the other industrial nations, is projected to age so rapidly that it will soon be among the oldest populations in the world.

The aged dependency ratio is suggestive of the financial implications of population aging.[8] Holding everything else the same, a doubling of the aged dependency ratio implies a doubling of tax rates required to support systems such as social security, or a halving of the level of support per beneficiary. In the absence of some significant realignment of public and private arrangements for the aged, taxpayers in such countries as the United States, Canada, Germany, and Japan can expect an increase in the per capita cost of public programs on the order of 50 percent or more between 2000 and 2025, even before taking into account the growing real burden and the changing mix of public programs likely to accompany the aging of the aged.

FIGURE 2 Population aging in various countries, 1950–2025

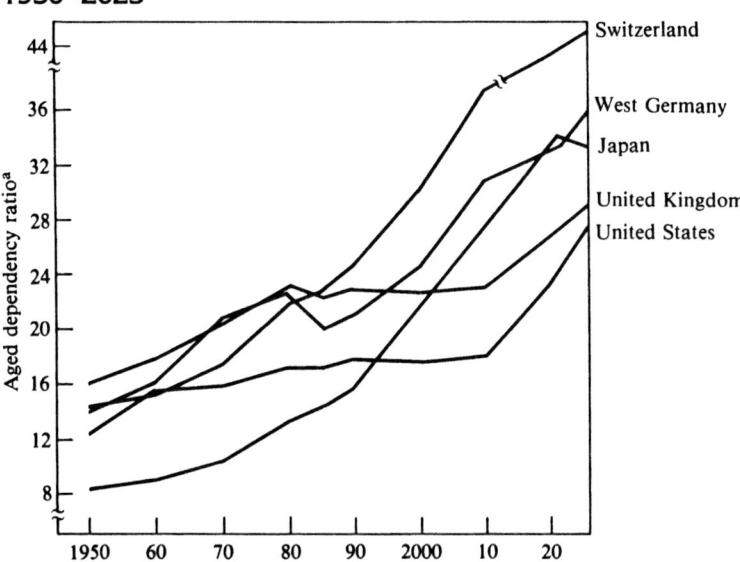

aNumber of persons aged 65 and older per 100 persons aged 15–64; UN intermediate assumptions.
SOURCE: United Nations (1985).

The aging of the aged

An important phenomenon obscured by these summary statistics is the aging of the aged. Whereas in 1950, 4.8 percent of the elderly population in the United States was 85 or older, that figure stood at 8.8 percent in 1980 and is projected to reach 14.7 percent in the year 2000 and 17.4 percent by 2010(US Bureau of the Census, 1984: 17). (Thereafter, the baby boom cohorts begin to swell the ranks of those aged 65–69.) Importantly, any apparent lull in the 1990s in the overall aging of the population will tend to be offset by the aging of the aged, whose needs will place great demands on health and welfare programs.[9]

The operation and aging of social security systems

Most of the world's social security systems are financed on a "pay-as-you-go" basis. Under such an arrangement, current benefits are financed by current taxes, or, roughly speaking, benefits to today's retirees are financed by taxes on today's workers. As contrasted with a funded pension scheme, in which assets are held against accruing liabilities, a pay-as-you-go system accumulates little or no reserves and thus leaves implicit virtually all of its debt.[10] Each generation effectively counts on the next generation for its support in retirement; there is no stockpiling of resources to help defray the cost of future benefits. From the standpoint of the economy and society's aggregate welfare, the desirability of such a system depends on the long-run relation between growth in population and productivity (which determines the rate of return on implicit social security debt) and the productivity of capital (which determines the rate of return on investments in real capital).[11]

To separate the effects of social security aging from those of population aging, consider first a very simple world in which all workers pay social security taxes at a constant rate fixed by law; all elderly persons receive benefits; and all taxes collected are spent concurrently. Let productivity (and real wages) and the population grow at some constant rate. In addition, let each age group grow at the same rate (i.e., the population is stable), ensuring that age composition remains constant over time.

Now, when a pay-as-you-go system is introduced, those who are already elderly fare extremely well. The proceeds of the tax applied to all workers are distributed to the currently retired, who, by assumption, have paid no taxes at all. The implicit rate of return on taxes paid is thus infinite for all those in the first generation that retires under the system. Over time, wage growth allows successive generations of retirees to receive higher benefits. These benefits will bear a constant relation to preretirement earnings, as measured by the "replacement rate" (i.e., retirement benefits as a proportion of earnings just prior to retirement), but a progressively less favorable relation to taxes paid.[12] Each subsequent generation spends a greater proportion of its worklife under the system paying taxes, and the implicit rate of return on tax payments falls. Ultimately, under a mature pay-as-you-go system, when everyone pays taxes over his or her entire worklife, the maximum rate of return payable is equal to the rate of growth of taxable wages, which is roughly equal to the rate of productivity growth plus the rate of population growth. In the United States, this is at most about 2 percent annually (Feldstein, 1976).[13]

What is noteworthy about how a pay-as-you-go social security system ages is that implicit rates of return fall for succeeding generations, meaning that the system inevitably becomes less "profitable" over time. This happens despite the fact that benefit levels are rising in accordance with earnings growth, and even if, as in the preceding example, the ratio of taxpayers to beneficiaries is stable, reflecting the underlying age composition of the population. Rates of return can be bolstered in the face of an aging system, but only on a temporary basis and only through expansionary tax increases.[14]

One element of the worldwide crisis in social security is already suggested—systems that have been around for a few decades simply cannot offer people what they provided in the past and may well offer lower returns than alternative financial arrangements, such as private investments.[15] Regardless of the goals of social insurance, governments will find it increasingly difficult to provide citizens with what they have grown accustomed to. If the rate of return that social security can ultimately offer is lower than the rate of return that could be earned were the taxes invested in real capital, the political and social crisis will embody a significant economic dimension as well. In this case, income and wealth opportunities are forgone.[16]

Now suppose an aging population is superimposed on an aging (or mature) social insurance system. For example, let us assume a decline in fertility that lowers the rate of population growth and leads to an increase in the ratio of elderly persons to working-age persons. This means the ratio of beneficiaries to taxpayers rises, total earnings grow more slowly, and, unless benefits fall automatically, fiscal insolvency results.[17] To restore solvency without raising taxes, benefits would have to be cut roughly in proportion to the decline in the ratio of taxpayers to beneficiaries. Alternatively, to maintain some given replacement rate, taxes would have to be increased roughly in proportion to the increase in the aged dependency ratio.

In either event, implicit rates of return fall to reflect the full decline in the rate of population growth.[18] Social security's profitability to society thus falls, and, to the extent that population growth and composition have a more significant impact on total wage growth than do any induced changes in the productivity of capital, the opportunity cost of pay-as-you-go financing rises.

The inherent instability of pay-as-you-go systems is highlighted by this example. Only one economic or demographic variable changed and it did so in a systematic way. Without allowing for any of the ups and downs we actually observe in, for example, the unemployment rate or productivity, or any other systematic changes in, say, longevity, government intervention is necessary if insolvency is to be prevented.[19] Only in perfectly stable environments are mature pay-as-you-go systems immune to the threat of insolvency.[20]

What kind of legislation is required to restore solvency in the face of a decrease in fertility? Because population aging occurs over many decades, maintaining solvency on a long-term basis will require either regular intervention to cut benefits or increase taxes, or long-range changes in the law that generate increased savings or revenues to match changes in future obligations. In other words, unless the government makes changes at the onset of the fertility decline, it will have to regularly address the social security solvency issue in the future. All the while, the rate of return that can ultimately be paid will be falling.

The importance of financial instability cannot be overstated as a source of deep political and economic concern. Adverse shifts in population growth (or productivity) force difficult decisions about how the risks of uncertain events are to be distributed across generations. A systematic policy of cutting benefits to restore solvency (as would be dictated under a defined contribution system) would shift all of the risk to retirees; a systematic policy of raising taxes (as under a defined benefit system) would shift all of the risk to workers. Neither approach produces optimal risk sharing among generations or an efficient distribution of welfare over time; neither is likely to be a viable approach in the longer term. Citing Richard Musgrave (1981):

> In all, the contingency of declining population growth leaves [a fixed replacement rate or a fixed tax rate system] a very uneasy foundation for the social security contract. At least it does so for those who take seriously the notion

that the system should be based on a contract that can be kept and not be formulated in a way that contains a built in potential for collapse.[21] (p. 103)

Ad hoc adjustments in taxes and benefits are certainly not the answer. Although such a strategy (if it can be called one) might well result in some sharing of the risks of uncertain events, it would introduce a new form of risk—that surrounding changes in the law. As Sherwin Rosen has observed (1984), "uncertainty about the law is peculiar to social security debt and does not promote efficient lifetime allocation of consumption" (p. 241).[22]

Unfortunately, there is nothing inherent in pay-as-you-go systems and certainly there are no ready answers in economic theory that would tell us how social security systems should be designed so as to properly distribute the risks of uncertain developments and thereby maximize aggregate welfare. One thing is clear, however: an intergenerational "contract," such as that embodied in a social security system, is seriously diluted in value if its terms are not knowable in advance and perceived to be enforceable.

The maturing and rejuvenation of pay-as-you-go systems

As suggested above, declining fertility and aging societies can have severe consequences for a mature pay-as-you-go system, depressing its profitability and undermining its financial base. Why, then, is the idea of a "crisis in social security" of relatively recent origin, dating only to the mid-1970s?[23] A look at the way actual social security systems have evolved over the years provides some important clues.

To begin, although social insurance systems emerged quite early—in Germany in 1889, France in 1910, and the Netherlands in 1913—some systems are much younger. Sweden, Canada, Finland, Norway, and Denmark, for instance, all enacted earnings-related social security programs in the 1960s; the Swiss program dates only to 1948.[24] Even among the early systems, major revisions were dictated by hyperinflation, monetary reform, and two world wars. For systems introduced or overhauled in the 1930s and 1940s, the US system included, only in the past ten years or so have people begun to retire who have paid taxes over an entire worklife.

Consider the development of benefit eligibility and coverage under a typical social security system. Rather than "blanketing in" the elderly, providing full benefits to all who are old when the program is created, benefit eligibility generally accrues over time.[25] Either the individual must work under the system for a certain amount of time to be eligible for benefits (and this requirement may increase as the system matures) and/or the benefit amount is tied directly to time spent under the system. In either event, it generally takes a number of years, possibly decades, before all of the elderly meet the eligibility criteria and are entitled to full benefits.[26] Along similar lines, the coverage of new social security systems is frequently not universal. The likelihood that individuals will move into covered employment and gain eligibility for benefits thus increases over time.

For both benefit and coverage reasons, therefore, the proportion of retirees eligible for full benefits is likely to be low in the early decades, with the result that the ratio of social security taxpayers to beneficiaries is artificially high relative to the underlying ratio of young to old.[27] One byproduct of this is substantial reserve accumulation in the early years of pay-as-you-go systems. Even quite modest tax rates are typically higher than necessary to meet current benefits. As costs rise to meet tax income, reserves are depleted and pay-as-you-go financing results.[28] In the meantime, excess reserves provide a ready alternative to tax increases as a method of financing expansion.

In addition to being chronologically young during most of this century, social security systems were also being expanded by legislation. Expansion of pay-as-you-go systems has effects that are fully comparable to the start-up of such systems. For example, an increase in the tax rate used to finance an across-the-board benefit increase—though it has no effect on the rate of return payable in the long term—generates windfall gains for all current retirees and bolsters rates of return for all those who will receive the higher benefits without paying the higher tax over their full work lives. Just as effectively, coverage can be expanded or the ceiling on taxable earnings can be increased to swell the pool of taxable resources and temporarily improve returns; reserves can be drawn down. Each such action tends to recreate the transitional gains to pay-as-you-go financing. In effect, the social security system is rejuvenated but at the expense of a permanently higher structure of liabilities and thus a permanently higher tax rate. Economic growth, such as characterized the industrial nations in the years following World War II, is similarly effective at rejuvenating social security systems.[29]

The effects of declining fertility can thus be masked for many years in young or expanding social security systems. During the transition years, rates of return are artificially high and bear no direct relation to underlying population and productivity growth; taxes are deceptively low, bearing no necessary relation to changes in the system's obligations or indebtedness. Ultimately, however, systems mature. As they do, rates of return for young workers fall toward levels sustainable by population and productivity growth, and the ratio of taxpayers to beneficiaries falls to that defined by the underlying age distribution.[30] It is then that adverse demographic shifts have effects that are both dramatic and highly visible.[31]

Recent developments in social security

Throughout the industrial nations, social security programs are reeling from the dual pressures of aging populations and sagging economies, which mature pay-as-you-go systems are poorly equipped to handle. Since the early 1970s, reserves have been depleted, taxes have been increased substantially, and, although outright benefit reductions are uncommon, efforts to scale back the growth of benefits have begun to surface. The rapid expansion of social insurance programs—an internationally shared experience during the 1960s and early 1970s—is no longer the norm; quite possibly, it is a thing of the past. Everywhere, funding the obligations already incurred has become a difficult task, and for the first time consideration is being given to proposals to modify those obligations—or to restructure how those obligations are met—so as to brace for the retiree bulge in the next century.[32]

Before looking at these developments in more detail, we should note that "social security" means different things to different nations, and cross-national comparisons must be interpreted with great caution. The International Labour Office provides perhaps the most comprehensive source of cross-national data, and its tabulations suggest the following. If broadly construed to include public programs of old-age, survivors, and disability insurance, workers' compensation, health insurance, unemployment compensation, and public assistance, "social security"—or what we might refer to as all income-maintenance programs in the United States—accounts (in 1980) for half or more of total government spending in West Germany, France, Austria, Sweden, Belgium, and the Netherlands; for 40 percent or more of spending in the United Kingdom, Japan, Canada, and Italy; and for 38 percent in the United States. In other words, "social security" spending amounts to close to one-fifth to one-quarter of gross domestic product (GDP) in most of these countries, West Germany and the United Kingdom included, and as much as a third of GDP in Sweden (as compared with 13 percent in the United States and 11 percent in Japan.)[33] Old-age, survivors, and disability insurance—which conforms to the US definition of social security (excluding Medicare)—accounts for 40–50 percent of this total. However measured, modern social security programs are huge, in some cases constituting the largest items in government budgets.

Table 3, which presents social security expenditures relative to gross domestic product for 12 countries, illustrates the growth of social security programs over the past two decades. Here (as elsewhere below) the narrower definition of social security is employed. As illustrated, spending on social security pensions (benefit payments only) as a fraction of gross domestic product increased in the United States and the United Kingdom by one-third during the 1960s and by half again in the 1970s, roughly doubling over the two-decade period. Spending also doubled in Austria and Belgium over the period and tripled in Switzerland, Sweden, and the Netherlands. In real per capita terms (per working-age person), social security expenditures more than doubled between 1960 and 1971 in Austria, Belgium, France, Germany, the Netherlands, Sweden, Switzerland, and the United States, and increased by half again in the next six years in every country but Austria (where real per capita expenditures increased 38 percent) (US Senate, Special Committee on Aging, 1981: 17).

Growth of this magnitude does not result from population aging alone. Systems were maturing at the same time governments were legislating a substantial amount of growth. As late as the 1970s, legislation was being enacted

TABLE 3 Social security pension payments as a percent of gross domestic product, selected countries, 1960–80[a]

	1960	1970	1980
Austria	4.6	7.3	8.8
Belgium	3.1	4.2	6.6
Canada	2.0	2.2	3.2
France	2.6	4.3	7.7
West Germany	5.9	6.9	9.5
Italy	3.3	5.9	—[d]
Japan	—[c]	—[c]	—[c]
Netherlands[b]	3.8	7.2	11.3
Sweden	3.6	5.3	9.7
Switzerland	2.1	4.2	7.5
United Kingdom	2.9	3.9	5.6
United States	2.3	3.1	4.7

[a] Benefit payments only: old-age and survivors insurance and disability insurance programs. Does not include military pensions, government employee pensions, or explicit public assistance for the elderly (although means-tested components of social security coverage are included).
[b] Figures include workers' compensation–type payments (which are otherwise excluded from table).
[c] Less than 1 percent.
[d] Not comparable due to reorganization of data.
SOURCES: International Labour Office (1985: Tables 8 and 9); Social Security Administration (1983: 74).

that lowered retirement ages or liberalized provisions for early retirement (in France, Germany, Italy, Austria, Sweden, and Switzerland, among others), expanded disability programs (in the United Kingdom, the Netherlands, and France), and granted outright benefit increases (in France, Italy, Japan, Switzerland, and the United States). By 1975, automatic cost-of-living benefit adjustments were in place in 20 countries.[34] Replacement rates for retired workers and spouses, moreover, were increased substantially in some countries. Between 1969 and 1980, the replacement rate for an aged couple, based on average earnings, increased 50 percent in the United States and Sweden—meaning that a couple retiring in 1980 received benefits that were 50 percent higher than a couple with the same earnings history who retired in 1969—and rose by a third in France, a fifth in Canada, and more than doubled in Japan (Aldrich, 1982). As a result of each of these changes, the size of present and future liabilities increased dramatically.[35]

Without unusually rapid and sustained economic growth or sharp increases in taxes, a nation simply cannot finance, on a long-term basis, higher replacement rates and expanded eligibility for an aging population. Sooner or later something has to give. The economic events of the 1970s turned out to be the straw that broke the camel's back.

In a number of countries, reserves were wiped out in the attempt to meet escalating benefit payments in the face of an eroding tax base. In the United States, for example, trust fund reserves amounted to a year's worth of benefits in 1970 and to half that in 1977, dwindling to one month's benefits in 1983[36] (Board of Trustees, 1985: 45). In Germany, reserves fell from the equivalent of nine months' benefits to 1.5 months' between 1974 and 1980; and in Belgium, reserves fell from 5.5 to 1.7 months' benefits in the period 1975–80. The effects of maturing systems, expanding benefit claims, and eroding tax bases were also felt in countries with substantial reserve funds such as Switzerland, where reserves fell from 4.5 years' to 1.2 months' benefits in the period 1966–75 and continued to deteriorate thereafter; and in countries with new social security systems that were still amassing large reserves such as Sweden, where the ratio of reserves to benefit payments fell from the equivalent of 32 times annual expenditures in 1970 to less than 18 times by 1980. By the 1970s, moreover, the coverage of social security programs was nearly universal.[37]

Short of explicit borrowing, the options were quickly reduced to only two—increase taxes or cut benefits. Virtually every country opted for the former. As illustrated in Table 4, between 1971 and 1979, payroll tax rates were increased 40–50 percent in France and Japan, 60–70 percent in Sweden, Switzerland, and the Netherlands, and nearly doubled in the United Kingdom. In most countries, taxes were increased again in 1981 and 1983.[38] For individuals with above-average earnings, effective rate increases were even more

TABLE 4 Social security payroll tax rates, selected countries, 1967–81[a]

	1967	1971	1975	1979	1981
Austria	16.5	17.5	17.5	19.5	21.1
Belgium	12.5	14.0	14.0	14.0	15.1
France	—	8.8	10.3	12.9	13.0
West Germany	14.0	17.0	18.0	18.0	18.5
Italy	15.7	19.0	—	23.8	24.5
Japan[b]	5.5	6.2	7.6	9.1	10.6
Netherlands[c]	—	16.7	21.1	28.1	32.5
Sweden	—	11.8	15.0	20.3	21.2
Switzerland	4.4	5.8	9.4	9.4	9.4
United Kingdom[d]	—	10.3	14.0	20.0	21.5
United States	7.8	9.2	9.9	10.2	10.7

[a] Figures represent the social security tax expressed as a percent of taxable earnings. For old-age and survivors insurance and disability insurance programs, the figures represent the combined employee–employer tax rate. The tax generally applies to a base amount of earnings, which averages roughly 150–160 percent of average earnings in manufacturing (as of 1979).
[b] Rates apply to men.
[c] Rates include cost of work-related injury payments. Cost of old-age and survivors insurance and disability insurance not separately available.
[d] Rates include cost of health insurance, unemployment compensation, and work-related injury payments. Cost of old-age and survivors insurance and disability insurance not separately available.
SOURCES: Social Security Administration (1967); Zeitzer (1983); US Senate, Special Committee on Aging (1981); Simanis (1980).

substantial than indicated by the table. During the 1970s, the amount of earnings subject to the payroll tax increased more rapidly than wages (or prices) in every country under review except France and Austria. In the United States, the United Kingdom, and Japan, for example, the ceiling on taxable earnings grew at twice the rate of growth of average wages. Where benefits were not already taxable as ordinary income, moreover, efforts were made to subject a portion of benefits to the income tax (in the United States, France, and Belgium) (Zeitzer, 1983).[39]

In more than one instance, tax increases were insufficient to stem the tide, and governments moved to shore up their systems by slowing the growth of benefits. The cost-of-living adjustment of benefits became a prime target: between 1975 and 1983, the annual cost-of-living adjustment was delayed (in France, Sweden, West Germany, and the United States), capped (in Canada, Italy, and West Germany), or otherwise revised (in Belgium, Finland, the Netherlands, Sweden, and the United States). In addition, benefit eligibility was tightened for secondary beneficiaries such as children and spouses of retired workers (in West Germany, Switzerland, and the United States); duplicate benefits were capped (in Austria, Switzerland, and the United States); the retirement test, which reduces or eliminates benefits on account of earnings, was tightened in several countries; and other technical changes were made to reduce program outlays (in West Germany, Switzerland, and the United States). In the United Kingdom and the Netherlands new spending programs were delayed.[40]

Short-term solutions to long-term problems

At best, the various pieces of legislation approved in the past five to ten years were in the nature of "damage control." Social security systems faced financing problems of immediate and potentially grave political consequence; governments responded with short-term solutions. Taxes were raised, benefits were trimmed, and government subsidies were increased just enough to ensure that benefit payments were not interrupted.

Remarkably little was done to deal with the explosion of benefit costs in the next century and other simmering long-range problems. The United States and Japan, in fact, are the only countries to have enacted legislation to bolster long-range solvency. Under legislation enacted in the United States in 1983, the social security retirement age will be increased from 65 to 67 between 2000 and 2027 (leaving early retirement benefits payable at 62), a portion of benefits became taxable under the federal income tax, the cost-of-living adjustment was delayed, tax rates were increased, and coverage was expanded to certain government employees (US House of Representatives, 1983).[41]

In Japan, among other significant changes in the law, the retirement age and the tax rate applied to women will be increased gradually to equal those applied to men, replacement rates will be stabilized at current levels rather than being permitted to continue rising as the system matures, and while the distribution of benefits will be made more favorable for spouses, aggregate benefit costs will be reduced. As a result of Japan's recent legislation, it is estimated that the tax rate necessary to finance benefits in the year 2025 will have been reduced by roughly one-fourth.[42]

The European systems, by contrast, have "no concrete, long-term plans to deal with the second cycle of an aging population"—and the accompanying social security deficits—anticipated in the early decades of the 21st century (US Senate, Special Committee on Aging, 1981: 38). In marked contrast to the United States and Japan, few countries even produce long-range financial statements for their social security systems; fewer still act on those projections to maintain or periodically restore long-range balance between the two sides of the fiscal ledger. At present rates of taxation, the retiree bulge in the next century spells long-range insolvency for social security systems around the world. According to at least one estimate, many countries face tax rate increases on the order of 50–100 percent to finance benefits in the year 2030 (Ross, 1979: 6). The taxes necessary to finance the cost of health care programs for the aged would be in addition to this.

In view of the desirability of announcing program changes well in advance of implementation, the failure of governments to enact long-range solvency plans is disturbing. It reveals a fundamental lack of consensus about the future of social security and about how to allocate the costs and rewards of future developments, both foreseen and unforeseen.

A word of caution is in order, though: it is difficult, if not impossible, to determine from a set of trust fund projections which countries are better or less well prepared to handle the retiree bulge in the next century. Periodic bouts of insolvency are inevitable with pay-as-you-go financing, just as miscalculations in projections are inevitable in an uncertain world. Beyond this, consensus now need not imply consensus later. As the age distribution changes, along with the economic and political opportunities for workers and retirees, political coalitions will inevitably change, as will public policies affecting the elderly. Nothing in a set of financial statistics can ensure that these changes in public policy will arrive without political strife.

At a minimum, one must remain skeptical that simple adjustments in tax or benefit formulas constitute a solution to what ails social security. If low fertility is here for the foreseeable future, so are poor rates of return, which can undermine political support among younger people—those upon whom the survival of social security systems depends. Moreover, if the current structure of social security, including tax, benefit, and funding provisions, adversely affects economic decisions—discouraging people from saving for their retirement or discouraging the elderly from continuing to work—then the growth of these systems in the years ahead may well undermine the economic performance upon which their financial viability depends. Then too, there is the practical consideration of whether the government can, even if it wishes to do so, advance fund the retiree bulge in any meaningful way. Investing excess social security revenues in government debt, which is the practice in the United States, may accomplish little more than a rearrangement of future tax liabilities.

A realistic assessment of social security—the problems and prospects of mature systems in aging societies—suggests that reform must address not only actuarial relations between projected benefits and costs, but also the implications of the present structure of social security for the economic and demographic choices made in future years. Reforms geared toward removing the obstacles to working and saving, improving the options open to young people, and, to the extent possible, reducing the dependence of future retirees on the government for support in old age would all seem to hold promise in this regard. The ability to meet the challenges posed by the changes in economic, social, and political life likely to accompany the "graying" of nations will almost certainly depend on the adaptability of social security programs.[43]

Conclusions

This article has examined two sources of worldwide crisis in social security: aging populations, stemming principally from long-term low fertility, and aging social security systems. To date, this crisis has been manifest principally in deficits. Societies in which retired populations are growing more rapidly than working populations, and in which a growing proportion of retirees claim benefits that are increasing in real per capita terms, inevitably have social security systems beset by financing problems.

As discussed above, the United States and Japan have recently reformed their systems in an effort to restore long-range solvency. Such efforts are important, of course, in view of the size and potential impact of social security systems around the world. A giant public program that transfers resources from workers to retirees, and among retirees as well, can hardly avoid altering lifetime decisions with regard to work, retirement, and savings. These long-term and ultimately irreversible decisions are best made by individuals (and most easily accommodated by markets) with a good deal of advance notice. The less disruption of plans, such as that occasioned by ad hoc or unexpected changes in public policy, the better. Taking the steps necessary to shore up social security for present and future generations poses a challenge of monumental importance to the industrial nations of the world.

But it would be a mistake to place too much stock in government actuaries' pronouncements of "long-range balance." Periodic bouts with insolvency are inevitable with pay-as-you-go financing, just as miscalculations in projections are inevitable with an uncertain future. Beyond this, the act of legislating tax rate increases today to be borne by workers in the future, or legislating benefit cuts today to be borne some time in the future, may or may not "solve" the problem. Whether it does will depend on the degree of consensus about the nature of the problem and the range of solutions, as well as on the effects social security has on economic and demographic choices made in the years to come.

Notes

1 The Bureau of the Census projects that the population aged 65 and older in the United States will hover between 11 percent and 13 percent for the better part of two decades, through 2000, before jumping to 21 percent over the next three decades. US Bureau of the Census (1984: 9), intermediate assumptions.

2 United Nations projection for 1980–85. Unless otherwise noted, the source of population data is the United Nations (1985), which contains historical data through 1980 as well as projections, made in 1982, for the period 1980–85 through 2020–25.

3 See Bourgeois-Pichat, in this volume.

4 On the definition and measurement of population aging, see United Nations (1956) and US Bureau of the Census (1984).

5 A decline in fertility, holding everything else the same, increases the "age" of the population. A change in mortality or net migration can increase or decrease population age depending on how the change is distributed along the age distribution. Throughout, changes in fertility should be taken to mean changes in the total fertility rate (the number of children an average woman will bear in her lifetime, assuming no mortality).

6 Compared with projections prepared by individual countries, the United Nations intermediate projections tend to understate the relative size of the elderly population in future decades.

7 Corresponding to total fertility rates of 1.6, 1.9, and 2.3, with intermediate assumptions for both mortality and net migration. This compares with TFRs of 1.8, 2.1, and 2.3 assumed by the United Nations.

8 It is worth noting that the aged dependency ratio does not take into account labor force participation (actual "worker–retiree" ratios are less favorable); the age of the aged (because hospital utilization increases with age, the dependency ratio may understate the growth of the burden); or the pattern of public and private programs, with all the incentives and disincentives they embody.

In most countries, the increase in the aged dependency ratio will be offset, but only partly, by a decrease in the child dependency ratio. UN projections show total (aged plus child) dependency ratios rising by a fifth in the United States, Austria, and France, a third in Japan and Belgium, and a half in West Germany and Switzerland (see United Nations, 1985). To the extent that supporting an aged person is more costly than supporting a child and/or the support of the aged is disproportionately financed publicly, per capita tax costs would rise even with no change in the total dependency ratio. For more on this, see Clark and Spengler (1980) and Preston (1984).

9 One of the important side effects of population aging is the increase in the number of generations in families and the emergence of a sizable generation of elderly people with (and potentially dependent upon) elderly children. As a rough measure of this development, the number of persons in the United States aged 80 and over per 100 persons aged 60–64 increased from 29 percent to 53 percent between 1950 and 1981; this ratio is projected by the Bureau of the Census to peak once, at 96 percent, in the year 2000, fall to 65 percent in the year 2020, then rise sharply again with the aging of baby boom retirees. In the year 2000, the typical family is projected to have four generations, while each elderly person is projected to have fewer descendants (US Bureau of the Census, 1984: 90–98).

On the social and economic implications of population aging in the United States, see Clark and Spengler (1980), Spengler (1978), Preston (1984), Easterlin (1978), and Davis (1984). Preston takes an interesting approach, analyzing the implications of population aging for the quantity and quality of support for children.

10 See Browning (1975), Rosen (1984), and Weaver (1982).

11 This argument is based on the view that social security taxes—which are not invested in real capital but spent on current benefits—are perceived as a substitute for savings. An increase in the social security tax, accompanied by an increase in present and future benefits, for example, induces the individual to reduce private retirement savings. An alternative view is that social security is perceived as a tax-transfer scheme, the effects of

which are neutralized by intrafamily transfers. Altruistic families are seen to redistribute income among members to offset the actions of government. For example, an increase in the income of parents resulting from a tax imposed on children induces parents to increase their savings (or, analogously, induces taxpayer-children to reduce their transfers to parents so as to maintain their savings).

On the other hand, some reduction in private savings and a cost to society of pay-as-you-go financing are predicted to result if at least some people: (1) are not altruistic in the way described above, (2) are unable to fully adjust family transfers in response to changes in government policy, or (3) are not part of multiple-generation families (i.e., they are childless or parentless). For more on these two views, see Feldstein (1976), on the one hand, and Barro (1974) and Becker (1981), on the other.

12 Literally, this statement holds for each generation, and for the relation between the total benefits received by each generation and the taxes paid, or for an "average" individual. Actual tax and benefit features of the law, of course, are structured so that particular individuals or groups of individuals fare better or worse than the generation as a whole.

In this hypothetical world in which the economy and the population grow at a stable rate, either a level tax rate or a constant replacement rate could be established in the law, and the system could operate on a financially sound basis without legislative intervention.

13 For some individuals, returns will be substantially higher and for others, they will be negative, as discussed below.

14 A tax hike increases rates of return for all those who have already retired or who spend only part of their work lives subject to the new higher tax rate.

15 Empirical estimates and projections of rates of return under the US system show a sharp long-term decline in rates of return and also a significant degree of intragenerational redistribution (with rates of return projected to be negative for many individuals now middle aged or younger). See, for instance, Hurd and Shoven (1983) and Pellechio and Goodfellow (1983).

16 This is Feldstein's central argument for funding social security; see Feldstein (1976).

17 This assumes, as is typical in social security programs, that the benefit formula and the tax rate are fixed in the law; legislative action is required to change either one.

The rate of labor productivity growth is assumed to be exogenously determined and independent of population growth so that the decline in earnings growth is attributable solely to the decline in population growth.

18 Assuming the decline in fertility is permanent, the lower rate of return will be experienced fully by those entering the workforce once the population has stabilized. If the decline in fertility is temporary, then all of the losses—which may be sizable—are transitory, being borne by those who are currently old or currently working, depending on whether solvency is restored by benefit cuts or tax hikes.

19 This assumes, of course, that either the tax rate or the replacement rate is fixed in the law and that the system is actually operating on a pay-as-you-go basis. A partial reserve fund, such as that held in a number of countries, may permit temporary adverse conditions to be weathered, as discussed below.

20 According to Stanford Ross (1979), "inherent strain and instability arise—and require strategic adjustment—whenever the ratio of contributors to retired persons is lowered substantially. All industrial countries have been experiencing dramatic demographic shifts that are destabilizing" (p. 6).

The idea of introducing "automatic pilots" into social security (triggered tax or benefit changes, for example) has generated considerable interest in recent years. The National Commission on Social Security Reform recommended a measure to provide for automatic adjustments in the retirement age, on a delayed and phased-in basis, in accord with changes in longevity. Another recommendation, approved by Congress in 1983, provides that the cost-of-living adjustment will be based on the lower of two increases—in wages or prices—when trust fund reserves are extremely low.

21 See also Weaver (1984).

22 As Rosen goes on to note, the importance of these issues of risk sharing in government programs may be nullified by the

actions of families and the private reallocations that take place among members adjusting to current and future changes in family wealth. For more on this, see Barro (1974) and Becker (1981). The ability of families to adjust, however, is influenced by the size of social security taxes and transfers and the nature of the changes in the law.

23 On the crisis in the US social security system, see Weaver (1982), Derthick (1978), Boskin (1977), Keyfitz (1980), Capra, Skaperdas, and Kubarych (1982), and Ricardo-Campbell (1984).

24 See Haanes-Olsen (1976) and, more generally, Social Security Administration (1984), a basic source on programs around the world.

25 An earnings-related program of old-age, survivors, and disability insurance, such as in the United States, now exists in all of the Western industrial nations, including Japan. Some European systems, however, also include a basic pension, which either is paid at a flat rate to all elderly persons without regard to work history (as in Canada) or is based on minimum coverage requirements (as in the United Kingdom) and it may or may not involve a means-test. These programs are typically general revenue–financed and preceded the introduction of earnings-related, payroll tax–financed programs. The United Kingdom, Canada, Finland, Sweden, Switzerland, and Denmark all provide a basic pension plus an earnings-related pension.

26 In Canada, the earnings-related program began paying full benefits only in 1976; full benefits will not be paid in Sweden until 1990, in Denmark until 1995, and in the United Kingdom (which in the late 1970s revamped its social security system) until 1998. More than half the increase in Sweden's replacement rates between 1969 and 1980 was due to this maturing process; see Aldrich (1982).

27 In the United States, the ratio of taxpayers to beneficiaries, now 3.3:1, was 42:1 in 1945 and 17:1 in 1950; Board of Trustees (1985: 65).

28 In the United States, Old-Age and Survivors Insurance and Disability Insurance reserves exceeded benefit payments by 12-fold in 1950. Since 1970, reserves have amounted to less than a year's expenditures; Board of Trustees (1985: 45).

Today, Sweden, Canada, and Japan have the largest reserves. In Sweden, reserves exceeded annual outlays (in 1979) by 18-fold and amounted to one-third of gross national product. Until 1976, in fact, interest payments alone were sufficient to cover benefits. These systems are not fully funded, however, and in each case reserves are falling relative to outgo as the populations and the systems age. In introducing its program in the 1960s, Canada, for example, anticipated that by the early 1980s annual expenditures would begin exceeding outgo (as they have) and that reserves would be depleted by the early part of the next century; see Haanes-Olsen (1976) and Social Security Administration (1979: 59–66).

29 If sustained, economic growth (due to, say, a permanent increase in the rate of productivity) recreates the transitional gains of pay-as-you-go financing and permanently improves returns, and does so with no change in tax rates. If temporary, however, economic growth may lead to benefit increases (and rejuvenation of the system) that cannot be sustained in the longer term without a tax increase.

30 Given the rate of labor force participation.

31 Except where social security systems are still quite young, actual taxpayer–beneficiary ratios are considerably less favorable than hypothetical worker–retiree ratios (such as the ratio of working-age persons to aged persons or the ratio of persons under age 65 in the labor force to aged persons). In West Germany, which has 4.4 working-age persons per elderly person, the ratio of taxpayers to beneficiaries is less than 2.1:1. In the United States, the corresponding ratios are 5.8:1 as compared with 3.3:1. The tax rate necessary to finance any given level of social security benefits evidently depends on the age of the system—and tax and benefit coverage—the age of the population, and actual labor force participation and employment. For data, see Zeitzer (1983) and Rosa (1982).

32 On developments around the world, see Rosa (1982), Social Security Administration (1979), Wartonick and Packard (1983), US Senate, Special Committee on Aging (1981),

Zeitzer (1983), Simanis (1980), and Boskin (1977).

33 Social security data are from the International Labour Office (1985: Table 2); government spending data (for all levels of government) are from OECD (1985: Table R7).

34 See Aldrich (1982), US Senate, Special Committee on Aging (1981), and Zeitzer (1983).

35 Even under the financial pressures of an aging population, in 1983 France lowered the social security retirement age from 65 to 60 for workers with long periods of covered employment. As of 1983, both West Germany and Denmark were considering reducing the age at which benefits are payable; see Zeitzer (1983).

36 For data on other nations, see Haanes-Olsen (1976) and US Senate, Special Committee on Aging (1981). A pay-as-you-go system such as in the United States requires reserves equal to about 1.5 months of benefits to meet monthly payments and at least a year or so to weather typical short-term economic fluctuations.

37 If not universal, the compulsory retirement program for, say, wage and salary workers is typically part of a system of programs that covers the entire workforce.

38 Comparisons across countries are clearly imperfect given that the tax is applied to different earnings bases, finances different programs, and accounts for different shares of program costs.

39 The United States, among other countries, met part of the social security deficits by increased reliance on general revenues rather than through outright tax rate increases. Countries relying heavily on general revenues include West Germany, France, Japan, Austria, and Switzerland, with 20–25 percent of old-age and survivors insurance and disability insurance revenues met in this way (as of 1980), and Canada at the high end, with 56 percent.

40 Data in this paragraph are from Wartonick and Packard (1983), US Senate, Special Committee on Aging (1981), and Copeland (1978).

41 It is important to note that even if all of the assumptions used by the Social Security Board of Trustees prove correct, including the relatively favorable fertility rate assumption, the trust funds will run substantial deficits after the year 2030. Only if the reserves the system is projected to accumulate in the next 20–30 years are "saved" and remain available to be spent in later decades can benefits continue to be paid as the baby boom cohorts move into retirement.

42 The social security retirement age in Japan is presently 55 for women and 60 for men. For more on these reforms, see Ozawa (forthcoming).

43 Scaling back long-range benefit promises—which at least in the United States are projected to be substantially higher in real terms than today—and allowing, if not facilitating, the development of private pensions and innovative financial arrangements such as reverse mortgages hold real promise in this regard. A number of countries have taken steps to promote private savings. In the United Kingdom, the Conservative Government recently presented to Parliament a discussion paper on social security reform that includes a proposal to eliminate the government program and replace it with mandatory private pensions based on defined contributions.

References

Aldrich, Jonathan. 1982. "The earnings replacement rate of old-age benefits in 12 countries, 1969–80," *Social Security Bulletin* 45, no. 11 (November): 3–11.

Auerbach, Alan J., and Laurence J. Kotlikoff. 1984. "Simulating alternative social security responses to the demographic transition," National Bureau of Economic Research Working Paper No. 1308 (March).

Barro, Robert J. 1974. "Are government bonds net wealth?," *Journal of Political Economy* 82, no. 6: 1095–1117.

Becker, Gary S. 1981. *A Treatise on the Family*. Cambridge: Harvard University Press.

Board of Trustees of the Federal Old-Age and Survivors Insurance and Disability Insurance Trust Funds. 1984 and 1985. *Annual Report*.
Boskin, Michael J. (ed.). 1977. *The Crisis in Social Security*. San Francisco: Institute for Contemporary Studies.
Browning, Edgar. 1975. "Why the social insurance budget is too large in a democracy," *Economic Inquiry* 13 (September): 373–387.
Butz, William P., and Michael P. Ward. 1979. "Will US fertility remain low? A new economic interpretation," *Population and Development Review* 5 (December): 663–688.
Campbell, Colin D. (ed.). 1984. *Controlling the Cost of Social Security*. Washington, D.C.: American Enterprise Institute.
Capra, James R., Peter D. Skaperdas, and Roger M. Kubarych. 1982. "Social security: An analysis of its problems," *Federal Reserve Bank of New York Quarterly Review* (Autumn): 1–17.
Clark, Robert L., and Joseph J. Spengler. 1980. *The Economics of Individual and Population Aging*. Cambridge, England: Cambridge University Press.
Coale, Ansley J. 1972. *The Growth and Structure of Human Populations: A Mathematical Investigation*. Princeton: Princeton University Press.
Copeland, Lois S. 1978. "Worldwide developments in social security, 1975–77," *Social Security Bulletin* (May): 3–8.
Davis, Kingsley. 1984. "Demographic dilemmas in the mid-1980s," in Moore (1984).
Derthick, Martha. 1978. "Why easy votes on social security came to an end," *Public Interest* (Winter): 94–105.
Easterlin, Richard A. 1978. "What will 1984 be like? Social implications of recent trends in age structure," *Demography* 15, no. 4: 397–432.
Federal Reserve Bank of Boston. 1976. *Funding Pensions: Issues and Implications for Financial Markets*. Boston.
Feldstein, Martin. 1976. "The social security fund and aggregate capital accumulation," in Federal Reserve Bank of Boston (1976).
Haanes-Olsen, Leif. 1976. "Social security funding practices in selected countries," *Social Security Bulletin* (May): 24–29.
Horlick, Max. 1979. "Mandating private pensions: Experience in four European countries," *Social Security Bulletin* 42, no. 3: 18–29.
Hurd, Michael D., and John B. Shoven. 1983. "The distributional impact of social security," National Bureau of Economic Research Working Paper No. 1155 (June).
International Labour Office. 1985. *The Cost of Social Security: Eleventh Annual Inquiry*. Geneva.
Keyfitz, Nathan. 1980. "Why social security is in trouble," *Public Interest* 58: 102–119.
Moore, John H. (ed.). 1984. *To Promote Prosperity: U.S. Domestic Policy in the Mid-1980s*. Stanford: Hoover Institution Press.
Musgrave, Richard. 1981. "A reappraisal of financing social security," in Skidmore (1981).
Organization for Economic Cooperation and Development. 1985. *Economic Outlook: Historical Statistics: 1960–83*. Paris: OECD.
Ozawa, Martha N. Forthcoming. "Social security reform in Japan," *Social Service Review*.
Pellechio, Anthony, and Gordon Goodfellow. 1983. "Individual gains and losses from social security before and after the 1983 social security amendments," *Cato Journal* 3, no. 2: 417–442.
Preston, Samuel H. 1984. "Children and the elderly: Divergent paths for America's dependents," *Demography* 21, no. 4: 435–457.
Ricardo-Campbell, Rita. 1984. "Social security: A mature system in an aging society," in Moore (1984).
Rosa, Jean-Jacques. 1982. *The World Crisis in Social Security*. Paris: Fondation Nationale d'Economie Politique and the Institute for Contemporary Studies.
Rosen, Sherwin. 1984. "Some arithmetic of social security," in Campbell (1984).
Ross, Stanford G. 1979. "Social security: A worldwide issue," *Social Security Bulletin* 42: 3–10.

Simanis, Joseph G. 1980. "Worldwide trends in social security," *Social Security Bulletin* 43, no. 8 (August): 6–9.

Skidmore, Felicity (ed.). 1981. *Social Security Financing*. Cambridge: MIT Press.

Social Security Administration. 1967 and 1984. *Social Security Programs Throughout the World: 1966 and 1983*, Research Report No. 59. Washington, D.C.: US Government Printing Office.

———. 1979. *Social Security in a Changing World*, HEW Publication No. (SSA)79-11948. Washington, D.C.: US Government Printing Office.

———. 1981. "Promoting subsidized savings in the Federal Republic of Germany," *Social Security Bulletin* 44, no. 10: 39–40.

———. 1983. *Social Security Bulletin, Annual Statistical Supplement*.

———. 1985. "Proposals for social security reform in the United Kingdom," *Social Security Bulletin* 48, no. 8: 45–48.

Spengler, Joseph J. 1978. *Facing Zero Population Growth*. Durham, N.C.: Duke University Press.

Torrey, Barbara B. 1980. "Demographic shifts and projections: The implications for pension systems," unpublished manuscript prepared for the President's Pension Commission.

United Nations, Department of Economic and Social Affairs. 1956. *The Aging of Populations and Its Economic and Social Implications*, Population Studies No. 26. New York.

———, Department of International Economic and Social Affairs. 1985. *World Population Prospects: Estimates and Projections as Assessed in 1982*, Population Studies No. 86. New York.

United States Bureau of the Census. 1984. *Demographic and Socioeconomic Aspects of Aging in the United States*, Current Population Reports, Special Studies, Series P-23, No. 138. Washington, D.C.: US Government Printing Office (August).

———, House of Representatives. 1983. *Conference Report on Social Security Amendments of 1983*, Report No. 98-47.

United States Senate, Special Committee on Aging. 1981. *Social Security in Europe: The Impact of an Aging Population*. Washington, D.C.: US Government Printing Office.

Wartonick, Daniel, and Michael Packard. 1983. "Slowing down pension indexing: The foreign experience," *Social Security Bulletin* 46, no. 6: 9–15.

Weaver, Carolyn L. 1982. *Crisis in Social Security: Economic and Political Origins*. Durham: Duke University Press.

———. 1984. "The evolution of executive–legislative relations in social security policymaking," unpublished manuscript prepared for the Center for Strategic and International Studies, Georgetown University.

Zeitzer, Ilene R. 1983. "Social security trends and developments in industrialized countries," *Social Security Bulletin* 46, no. 3 (March): 52–62.

Comment: Thomas Gale Moore

Carolyn Weaver's article considers the twin problems of an aging population and an aging social security system. Weaver measures only the cost of supporting the elderly, however. A different picture emerges from a focus on total dependency ratios, which include children as well as the aged. The rise in the cost of programs for the elderly is at least partly and may be totally offset by declines in costs of supporting fewer children. Fewer children mean less crime and lower education costs. More elderly mean larger medical costs. A full accounting would involve comparing the costs of housing for children versus housing for the elderly; food for children versus food for the elderly.

It is worth noting that Table 2 in Ansley Coale's article in this volume shows that, in the long run, the proportion of the population in the 20–64 working age group is almost invariant to fertility rates. Thus the total dependency ratio is unaffected; if the costs of children are equal to the costs of maintaining the elderly, the burden of below-replacement fertility is no greater than the burden of a rapidly growing population.

Some scholars consider children as consumer goods and so discount the burden of supporting them. But the welfare of elderly parents also enters into the utility function of their children. Moreover, children were once a form of social security for adults. When "social security" was socialized, parents were able to save on children, thus freeing resources for caring for the elderly. Consequently, it is important to include the savings on children in any calculation of the costs of below-replacement fertility.

While any pay-as-you go plan is subject to shock waves, it is certainly plausible that a sufficient margin can be built-in which can lower the probability of default, or even reduce it to zero. A stable, below-replacement age distribution still can be financially feasible. On the other hand, below-replacement fertility can be offset with innovative immigration policies; for example, open entry for people ages 18 through 25 could increase the work force and hence the funding of retirement programs, without the cost of educating the young.

US Social Security Under Low Fertility

Rita Ricardo-Campbell

It is sometimes not recognized that social security systems generate tradeoffs between societal gains and losses. The gains derive from the reduction in risks related to individuals' incomes at later stages of the life cycle. The losses derive from the potential effects of social security systems on overall economic growth and levels of human reproduction.

Focusing on existing social security programs in the United States, this article discusses ways to minimize their negative societal impacts and to cope with emerging below-replacement fertility. Inasmuch as the very survival of social security systems depends on the levels of reproduction, this article considers probable adjustments of social security under conditions of below-replacement fertility.

Social security systems and their bite

Social security systems create distortions in the labor supply and savings rate that reduce the potential size of a country's gross national product. Social security is believed to depress private savings because the government, through tax revenues, promises a steady income during one's old age, reducing the need for individuals to save. Economic growth and employment become depressed because less capital is available for investment. Social security encourages early retirement by assuring monetary income or benefits at a specific age. The shorter the individual's work life, the smaller is his contribution over his lifetime to the gross national product.

If a social security system is not funded, workers pay heavy taxes to support the benefits. Faced as well with other taxes on income to support various government programs, the worker perceives his diminished discretionary after-tax income as inadequate to support a family; hence more wives enter the labor force, resulting in lower birth rates than would otherwise occur. As the retirement age and birth rate fall, there are fewer workers to support older nonworkers. As a result, taxes are usually increased. Benefit growth is rarely restrained.

The situation in the United States illustrates this general thesis. The actual average age of male retirement is 63 (Rones, 1985, pp. 47–48). In 1983, life expectancy at age 65 promised an additional 18.6 years of life for women and 14.5 years for men. Costs of social security benefits per person rise as life expectancy increases. The US system is not funded. The fund's balance as a proportion of the annual payout was less than 20 percent as of 31 January 1986. To support the benefit load, taxation on the worker's first dollar of earnings gradually rose from an initial one percent on a $3,000 base to 7.15 percent on a base of $42,000 in 1986. This contribution is matched by an identical tax on the employer's payroll on the same base. The self-employed pay both taxes, although there is a small tax credit that is being gradually phased out. Over 20 percent of the US budget is used to pay for social security benefits.

While the working individual's discretionary income is lessened by rising taxes, his or her expectations for home ownership, sending children to college, luxury vacations, and a higher standard of living have not lessened. Thus, married women increasingly work outside the home. In 1984, not only were 70 percent of women aged 20–44 years and 66 percent aged 45–49 working, but there was no drop in the percentage of women who worked during their prime childbearing years. During the 1970s, women still took time out from the paid labor force to bear and rear children. Today, women combine working and having children during the same period of their lives. The small number of births is shrinking the future tax base of worker incomes.

The ratio of all persons aged 20–64 years to those aged 65 and above was nearly 9 in 1940, fell to 5 in 1980, and is estimated by the federal government to decline to 4.5 by 2000, and to 2.6 by 2040. The effective age of retirement has also been falling. The actual number of workers available to support the benefit load of all types of beneficiaries—the aged, the disabled, and dependent children and dependent parents—has gradually declined from 5 in 1960 to 3.3 in 1985 and is estimated to decline to 2 by 2030 (Office of the Actuary, 1984, p. 41; OASDI Trust Funds, 1986, p. 72).

Demographics rule the long-run financial balance of the major trust funds of the Old-Age and Survivors and Disability Insurance (OASDI). To a lesser degree, demographics also influence the financial balance of the Hospital Insurance Trust Fund.

Although social security in the United States encompasses four programs (namely the Old-Age and Survivors Insurance, or OASI; Disability Insurance; Medicare part A, Hospital Insurance; and Medicare part B, Supplementary Medical Insurance, each with separate funds), subsequent discussion in this article, unless a specific exception is made, refers only to the OASI program.

This program is usually what the media refer to as "social security," and it most clearly illustrates the impact of the demographic trends.

The OASI program, women, and retirement

OASI provides monthly benefits to retired workers, their spouses, dependent children, and surviving parents, if any. Several benefits can be paid against the earnings and payroll taxes of one worker. Spouses' benefits were added without any tax increase, on the basis of presumed need in 1939, when only about one-fourth of women worked.

The structure of the social security system of taxes and benefits actually discourages women from working. Most women, well over 90 percent, marry at some point in their lifetime. Any woman who has been married ten years to one worker who becomes entitled to a retirement benefit has a substantial claim on the system even though she may never have worked or paid social security taxes. If she is a surviving spouse she may receive 100 percent of the earned benefit at age 65. The system is "saved" financially, because no one may receive more than one benefit. This rule works against married women who have in their own right earned a benefit through working and paying taxes (Ricardo-Campbell, 1984).

Although the US social security system discourages women from working by taxing at a significant rate the first dollar of their earnings and by direct economic penalties hidden within the complexity of the benefit structure, these factors have not offset the long-run forces that push an increasing number of women to enter the labor force. The social security benefits that favor *nonworking* married women are received at age 60 or often later—far beyond the age of bearing children—while the taxes are paid by young women on their first dollar of earnings.

In the United States, after-tax income per capita is higher among those 65 years and older than among those under age 65. Among new retirees in 1982, 83 percent of married men and their wives and 69 percent of unmarried persons had income from assets; and although the amounts were relatively small for most, over half also had pension income, and these amounts were larger: married couples' median monthly pensions were $490; unmarried men received $400, while unmarried women received only $253. Total monthly income for the newly retired in 1982 averaged $1,956 for married couples and $1,024 for unmarried persons[1] (Maxfield and Reno, 1985, pp. 7–13).

Persons 65 years and older in the United States were, through 1986, given a double exemption under the income tax law. Even when taxes are not considered, "the per capita family income of the aged exceeds that of families headed by persons aged 25–44 years"[2] (Grad, 1984, p. 17). The latter group constitutes the parents of our future generations.

Originally, US social security benefits were intended to act as a "floor," serving as only one leg of a three-legged stool that would provide cash flow in old age. Private savings and pensions were the other two legs. Although the latter two have increased in importance, for some people the stool still balances on only one leg—social security.

Built into the US social security system are factors that dictate a gradual increase in the level of social security taxes. These include the cost-of-living adjustment applied to benefits and a generous award based on 100 percent of an earner's benefit to surviving spouses at age 60.

Health care programs

The US social security program includes Medicare, with its Hospital Insurance Trust Fund and Supplementary Medical Insurance Trust Fund. Although these programs are not discussed in detail here, their financing is briefly described to give a picture of the total tax burden of the social security system and the increasing burden of the taxes that support it. The hospitalization program pays for inpatient hospital care for those aged 65 years and over and for the long-term disabled. It is supported by a 1.45 percent tax on annual earnings up to $42,000 (1986), levied against each employee and his or her employer. There are few exclusions except among government workers. The self-employed rate is double, prior to a gradually phased-out tax credit. These rates are usually added to the OASDI tax rates to give the customary, loosely referred to social security tax of 7.15 percent for the employed and matched by the employer, and 14.3 percent for the self-employed in 1986. The maximum taxable annual earnings base for all rates is indexed annually to the average of total wages, which has consistently risen. The assets of the Hospital Insurance Trust Fund were $20.5 billion at the end of 1985, or about 32 percent of its annual payout. Even though the OASI Trust Fund made final repayment of its loan from the HI Trust Fund on 31 January 1986, under all sets of Social Security Administration actuarial assumptions the Hospital Insurance Trust Fund is expected to be exhausted during the 1990s.

General revenue taxes supply most of the income to the Supplementary Medical Insurance Trust Fund, out of which physicians' services and outpatient hospital services for those 65 years and over and the long-term disabled are largely paid. In fiscal year 1985, 73.0 percent of this fund's income came from general revenues and only 22.4 percent from the participants; the remaining 4.6 percent was earned interest payments. Many physicians charge more than the federal government reimburses, and their Medicare patients pay the excess charge out-of-pocket or through supplementary insurance.

In the United States in 1980, there were 10.6 million persons aged 75 years and older; by 1990 it is estimated that they will number 13.7 million and by 2000, 15 years hence, 17.2 million.[3]

The costs of medical care for the aged and the disabled are expected to continue to rise as more persons live longer, some with impairments from accidents and strokes who 20 years ago would have died from such causes. Additionally, third-party payments create little incentive for patients to seek less costly medical care in a world in which increasingly expensive medical technology may promise longer life and better quality of life.

Social security's Disability Insurance Trust Fund (DI) is financed by a one percent tax on earnings and payroll combined, applied to the same indexed, maximum-earnings base. The benefits payable to those with long-term disability are similar to OASI benefits, but generally the levels of disability benefits are a bit larger than OASI benefits based on the same earnings. The administrative difficulties of objectively applying across 50 states a medical criterion of "permanent disability," defined as sufficient to prevent one from working, are great. The rates of permanent-disability awards, corrected for age per 100,000 persons, vary widely among the 50 states. Recent legislative debate is replete with examples of administrative control problems that led to the 1984 reform legislation.

The DI Trust Fund has been paying out more than it takes in. Its balance as of 31 January 1986 was $6.4 billion, or about one-third of the fund's annual payout, an amount that appears insufficient in view of the increasing numbers the program will cover as more impaired, and young, victims of accidents and disease are kept alive. Additionally, the later entitlement age in 2009 for the full social security retirement benefit will add to the number of those who at age 65 will be eligible for a disability benefit, but not for a full retirement benefit.

Demographic projections and the future of social security

It is reasonable to believe that the social security system's actuaries, in making their 75-year demographic projections, may be underestimating future life expectancy and overestimating the future total fertility rate of women in the United States. If their demographic assumptions are thereby too "optimistic," then the projected tax rates and base will be too low in relationship to the projected benefits. If the demographic assumptions behind the estimated, long-run costs (Intermediate II-B assumptions)[4] are wrong, either the taxes will have to be increased further or the level of benefits constrained, or both. Net immigration alone—legal and illegal—is unlikely to make a substantial difference.

Alternatively, if future births and, only secondarily, the number of immigrants are much greater than projected, it might be possible to break out of the current circular pattern of higher taxes, more women working, fewer children, a shrinking tax base, and even higher taxes.

The mortality projections

The Social Security Administration's (SSA) assumptions in its 1985 trustees report, used to estimate future mortality rates, are more defensible than those the SSA made in previous years, when critics (myself included) protested that they were too "optimistic." The SSA's 1977 predictions of life expectancy for the year 2000 of 14.6 additional years at age 65 for men and 18.9 for women were almost attained in 1985, 15 years earlier than expected. The SSA had estimated that the mortality rate would decline by only half the 1900–1978 annual average rate of decline. The rate was closer to three-fourths. I have argued, then and now, that life expectancy at age 65, not life expectancy at

TABLE 1 1985 OASI actuarial estimates (Intermediate II-A and II-B combined)[a] of life expectancy at age 65 for males and females

	Male	Female
Past experience		
1981	14.2	18.6
1982	14.5	18.8
1983	14.3	18.7
1984	14.4	18.6
1985	14.4	18.8
Projected		
1990	14.9	19.4
1995	15.3	19.9
2000	15.6	20.3
2010	16.0	20.8
2020	16.3	21.3
2030	16.7	21.8
2040	17.1	22.2
2050	17.4	22.7
2060	17.8	23.2

[a] SSA actuaries use a range of estimates. The most "optimistic" in terms of costs (I) assumes high mortality rates; the most "pessimistic" (III) assumes low mortality rates. In recent years the most commonly accepted estimate has been the Intermediate II-B. In 1986, the actuaries combined the Intermediate II-A and II-B assumptions.
SOURCE: OASDI Trust Funds, 1986, Table 11, p. 35.

birth, is the more relevant data series. The 1986 report shows data on additional years of life for men and women at age 65, reproduced in part here as Table 1.

It is difficult at best to predict age-sex-specific death rates in the long term. Although extrapolation of such rates is often attempted, it is better to take account of changes in the causes of death, such as changes in lifestyle, the environment, new diseases, and biomedical advances, including the potential for genetic engineering. The SSA actuarial report, describing its revised method beginning in 1984 for predicting mortality, briefly notes past trends for ten disease categories, lists several factors in the areas of lifestyle, environment, and biomedical technology, and then states:

> After considering how these and other factors might affect mortality, we postulated a set of ultimate annual percentage improvements in central death rates for each alternative by sex and cause of death. . . . The assumed annual improvements applied during 1983–2008 were calculated by a logarithmic formula designed to gradually transform the improvement applied to obtain the 1983 levels into the postulated ultimate annual improvements. The ultimate improve-

ments were assumed to apply during 2008–2080. (Office of the Actuary, 1984, pp. 8, 9)

Arithmetic rationalization yields precise projections.

Recent estimates place the proportional contributions of one's lifestyle—habits of exercise, proper diet, stress management, and so on—to premature mortality at about half, environmental and heredity factors each at about 20 percent, and medical care at only about 10 percent ("Heredity vs. lifestyle," 1981). What would happen to the realized future life expectancy if, say, the number of persons who smoke changed rapidly?

In 1983, US life expectancy at birth was 75 years, but at least eight other industrialized countries already enjoy a greater life expectancy (World Bank, 1985, p. 175). As of 1985, the SSA actuaries apparently do not believe that the United States will catch up with other industrialized nations even by 2060, the last year of their 75-year projections.

Although by 2009 entitlement to the full OASI benefit will require the beneficiary to be age 66 (not 65 as currently), it is unlikely that this legal change alone will induce later retirement. Men retire on the average today at age 63. The 8 percent (rather than the current 3 percent) increase per annum in benefits for each year of delay in receipt of benefits after age 65 (starting in 1990) may be effective in delaying retirement, but large companies' private pension plans that are integrated with social security will reduce that effect. By 2020, when a significant proportion of the baby boom generation will have retired, the SSA assumes that life expectancy at age 65 will be nearly 2 and 2.5 years greater for males and females, respectively, than today.

Whatever the future holds in terms of mortality rates, and irrespective of the accuracy of the SSA's forecasting models, the long-range costs of the system are quite sensitive to errors in mortality predictions. Lower death rates than government demographers anticipate will increase both the income and the payout of OASI, but the increase in expenditures will substantially dominate. If the death rates of 1984–2060 were to fall by 60 percent rather than the predicted 39 percent, the SSA estimates that the actuarial balance would shift from −.44 to −1.30 (OASDI Trust Funds, 1986, p. 99). In the future this would require greater tax revenues to pay for benefits. Higher taxes are likely to depress fertility rates still more.

The fertility projections

The sensitivity of the social security system to overestimates of the fertility rate is even greater than to underestimates of longevity at old ages. The 1986 intermediate cost estimate assumes that a stable total fertility rate of 2.0 children per woman will be reached in 2010, up from the 1983 level of 1.76 births per woman, and will remain at 2.0 from 2010 until 2060. SSA actuaries give little weight to the 200-year secular decline in US fertility.

> We believe that the total fertility rate will ultimately exceed the present low level because such a total fertility rate has never been experienced in the United

States over a long period of time, and because such a total fertility rate is well below that needed to replenish the population. We believe that the total fertility rate will not return to the high levels observed in the past because of the shift in the status of children within their families from economic assets to economic liabilities, because of the increased availability and use of birth control methods, because of the changes of the roles of women in our society, because of the increasing prevalence of divorce, and because of the increased tendency toward postponement of marriage among young women. (Office of the Actuary, 1984, p. 5)

The SSA further cites 1975 total fertility rate data (lowest 1.6) for foreign countries. In 1983, both West Germany's and Denmark's total fertility rate was 1.4, a decline in the latter country of 12.5 percent over an eight-year period (World Bank, 1985, p. 213). The SSA seems to be unaware of the implications of recent total fertility rate data.

Although the World Bank's estimates of total fertility rates for the industrialized market countries support the SSA's projections, these rates were estimated as follows:

In some countries, fertility is already below replacement level or will decrease to below replacement level during the next five to ten years. Because a population will not remain stationary if its net reproduction rate is other than 1, it was assumed that fertility rates in these economies would regain replacement levels in order to make estimates of the stationary population for them. For the sake of consistency with the other estimates, the total fertility rates in the industrialized economies were assumed to remain constant until 1985-90 and then to increase to replacement level by 2010. (World Bank, 1985, p. 238)

This assumption was made without regard to whether such rates plausibly might occur.

The SSA admits that a total fertility rate of 1.6 children per woman is "plausible" for the United States and also notes that the US Bureau of the Census uses 1.9 as its intermediate estimate.

Primarily on the basis of the business cycle, a short-run phenomenon, some scholars in addition to the SSA actuaries are predicting that the current rate of 1.8 children per woman will slowly rise in the United States to 2.0 or higher. There was an upswing in real income per capita in 1983 and 1984 and a slight increase in fertility rates. Women now entering their childbearing years and their husbands belong to a smaller age cohort than the baby boomers. It is likely that their economic rewards will rise to reflect the anticipated comparative shortage of labor, beginning about 1990. Richard Easterlin (1980) theorizes that this will probably result in women bearing more children, sufficient to make up for the earlier smaller numbers of children born.

However, this simple scenario is not assured. Deep-seated worldwide forces lie behind the long-run downward trend in fertility in the industrialized market countries. Additional considerations are thus relevant.

Sociologists stress the male role in the acceptance of birth limitation (Inkeles et al., 1983, p. 221). In many European countries as well as in the United States, however, the dominance of male decisionmaking in this area has weakened, and in most families, even in male-dominated societies, the decision whether or not to have a child is jointly made. Increasingly, women are becoming the dominant decisionmakers in this area of personal affairs in which women bear greater costs than men.

> Because of the change in technology in respect to birth control, it is the woman, and not the man, who decides for the first time in history the number of children a woman will bear. Because of this factor, it is impossible to predict on the basis of experience, future birth rates, and the statistical data available appear to support this conclusion. (Ricardo-Campbell, 1977, p. 184)

It is quite plausible that some married women use oral contraceptives without informing their husbands. A review of a 1985 television program poses the question: "And will Paul Williams find the birth control pills that his dynamic pop-singer wife, Lauren, has been taking secretly because the baby he wants doesn't fit into her career plans?" (*The Wall Street Journal*, 18 September 1985, p. 22).

The nearly 50 percent decline in use of oral contraceptives by married women aged 15–44 over the period 1973–82 is likely to be reversed in the near future. The decline was due primarily to widely publicized, inaccurate assessments of potential adverse side effects. The early medical studies linking oral contraceptives in their various forms to increased risks of cardiovascular disease and ovarian and endometrial cancers were based on *retrospective* data. The first major *prospective* study—which is statistically more acceptable—found no evidence of increased risk of cardiovascular disease among women who used an oral contraceptive and did *not* smoke, and no evidence to link oral contraceptives to endometrial and ovarian cancers[5] (Ramcharan, 1980).

By 1986, medical studies had accumulated evidence supporting the contention that the low-dose oral contraceptive *protects* against ovarian and endometrial cancers, prevents osteoporosis, and may prevent rheumatoid arthritis and lessen the risk of heart disease. Conflicting epidemiological studies on whether estrogen (a major component of oral contraceptives) as used by nonsmoking postmenopausal women increases or decreases the risk of heart disease were published in the *New England Journal of Medicine* in the fall of 1985 (Wilson et al., 1985; Stanpfer et al., 1985). The potential interdependent impact on fertility rates of a future rising rate of oral contraceptive use (as its benefits become more widely known) and currently rising rates of irreversible surgical sterilization could be substantial.

The immigration projections

Immigration, legal and illegal, by populations that have relatively high birth rates offsets lower birth rates of US residents, at least until the birth rates of the immigrants fall to the average US rate and/or the net flow into the country stops. Estimates of the number of illegal immigrants living in the United States vary from the 1980 Census estimate of 2 million to as high as 6 million.[6] The annual flow is unknown. Newly arrived illegal immigrants are primarily young adults who pay social security taxes on their first dollar of earnings. If they remain and establish residence, many will also probably collect social security benefits. To the degree that they are low-paid earners, their benefits will reflect the heavier weights that favor such earners. The SSA's 1985 estimate of future annual net immigration of 400,000, based on 1970 data, is judged to be too low. Their recently released 1986 intermediate assumption is 500,000 (OASDI Trust Funds, 1986, p. 34). If these immigration projections are too low, the projections of short-run fertility rates may also be slightly too low.

Social security policy and demographic change

Social security and family policies

Government policies directed toward the specific goal of increasing the fertility rate are unlikely to succeed dramatically, as the history of family allowances worldwide illustrates. Almost all the industrialized market economies of Europe have family allowances awarded primarily for compassionate reasons to help with the costs of raising children. These non–means-tested amounts, which help with expenses after a child is born, are insufficient to pay for the increase in family costs incurred in having a child. It is possible that such pronatalist policies have slowed the decline in fertility rates in some countries, but it is difficult to prove causation in such cases.

The United States does not have family allowances, and the income tax deduction allowed for each child is very small relative to a family allowance benefit. Further, the US social security system even works in subtle ways to discourage births; for example, sizable social security benefits enable older persons to live apart from their children. Frequent babysitting by grandparents and maiden aunts has become passé. Except for special occasions, grandparents are rarely available to babysit, and the number of reliable daycare centers is low. While technological advances decrease women's household labor, they do not take care of young children. These factors also depress the fertility rate. Whatever the degree of importance of the many interdependent factors, the underlying trends that result in the long-run decline in the fertility rate are unlikely to change direction.

Singapore has recently instituted a differential family allowance that creates economic "incentives to college-educated women to marry and have more children," in the belief that this will increase the quality as well as the quantity of future children (*New York Times*, 21 December 1984, p. 6). Singapore's government even has a Social Development Unit to foster romance among the well-educated. But as the *New York Times* reports, "Many educated Singaporean women say they have no intention of marrying in a hurry, if at all, because the society is still far from enlightened in its treatment of them. . . . A young woman in a high civil-service job said that if she married, 'that would be the end of my freedom.' 'Because I couldn't work these hours,' she added, 'that would be the end of my career, too' " (*New York Times*, 11 April 1985, p. 2). These comments could be attributed as well to many increasingly well-educated women in the United States.

Family allowances, broadly defined to cover housing and daycare subsidies, once in place are politically difficult to remove and, if substantial enough to be effective, would be so costly that they would significantly redistribute income. The costs of bearing and rearing a child include not only the direct costs of their care and the indirect costs of possible loss of current earnings of the mother, but also a reduced level of her future earnings and income because work continuity necessary for promotions, social security, and sometimes pension credits may not be maintained.

A simple, comparable, but less costly and possibly as effective an approach as specific benefits to help in the cost of rearing children would be to award two years of earnings credit for each child born in computing a social security benefit. The US social security system requires ten years of covered earnings for entitlement to a worker's benefit. The two years of credit would increase the level of working women's benefits and enter into the computation of the benefit whether or not the woman temporarily leaves the labor force. It increases the benefit level by decreasing the number of zero- or low-earning years in computing the average earnings on which a benefit is based.

The two years of earnings credit that recognizes a mother's unique contribution to society is a long-overdue reform that would cost an estimated 0.07 percent of "payroll," as defined by the SSA.

A working woman in the United States receives one social security benefit: either an earned benefit at retirement at age 62 or a derivative benefit equal to half of her husband's benefit, if he is retired, whichever is larger. If a married woman survives her husband, she may receive a derivative benefit at age 60, which is based on the full amount of her husband's benefit, *or* at age 62 she may receive her own earned benefit, whichever is the larger. Ten years of covered earnings and concomitant payment of social security taxes are required for entitlement to an earned or primary benefit.

A government's goal in taxation of personal income, whether to support social security or other expenditures, should be primarily to raise revenues— not to affect social decisions by individuals. Under the personal income tax, existing (1986) levels of deductibles and credits for daycare expenses are minimal in comparison with additional family expenses related to having children. If the government increased such economic benefits to a level sufficiently high to affect birth rates, large amounts of income would escape taxes, and revenues would become less adequate to support other government programs.

Even the choice by the government to tax *either* family *or* individual income already affects an individual's social decisions. If a working woman compares her social security tax to her benefit package, it seems that she is being encouraged not to work for pay outside the home. Yet women in substantial numbers enter and remain in the labor force and pay increasing taxes on first-dollar earnings to support the social security system. About 3.5 percent of the long-run payroll costs come from the "nonused" portion of the married, working woman's tax. Additionally, when a working woman marries, a higher marginal rate of income tax is imposed on her earnings than when she was single, or on her husband's earnings if he earns less than she. Marriage may be postponed or cohabitation replace marriage, in part for this reason. In this circumstance, the fertility rate is likely to be lower than within marriage. Heavy taxes on two-worker families have resulted in a decline in the marriage rate, fewer children being born, and an increase in the divorce rate.

The United States has the highest divorce rate in the world. Married women who work have a source of income apart from their husband's and are more independent and more willing to "risk" the economic consequences of divorce. In other industrialized countries with lower divorce rates, women are also working. In comparison with the social insurance systems of other countries, the US social security system sets the stage for divorce by imposing increasingly heavy taxes on the first dollar of earnings and by its generosity in awarding benefits to divorced persons. In the United States a person divorced after ten years of marriage may receive a derivative benefit even if the earner has not yet retired, and, upon the death of the earner, may receive 100 percent of the worker's earned benefit, while a surviving spouse's benefit in most countries is only 60 percent. Other countries may have more liberal entitlement requirements for spousal benefits, but few countries pay any benefits to a divorced spouse. In Switzerland, for example, generally a divorced spouse must have borne a child to receive benefits; other social insurance systems also favor in other ways women who have borne a child. Such a pronatalist policy has not (to the author's knowledge) even been discussed in the United States.

Part-time female employment and fertility

Despite its tax and benefit structure, the US social security system has not offset the secular trend of increasing female employment. The negative relationship between female employment and fertility rates is documented as being mutually interdependent. "Current fertility decisions . . . are affected by the current employment decisions," and cumulative fertility or the number of children a woman has also affects her current employment decisions (Michael, 1985, p. S144; see also Jones, 1981, p. 172). The scarce resource of time dominates women's fertility decisions. Gary Becker's allocation-of-time approach should be applied in analysis of *part-time* female employment (Becker, 1985, esp. p. S43).

Data from the state of Utah illustrate how fertility differentials interrelate with cultural and religious values and specific economic conditions to affect the degree of part-time female employment. In 1983, the US fertility rate per thousand women aged 15–44 was 65.8, whereas the fertility rate in Utah was

107.0, or 63 percent higher. Mormon precepts encourage traditional families, the birth of children, and intensive church involvement. In Utah, 75 percent of the population is considered to be "Christian church adherents," mostly Mormons, while for the United States as a whole the proportion is 49 percent[7] (US Bureau of the Census, 1984a, p. 52). Yet the labor force participation rate of women in Utah is about the same as for all white women in the United States. On the other hand, the percentage of Utah women who work part-time is nearly double that of women in the country as a whole (US Bureau of the Census, 1983b, Table 213, p. 68; Utah Department of Employment, 1985, pp. 2–4). Children and part-time work may be a more viable option than children and full-time work.

In the United States about 20 percent of all women workers are employed part-time (US Bureau of Labor Statistics, 1985, Table 7, p. 162). This is a much lower percentage than in the other industrialized market economies of the world. "Part-time work in the United States does not pay well whether the worker is a man or a woman. Part-timers are usually confined to the lowest-paying jobs. Women who work part-time may have the same amount of human capital as women working full-time, but many of them wish to combine, more easily than full-time permits, marriage, children and a job" (Ricardo-Campbell, 1985, p. 6). Availability of part-time work, except for the self-employed, is very limited.

The expansion of women's labor supply during the 1970s in many other industrial countries took place predominantly among part-time workers. In many of those countries, hours to shop outside of a normal working day and on weekends were very limited, thus discouraging women from working full-time. The United States has some stores that are open 24 hours a day. If more women in the United States worked part-time rather than full-time, would they have more children?

One can argue that part-time female employment can alleviate the difficult choice between working and having children. All women do not view as alternatives a job and a child, but rather recognize combining them to be a viable way of life.

Obviously, such a choice involves tradeoffs. The marginalist nature of such tradeoffs as between specific amounts of time worked and specific levels of fertility, or between incremental changes in income and incremental changes in expenditures, is part of individual decisionmaking about fertility. Many women deliberately choose work and children and try to have both a career and a family simultaneously. Such a woman is sometimes labeled "super-woman." Her tradeoffs involve additional variables that have not been analyzed or even discussed here.

Economists stress the indirect costs of forgone earnings if women quit work to bear and rear children. Many women in the United States choose not to follow this path—they have children and continue to work. The percentage of women in the childbearing years who are working is not lower than the percentage in other age groups. In 1983, among ever-married women aged

30–34, 16 percent were childless, or double the percentage in that age group in 1970 (US Bureau of the Census, 1983a, p. 5). Within a recent 13-year period, 1970–83, birth rates per thousand women for the first and second child dropped by 15.6 percent, but for the third and fourth child by 33.7 percent and for the fifth, sixth, and seventh child by about 67 percent (National Center for Health Statistics, 1985, p. 19). The large family is disappearing.

Dilemmas in US social security policy

Several questions must eventually be faced.

Is it desirable for the federal government to attempt to influence the birth rate by changing the economic balance between the rewards for having and not having a child? Some persons believe that the United States is overpopulated within the context of the world's population and the balance of natural resources. Others believe that every society should aim to replace itself and not permit a long-term decline toward extinction without trying to influence the personal decisions involved. Whatever the structure of taxes and benefits used, social security is likely to influence such decisions.

Can any government action, or several actions taken together, be effective in significantly raising the prevailing birth rate of modern countries? If so, would this be accomplished through tax systems that transfer income from persons who are not currently parents of young children to those who are, irrespective of income level? Examples of tax-financed benefits of this nature are child allowances, daycare centers, and special housing subsidies aimed at directly lessening the cost of bearing and rearing children. Other market-oriented, industrialized countries that already have some combination of these and similar benefits also have below-replacement fertility rates, often ones below that of the United States.

Would it be more effective to reduce the current transfer of income between generations, which under the US social security system favors old over young and favors them without consideration of need? Although the United States and Japan tax away less than 40 percent of gross national product while other countries such as Sweden and the Netherlands tax away over 60 percent, it appears likely that even our lower level of taxation is depressing birth rates. France, in an attempt to lessen the social insurance tax burden on its young, has recently introduced a means test for receipt of spouse's benefits.

Is it desirable for the government to create a climate of opinion that would foster creation of more part-time job opportunities during the probable "labor shortage" beginning in the 1990s, when the low birth rates of the 1960s will be reflected in fewer persons entering the labor force, and at the turn of the century, when the baby boomers start to retire? The expanding service sector lends itself more readily than manufacturing to part-time work. Employers would need to develop an acceptable system for prorating fringe benefits. The lower wage rates and fringe benefits in many part-time as compared with full-time jobs make them economically less attractive, but the reduced number of hours per week make work and child care mutually more compatible.

During recent years the US federal government has spent on social insurance and welfare programs (depending on the classifications used) 14 to 16 percent of gross national product, and at all government levels about 20 percent. The federal government spends less than 3 percent of the GNP on means-tested programs, while spending most of the remainder on various indexed retirement benefits. The latter are not funded but function on a pay-as-you-go basis, thus effectively redistributing income from young to old. It is now true that nearly everyone has a close relative who receives some type of social security benefit—hence the political difficulty in containing increases in these benefits. But the widespread, below-replacement fertility rates among the market-oriented, industrialized countries—as low as 1.3 births per woman in West Germany—portend the eventual demise of the welfare state.

It is questionable whether governments can effectively encourage more births than otherwise would occur even if they change substantially the cost/benefit ratio of bearing and rearing children. Such a ratio includes the nonmeasurable psychic costs and benefits of having a child. For example, parents derive a psychic benefit from having a child or grandchild to carry on the family name and traditions.

The strength of the underlying socioeconomic forces is great. Children are no longer considered investments, but rather consumption expenses, and the appeal of a high standard of living as dramatized on television and elsewhere is overwhelming. Two-worker families have more discretionary income than one-worker families; similarly, childless families have more discretionary income than families with children. "Children have become the primary symbol of leisure-class status. . . . [B]y having children, you're announcing that you can afford the luxury of raising them" (Kahn, 1985, p. 181).

The last few decades have witnessed a shift away from its being more socially desirable in the United States to have children to its being more desirable to have a career. Can governments really change this new ranking of values?

It seems inadequate for societies with an aging population, such as the United States, merely to acknowledge that the downward trend in the birth rate has been induced by heavy transfer payments. Some positive reinforcement that bearing and rearing children have value in our society is needed. Two years of earnings credit toward a social security benefit for each child born is a minimal step in this direction. Also desirable is planning ahead for the anticipated labor shortages of the 1990s and beyond. In order to yield an optimum supply of workers, a variety of job opportunities in respect to hours as well as skills is needed. As I have written in another context:

> The government could create an economic climate through provision of information for private employers to provide part-time jobs and work-sharing by two persons of one job.
>
> There may be a multiple public policy payoff if this approach can be realized. If some married mothers of young children switch from full-time to part-time

work the stability of family life probably increases. With more part-time jobs available more older persons will work over a longer period of their lives and lessen the drain on the social security system. (Ricardo-Campbell, 1985, p. 25)

And more women may find it increasingly desirable both to have children and to work rather than to forgo children in favor of a career.

Notes

1 The medians were $1511 and $775 respectively.

2 However, incomes of aged persons not living in families were lower.

3 Data for 1980 are from Arnett et al. (1985, p. 4); data for 1990 and 2000 from US Bureau of the Census (1984b, pp. 54, 74).

4 The Social Security Administration has at least four sets of alternative assumptions: I (the most optimistic), II-A, II-B (the most commonly accepted), and III (the most pessimistic).

5 The study followed some 18,000 women aged 18–54 over several years. For a more recent prospective, controlled study see the Cancer and Steroid Hormone Study of the Centers for Disease Control and the National Institute of Child Health and Human Development (1986).

6 For a good discussion of illegal immigrants, see Chiswick (1985).

7 The Mormon religion, which is dominant in Utah, is classified by the government as a Christian religion. Reported church and synagogue attendance in the United States has declined from 49 percent in 1958 to 40 percent in 1983; the decline has been much greater among persons less than 50 years old.

References

Arnett III, Ross H., et al. 1985. "Health spending trends in the 1980s: Adjusting to financial incentives," *Health Care Financing Review* 6, no. 3 (Spring): 1–26.
Becker, Gary S. 1985. "Human capital, effort, and the sexual division of labor," *Journal of Labor Economics* 3, no. 1, Part 2 (January): S33–S58.
Cancer and Steroid Hormone Study of the Centers for Disease Control and the National Institute of Child Health and Human Development. 1986. "Oral-contraceptive use and the risk of breast cancer," *New England Journal of Medicine* 315, no. 7 (14 August): 405–411.
Chiswick, Barry R. 1985. "Illegal aliens: A preliminary report on an employee–employer survey," Working Paper in Economics No. E-85-23. Stanford, Calif.: The Hoover Institution.
Easterlin, Richard A. 1980. *Birth and Fortune: The Impact of Numbers on Personal Welfare.* New York: Basic Books.
Grad, Susan. 1984. "Incomes of the aged and nonaged, 1950–82," *Social Security Bulletin* 47, no. 6 (June): 3–17.
"Heredity vs. lifestyle—What determines your risk of heart attack." 1981. Report to participants in the Stanford University Employee Heart Disease Risk Project. Stanford, Calif.: Stanford University, February, unpaginated.
Inkeles, Alex, et al. 1983. *Exploring Individual Modernity.* New York: Columbia University Press.
Jones, Elise F. 1981. "The impact of women's employment on marital fertility in the U.S., 1970–1975," *Population Studies* 35, no. 2 (July): 161–173.

Kahn, E. J. 1985. "Stress at an early age," *Boston Magazine* 77, no. 12 (December): 178–182; 255–257.

Maxfield, Linda Drazga, and Virginia P. Reno. 1985. "Distribution of income sources of recent retirees: Findings from the new beneficiary survey," *Social Security Bulletin* 48, no. 1 (January): 7–13.

Michael, Robert T. 1985. "Consequences of the rise in female labor force participation rates: Questions and probes," *Journal of Labor Economics* 3, no. 1, Part 2 (January): S117–S146.

National Center for Health Statistics. 1985. "Advance report of final natality statistics, 1983," *Monthly Vital Statistics Report* 34, no. 6, Supp. DHHS Pub. No. (PHS) 85-1120 (September). Hyattsville, Md.: Public Health Service.

OASDI Trust Funds. 1986. *The 1986 Annual Report of the Board of Trustees of the Federal Old-Age and Survivors Insurance and Disability Insurance Trust Funds*, 99th Congress, 2nd Session. Washington, D.C.: US Government Printing Office.

Office of the Actuary, Social Security Administration, Alice H. Wade. 1984. "Social security area population projections, 1984," Actuarial Study No. 92, SSA Pub. No. 11-11539 (May).

Ramcharan, Savitri. 1980. *Walnut Creek Contraceptive Drug Study*, Vol. 3, Interim Report. Washington, D.C.: National Institutes of Health, US Government Printing Office, Chapters 3 and 5.

Ricardo-Campbell, Rita. 1977. *Social Security: Promise and Reality*. Stanford, Calif.: The Hoover Institution Press.

———. 1984. "Social security reform: A mature system in an aging society," in *To Promote Prosperity: U.S. Domestic Policy in the Mid-1980s*, ed. John H. Moore. Stanford, Calif.: The Hoover Institution Press.

———. 1985. *Women and Comparable Worth*. Stanford, Calif.: The Hoover Institution Press.

Rones, Philip L. 1985. "Using the CPS to track retirement trends among older men," *Monthly Labor Review* 108, no. 2 (February): 46–49.

Stanpfer, Meir J., et al. 1985. "A prospective study of postmenopausal estrogen therapy and coronary heart disease," *New England Journal of Medicine* 313, no. 17 (24 October): 1044–1049.

United States Bureau of the Census. 1983a. *Fertility of American Women: June 1983*, Current Population Reports, Series P-20, No. 395. Washington, D.C.: US Government Printing Office.

———. 1983b. *1980 Census of the Population*, Vol. 1, Detailed Population Characteristics, Part 46 (Utah), PC 80-1-D46. Washington, D.C.: US Government Printing Office.

———. 1984a. *Statistical Abstract of the United States: 1985*, 105th ed. Washington, D.C.: US Government Printing Office.

———. 1984b. *Projections of the Population of the United States, by Age, Sex, and Race: 1983 to 2080*, Current Population Reports, Series P-25, No. 952. Washington, D.C.: US Government Printing Office.

United States Bureau of Labor Statistics. 1985. *Employment and Earnings* 32, no. 1 (January).

Utah Department of Employment. 1985. *Utah Labor Market Report* (October).

Wilson, Peter W. F., Robert J. Garrison, and William P. Castelli. 1985. "Postmenopausal estrogen use, cigarette smoking, and cardiovascular morbidity in women over 50," *New England Journal of Medicine* 313, no. 17 (24 October): 1038–1043.

World Bank. 1985. *World Development Report 1985*. New York: Oxford University Press.

Comment: Annelise Anderson

This comment draws on the article by Rita Ricardo-Campbell but also looks more generally at the implications of below-replacement fertility for public policy in the context of the United States.

Many observers see the change in value orientation firmly set, and its consequences for fertility difficult to change short of coercive measures. According to Paul Johnson, the historian:

> At the beginning of the 1920s the belief began to circulate, for the first time at a popular level, that there were no longer any absolutes: of time and space, of good and evil, of knowledge, above all of value. . . . [T]he public response to relativity was one of the principal formative influences on the course of twentieth-century history. It formed a knife, inadvertently wielded by its author, to help cut society adrift from its traditional moorings in the faith and morals of Judeo-Christian culture. (1983, pp. 4–5)

E. O. Wilson, the sociobiologist, puts it this way: "The first dilemma, in a word, is that we have no particular place to go. . . . [T]he danger implicit in the first dilemma is the rapid dissolution of transcendental goals toward which societies can organize their energies" (1979, pp. 3, 5).

The consequence of this basic change in our world view is that while values of different groups will no doubt vary over time, overall we cannot expect the problem of below-replacement fertility to be solved by waving the flag about motherhood. The efforts of groups like the New Right in America can be seen as an attempt to bring back more structured times, when we knew why we were here and what our proper roles in life were. But such attempts are not likely to succeed.

As Alison McIntosh demonstrates later in this volume, the financial incentives of the type tried by Western European governments also offer little hope for success. Tinkering with child allowances does not seem to be the answer. The problem is that such policies are directed toward making children cheaper, instead of reducing the costs to the prospective mother.

Rita Ricardo-Campbell has offered an insight that may provide the touchstone for public policy on fertility: "Increasingly," she says, "women are becoming the dominant decisionmakers in this area of personal affairs" (p. 304). If it is true—and I think it is—that women are increasingly the decisionmakers with respect to the number of children they choose to bear, we need to look more closely at the situation of women in the modern world. There are two essential characteristics of this situation:

— First, women have more opportunities open to them than they have ever had before, in the marketplace, the political arena, virtually everywhere.
— Second, the risk of having children—and I am not speaking here of the physical risk—is greater than it has ever been. Motherhood is no longer a secure profession. A woman has no assurance that the father of her children will stay around to provide for them while they are growing up or for her in retirement.

In other words, the developments of modern times have destroyed the security of marriage as an institution, and with it the partnership of a man and a woman in the division of labor that can result in the building of larger families.

The major source of economic security for most women in the modern world is their own earning power and, for retirement, their own pensions. In this situation, it is not surprising that women are turning increasingly to the marketplace. They are doing so in spite of some disincentives to work, as Ricardo-Campbell notes. In the United States, as second workers in a family, women may not benefit fully from their social security contributions; and US marginal tax rates on the second earner's income are high. In fact, were we to seek reasons for a failure of women to enter the labor market, we could easily cite the economic disincentives for the second worker in a family. Nevertheless, women *are* working. The economic security of their own earning power is a major reason for employment, but so are nonpecuniary benefits. In fact the extent of women's entry into the labor force may suggest that the answer to Freud's old question—whatever is it that women really want?—is that women want the same thing men want: a piece of the action. It will be difficult to take that away in societies where women have the vote.

In this context the decision to have fewer—or no—children makes sense as well. The critical questions a woman faces are whether she will be able to support her children and provide for herself in the event her husband leaves her, and whether she will be able to resume her career even if he does not. Children have consequences: they may take a woman out of the labor force or necessitate part-time work or work at a job that, probably lower paying, enables her to fulfill responsibilities to human beings who are dependent on her. And having more children has more consequences for a longer period of time. One or two may be possible; three or four may be unmanageable.

Daycare and labor-saving devices are of course helpful, but go only so far if one of the major benefits of children is derived from watching them grow—especially if one believes that parental time has some influence on how they turn out, that is, on their quality.

Consider again the words of E. O. Wilson, referring not only to human beings but to the majority of animal species:

> [I]f males are able to court one female after another, some will be big winners and others will be absolute losers, while virtually all healthy females will succeed in being fertilized. It pays males to be aggressive, hasty, fickle, and undiscriminating. In theory it is more profitable for females to be coy, to hold back until they can identify males with the best genes. In species that rear young, it is also important for the females to select males who are more likely to stay with them after insemination. (1979, p. 129)

With a divorce rate of over 50 percent, having children is indeed a perilous enterprise. The birth rate might be even lower except for the possibility that women overestimate the likelihood that they will remain married.

Social and institutional arrangements that reduce the risks of loss of current and future income to the prospective mother and improve her chances of reentering the labor force are already under way in the United States:

Current income Some firms are developing more generous policies for maternity leave. This trend is likely to continue as smaller cohorts enter the labor force and firms become more eager to retain experienced workers. Computer technology, making it possible to perform some work from a computer terminal at home, should also help.

Earning power Maintaining earning power and the ability to re-enter the labor force may be extremely important. Again, the smaller cohorts entering the labor force should be an incentive for firms to arrange part-time work or retrain valued employees. If we must have a government-funded program, one directed toward increased fertility and dealing with the problem of entry or reentry could be modeled on the GI bill's education benefits: government-financed education or retraining for women who have had three children. Such a program might encourage women to have a family on graduation from high school or college and return for higher education after the children are older. (The problem of "having it all"—children and a career—is a very common topic of discussion among women. As a matter of public policy to encourage higher fertility, we may want to encourage "having it all" sequentially, the children early and the career later.)

Retirement income Ricardo-Campbell has proposed two years of social security earnings credit for each child a woman has. My concern with this proposal is that it would apply to mothers of illegitimate children on welfare as well as tax-paying couples, and standing alone is likely to have little effect. I would go further, and institute earnings sharing. The social security tax would be levied on husband's and wife's paychecks, and the amounts would be split for purposes of credit equally between husband and wife. This could be accompanied by requiring—or permitting—taxation of up to double the base for married couples with only one earner. It would create a separate and portable social security account for every person, and spousal benefits could be eliminated; one could get divorced after nine instead of ten years without damage to one's future.

I agree that US social security tax rates are too high, and I suspect Ricardo-Campbell is right in attributing some portion of low fertility to these taxes. In the United States there is an opportunity to lower these rates by appealing to the baby-boomers now in the labor force to accept reduced benefits in return for reduced taxes, while maintaining current benefit levels for those now retired or close to retirement age. Such a change would hold those now retired harmless, while benefiting those now working and their children, on whom the high taxes to support the retired baby-boomers will fall if the benefit levels are not changed.

A second critical component of retirement income is the private pension. Since the 1970s pension rights have increasingly been considered property for purposes of US divorce settlements, and the 1984 Retirement Equity Act clarified the conditions under which a woman could gain rights to some portion of her husband's future pension (and vice versa, of course). Considering pensions as part of the property to be split up in a divorce should help to provide the retirement security women might need to make childbearing and childrearing more acceptable—that is, less risky—as women become more aware of the developments in the law.

These changes, along with the increasing use of the concept of common property in divorce proceedings, should reduce the financial dependency that accompanies the nonmarket labor of bearing and raising children, whereby women risk being left with neither marketable labor skills nor retirement security after years spent in the home. The alternative to developments such as these, in which access to the labor force and economic independence is made easier—the very developments that may be partially responsible for low fertility—is to go backward, by instituting coercive measures to deny access to contraception, creating punitive damages for divorce, or, worst of all, limiting the access of women to the working world; in other words, keeping them barefoot and pregnant. Politically such measures are unattractive and unlikely to gain acceptance, especially in countries where women have the vote.

Nevertheless, economic growth increases opportunities and makes the world's work more interesting. The pull of the workplace is likely to remain strong. The two-adult family may be an inefficient size for raising enough children for replacement fertility. The two-adult family—even more so, the one-adult family—is not the norm for human social organization. E. O. Wilson, commenting on the precipitous decline in the American birth rate, suggests that the family is not a cultural artifact destined for extinction; rather, the family remains one of the universals of human social organization. But he defines the family more broadly, as a set of closely related adults and their children (1979, p. 141).

Perhaps three adults with four children would be more efficient than two with three; or perhaps four adults with five children, or a line marriage in which men and women are alternately added to the population as needs arise. I am not suggesting that we promote such arrangements, but only that we not foreclose the possibility of three or more adults entering into a legal partnership to pool earnings and divide up assets and financial responsibility for children in the event of the dissolution of the partnership.

Finally, immigration is a partial and flexible solution. The great problem with immigration is apparently xenophobia. The effort in the United States to restrict illegal immigration through legislated employer sanctions is a displaced policy: the best data available suggest that our perception of foreigners among us is a result primarily of legal rather than illegal immigration (see Levine, Hill, and Warren, 1985; Anderson, 1986). A recent article in the French magazine *Le Figaro* raises the specter of a threat to French identity and culture from immigration (Miller, 1985). Clearly, there is no shortage of people in the world, but there is a shortage of appropriate immigration policies. More important, we lack *naturalization* policies that can lead to the acceptance and acculturation of immigrants into the societies of the modern world.

References

Anderson, Annelise. 1986. *Illegal Aliens Employer Sanctions: Solving the Wrong Problem.* Stanford: Hoover Institution Monograph Series 5, The Hoover Institution, Stanford University.

Johnson, Paul. 1983. *Modern Times: The World from the Twenties to the Eighties.* New York: Harper & Row.

Levine, Daniel B., Kenneth Hill, and Robert Warren (eds.). 1985. *Immigration Statistics: A Story of Neglect.* Washington, D.C.: National Academy Press.

Miller, Judith. 1985. "French article touches off furor about the effects of immigration," *New York Times*, 3 November.

Wilson, E. O. 1979. *On Human Nature.* New York: Bantam Books.

Recent Pronatalist Policies in Western Europe

C. Alison McIntosh

Twenty years after the onset of declining fertility in Western Europe, governments are still uncertain how it will affect their countries and what they should do about it. Demographers, mindful of past forecasting mistakes, are reluctant to rule out a return to higher fertility, especially since at least one economic theory has been advanced to explain how this might come about (Easterlin, 1980). Still, most analysts believe that current trends in marriage and family formation make an early and spontaneous return to higher birth rates unlikely (Westoff, 1978 and in this volume).

In terms of consequences, the prospects for continued economic growth are also unclear. Within the last decade, analysts seem to have reached a guarded consensus that adjustments can be made that will keep economies growing (Hansluwka, 1980, p. 310; Council of Europe, 1978, p. 242; Espenshade, 1978, pp. 667–668). Geoffrey McNicoll (in this volume) is somewhat less sanguine, citing little-researched factors of distribution and international economic relations that could nullify the necessary internal adjustments. There is greater agreement on the need for a major restructuring of the welfare state in these aging societies to avoid what many politicians see as a threat to the social contract between the generations (see, e.g., Eversley and Köllmann, 1982; Kaufmann and Leisering, 1983). One possible mitigating step, reopening the door to mass immigration, is widely rejected on the grounds that its social and political costs would outweigh the advantages of a larger labor force and a more substantial tax base. Since rates of infant and child mortality are already low in the industrialized countries, improvements in mortality control would simply add more elderly dependents to the population. Thus, many political leaders in Western Europe are looking for ways to reverse fertility trends.

Many Western European governments have increased their financial assistance to families (United Nations, 1984). Only France and Luxembourg, however, appear to have adopted a specific demographic target—the return to replacement-level fertility. Some countries, like the Netherlands, with high population densities, profess to welcome the prospect of a decrease in population size. Others, like Great Britain, have always resisted the idea of population policy. Because of the diversity of opinion, members of the European Economic Community rejected France's 1983 proposal for a joint pronatalist initiative (Tomlinson, 1984, p. 111).

Without in-depth study, it is not easy to judge a country's position on population. Governments are not monolithic and there is commonly a range of opinion, even at the center. Furthermore, even democratic governments are sometimes reluctant to disclose their intentions, for population policy often raises sensitive and potentially divisive issues. In some instances, a policy is announced but suitable measures and effective institutions are lacking, or the budget is inadequate for the task. In 1976, France adopted a demographic target—replacement-level fertility or a little above—but it has taken years to bring the institutional structure for policymaking up to its level in 1945, when pronatalism was at its peak, and, to date, financial appropriations have been modest. Still, France's persistent efforts over the last ten years seem to imply a genuine commitment to pronatalist policy. Likewise, a determination to act appears to be developing in West Germany, although a coordinated set of measures has yet to be designed and no formal pronatalist policy has been announced.

It is the thesis of this article that a key to the cautious response of low-fertility nations lies in three factors that shape the way political elites perceive demographic trends and possible solutions. First, and most importantly, public demand for population policy is weak. Historically, European pronatalist policies were associated almost exclusively with centralized and authoritarian states and somewhat monistic societies (Finkle and McIntosh, 1979, pp. 278–281). Today, by contrast, democratic governments in pluralistic societies must be responsive to the numerous and diverse interest groups that have gained access to the political process. Second, there is a lack of confidence in any of the pronatalist measures that have been proposed. Western European governments today do not have the option of addressing the birth rate directly by restricting access to contraception or legal abortion. They recognize that financial incentives have not prevented the decline of fertility; moreover, the broader measures they are now considering are both imprecise and difficult to formulate. Finally, the rationale for pronatalist policy is not compelling. In the past, pronatalist sentiment was largely based on the belief that a nation's military power and diplomatic influence derived from the size and growth rate of its population.[1] Today, demographic factors carry less weight. The wealth of a nation, the quality and education of its population, as well as its capacity to form and maintain alliances, are considered more important sources of national power (Wright, 1955, p. 362; Russett and Starr, 1985, pp. 127–161). Furthermore, although political leaders concur that low-fertility countries face difficult problems of adjustment to the changing age structure, there is a general expectation that the adjustment can be made. Governments appear loath to use the possibility of future crisis as the justification for measures that do not command broad popular support.

In the pages that follow I examine some of the features of the policy-making environment that impede the actions of Western European governments in the field of population policy. The discussion draws primarily on the examples of France, West Germany, and, to a lesser extent, Sweden.[2] These countries are of particular interest in that all three introduced pronatalist policies in response to the low fertility of the late 1920s. In France and Germany, especially, both attitudinal and institutional residues from that time still color perceptions of population questions. Sweden cannot accurately be described as "pronatalist," but that country has consistently led the way in developing social policies that have informed the population policy discussions of other nations. While France and Germany may have gone further than other Western European countries in developing their policy responses to below-replacement fertility, they do not differ significantly from other countries in their main lines of thinking.

The context of population policy

Recent years have witnessed some evolution in the way in which government leaders approach population questions. Less than a decade ago, the starting point for discussion was a country's earlier experience of fertility decline: France's pronatalism, Germany's revulsion against population policy, and Sweden's concern for social welfare and equality provided the backdrop against which contemporary trends were assessed (McIntosh, 1981). Today, policymakers seem to have come to terms with the past. While these characteristic orientations to population trends lie just below the surface and account for many of the differences among countries, policy discussions now seem to be much more firmly based on contemporary experience. In addition, because of the accumulation of research on the dynamics of low fertility and on its likely societal consequences, today's debate is more fully informed and better grounded in empirical reality.

The attitudinal context of policymaking has also been affected by the arrival at the middle and upper levels of government of individuals who have no personal recollection of either the fertility decline of the 1930s or the pronatalist policies of the 1940s and 1950s. Many people in France see the upheavals of 1968 as a watershed; since that date, they say, young people have shown little interest in population growth—a perception shared by many government officials. This lack of interest among officials brings a certain ambivalence into the heart of policymaking circles. Thus, early in 1985, Pierre Laroque, now Vice-President of the High Committee for Population, told this writer: "[President François] Mitterrand is serious about population. So is the Ministry of Social Affairs. Everyone else in the present government is Malthusian'' (interview, 1985). In Germany, the gradual passing from the scene of those who remember National Socialism should help to desensitize the question of population policy; yet, in Germany too, some officials who influence the policy process share the public's lack of interest. This was exemplified when a member of the interministerial working group that is examining the consequences of population decline commented: "The question that bothers me is why are demographers so worried about declining fertility? Germany is so overcrowded. We would be much better off with fewer people'' (interview, 1985).

These remarks are not intended to suggest that policymakers are less than conscientious in their search for a solution to a difficult problem. What they do imply is that many of the bureaucrats to whom high-level decisionmakers look for ideas and advice, who write the reports and draft the proposals for policy, are not themselves fully convinced of the gravity of the demographic situation. The analyses they prepare and the proposals they advance are likely to be tempered by alternative values that they consider equally or more important.

The economic context

For roughly a decade, the development of population policy has been severely constrained by financial difficulties originating both in the oil crises of 1973 and 1979 that precipitated the economic recession, and in age-structural changes resulting from low fertility. The escalating cost of health care, especially for the elderly; the demographically inspired increase in the number of claimants of old-age pensions; and the feeble rate of economic growth, which has raised the demand for unemployment benefits and retirement pensions while it has reduced the number of workers contributing to the funds—these are only the most obvious elements. Because of these financial constraints, governments in many Western European countries have had to hold the line on—or even cut—their assistance to families.

Neither France nor Germany has been able to avoid the cuts. In 1982 Germany's Christian Democratic/Liberal government was forced to reduce the budget for family policy as part of an emergency restructuring of the social security system. This was mainly effected by reducing the child allowance (*Kindergelt*) for middle and upper income families, but the cuts also included a reduction in the benefit payable for the six-month maternity leave, and elimination of the education allowance for children of school age.[3] This was an embarrassing experience for a government that had campaigned for office on the basis of the opposition's "neglect" of the population issue.

In France, likewise, the egalitarian but expensive family policy proposed by the Mitterrand government in 1981 had to be abandoned a year later when the social security funds were found to be in deficit. The new policy would have greatly reduced the special allowances introduced by President Valéry Giscard d'Estaing for the third child, increased allowances for second children, and gradually extended them to the first child. After the crisis, the socialist government returned to a less expensive policy that directed most of its assistance to families in greatest need—including three-child families (Hecht, 1982, p. 221). In 1982, moreover, as part of a broader economic policy, the Mitterrand government proposed taxing family allowances. This was the first time such a proposal had been made by a socialist government in France (ibid., pp. 212–214).

Recovery from the world economic recession is taking place more slowly in Europe than in the United States. It is all the more remarkable, then, that at the end of 1984 the West German government announced its intention to restore and increase its assistance to families beginning in 1986. The duration of compensated postmaternity leave is to be extended to a full year, with the benefit to be payable whether or not the woman participates in the labor force. The income tax deduction for dependent children is to be dramatically increased, from DM 432 to DM 2484 (from approximately US$215 to $1238), and a small increase is also scheduled in the deduction for dependent adults. In addition, education allowances for school children will be raised. Further small changes in the income tax structure are to be introduced in 1988 (*Bulletin*, January 1985, pp. 13–14). In the opinion of Rita Süssmuth, a family sociologist later appointed Minister of Youth, Family, and Health, expenditures of this magnitude would not have been considered at such a time in the absence of serious concern over the birth rate (interview, 1985).

The institutional context

The official policy statements collected by the United Nations (1984) indicate that Western European governments are relying to a great extent on family policies to address the decline of fertility. This is not surprising, since these well-entrenched and popular programs provide governments with a ready-made instrument for tackling the fertility problem indirectly while maintaining some distance from the sensitive issues surrounding population policy. Additionally, since many people, especially on the political right, associate the fertility decline with the spread of "destructive" social practices—abortion, divorce, cohabitation outside of marriage—family policy appears to them an appropriate vehicle for reform.

In some ways the use of family policy to stimulate the birth rate is a carryover from the 1930s and 1940s. Although the history of child allowances as an income-maintenance device can be traced back to the mid-nineteenth century (Glass, 1940, pp. 99–100), family policy was primarily developed as a response to the widespread poverty and low fertility of the 1930s (Glass, 1940; A. Myrdal, 1941). Since that time it has been greatly elaborated, and the social welfare objective has come to dominate the pronatalist aim. Indeed, the politics of family policy today is largely concerned with ways of revitalizing the demographic aims.

Family policies vary widely in their scope and in the number and complexity of their measures. As a minimum, however, most countries now provide the following as part of their social insurance programs:

— medical care during pregnancy and child birth
— a mandated period of compensated pre- and postmaternity leave
— health supervision of infants and young children
— cash allowances for families with children up to school-leaving age, or beyond it if the child is obtaining job training or higher education
— assistance in obtaining and paying for suitable housing—either low-cost loans for purchasing or furnishing a home, or subsidies for rental accommodation
— some form of income tax relief for dependent children.

More recent additions to family policy include the right of access to contraceptives and legal abortion, and measures intended to reconcile the demands of parenthood with those of participation in the labor force. In introducing the latter, many governments have had the birth rate in mind; measures include the provision of daycare and leisure-time centers for children, and extended periods of maternal or parental leave that may be taken after the expiration of maternity leave. Such leave may or may not be compensated but usually includes the right to return to the same or a similar job, and the protection of seniority. In some countries parental leave may be counted as work in fulfilling the eligibility requirements for an old-age pension (social security).[4]

Despite its popularity, family policy is an imperfect instrument for stimulating fertility. Reliance on family policy tends to divert attention from the consideration of other approaches, and it manifestly has not prevented the decline of fertility. Although no one can tell what the level of fertility would be in the absence of family policy, most analysts believe that new or increased family incentives have at most a temporary effect on the *timing* of births and do not influence the *size* of the completed family. Not all scholars agree with this assessment, however. In France, Gérard Calot and Jacqueline Hecht (1978) estimated that approximately 10 percent of French fertility in the late 1940s and 1950s could be attributed to pronatalist family legislation. More recently Jean-Claude Chesnais (1985), on the basis of correlations between the magnitude of social transfers to the family and fertility levels in several countries, has argued that family policy can be effective in raising fertility.

The pronatalist effect of family policy is weakened by the dual, and frequently contradictory, objectives of welfare and pronatalism. Within a family ministry, demographic policy has to compete with many other programs for both funding and visibility. In France, for example, population policy is a subsection of family policy, which is only one of the responsibilities of the social security administration. Under the socialist government, social security itself constituted only one division among many in an umbrella Ministry of

Social Affairs and National Solidarity with still broader responsibilities. Indeed, family ministries are almost invariably embedded in multifunctional ministries of wider scope. Inevitably, in such circumstances, the focus of some proposals may be lost as they are shaped to conform with overall policy, or measures introduced in one department may conflict with those of another.[5] Processes of this kind account for much of the incoherence of family policy, as well as a weaker demographic impact than was intended by pronatalists.

The almost universal tendency to assign responsibility for family welfare to large composite ministries reflects not only the broad scope of family policy, but also the low status accorded family departments within the government hierarchy. Low status means that family ministries are likely to have tenuous access to the centers of government power; just as important, they have little capacity to influence or coordinate the activities of other government agencies. The need for such coordination is particularly acute in the formulation of population policy, as demographic trends are widely thought to be affected by conditions that cut across several sectors of a government's economic and social policy. Immigration and labor policy are two such sectors to which we return presently. However, even within the central core of population/family policy itself, new ways of defining the field are making the problem of coordination more complex.

In a major change from the philosophy of the 1940s, policymakers in today's more affluent world have come to doubt the efficacy of financial incentives as a means of encouraging women to bear more children. Uncertain about what would be more effective, governments are turning to a broader concept of family policy that has emerged since the 1970s. Much policy discussion today is focused on ways to create a social environment that is more closely adapted to the needs of parents and children. Advocates of such an approach have in mind not only improvements in working hours and conditions for parents of young children, but also such proposals as better integration of different age groups in housing areas; provision of more recreational facilities in the suburbs; better public transportation between the home, work, daycare centers, and shopping areas; traffic-free streets in residential areas; more parental involvement in daycare and nursery centers; the right to stay at home with sick children without loss of wages; and a host of similar measures.[6]

From a demographic perspective, the trouble with these proposals is that they are indirect and nonspecific with respect to fertility, and their introduction would require the collaboration of a diversity of interest groups as well as governmental and nongovernmental agencies at both central and local levels. The multiplicity of both actors and objectives makes the formulation of a coherent set of measures difficult. Even France, with its pronatalist past and institutions with extensive experience in population policy formulation, has encountered problems of this sort. Throughout the 1980s, members of the High Committee on Population, the principal institution for advising on the formulation of population policy, have had difficulty in reaching agreement.[7] Members of the committee interviewed in 1985 attributed the problem, in part, to the size and diverse interests of the membership since its reconstitution in 1979. In an effort to create a more effective working environment the committee was again reorganized in 1985 and its membership reduced in number. Like his predecessor, Charles de Gaulle, President Mitterrand has assumed the presidency of the committee, ensuring once again that its advice reaches the highest political level (*Bulletin Quotidien,* 1985, pp. 13–14).

The range and scope of family policy proposals are likely to be even greater impediments to the elaboration of coherent policy in West Germany, where specialized institutions for population policymaking are lacking and where responsibility for policy formulation and implementation is divided between the federal and state governments (McIntosh, 1983, pp. 202–207).

Labor and immigration policy

Even a brief discussion of institutional coordination would be incomplete without some consideration of where labor market and immigration policy fits within the broader context of pronatalism. In the search for ways to reconcile the conflicting demands of parenthood and work, the introduction of the right to an extended period of postmaternity leave seems to have been one of the few successes. Early attempts to provide mothers with longer maternity leave, or to allow them to work shorter hours for the same pay, were frequently opposed by feminist groups and trade unions, which feared this would reinforce the marginalization of women in the labor market; the idea became more acceptable when the right was extended to either parent. However, unions still express opposition to attempts to provide more flexible working hours. In France, the government recently reached agreement with unions and employers over working conditions for parents, but the proposal was rejected by the majority of workers (interview, 1985). According to informants in both France and Germany, employers are generally more receptive than unions to the idea of change; nevertheless, while not strongly opposed to making working conditions more compatible with parental responsibilities, employers tend not to actively promote the necessary changes since these make the task of management more difficult.

To this writer's knowledge, Sweden has elaborated the only really successful labor market policy for parents. But that country instituted the parental insurance scheme as part of a national effort to bring about equality between the sexes, several years before the problem of low fertility was recognized. One of the guiding ideas of this policy was that every adult—man or woman, with children or without—should be responsible for his or her own economic support, and the unions cooperated with employers and government to make this possible (Reimer, 1986). Most of the unions, both for professionals and workers, now have well-established departments to look after family interests.

In many ways, however, Sweden is a special case. The society and its institutions are small, and there is a long tradition of cooperation between workers and employers and between government and societal organizations in general (Anton, 1980). While these conditions for coordinated policymaking have no parallel elsewhere in Western Europe, even Sweden's extensive provisions in the field of work and family have not prevented the continued decline of fertility.

Western European nations have long relied on immigration to supply their need for labor in times of economic prosperity. Today, however, immigration policy has become separated from population policy in general and is no longer regarded as even a partial solution to the problem of low fertility. The protracted economic recession in Western Europe has exacerbated the problem of assimilation, and governments that closed their borders to newcomers in the early 1970s are now trying to send unemployed immigrants home. Although a racist attitude is currently evident in several countries, it is difficult to believe that Europeans will not reconsider their immigration policies once prosperity returns—particularly countries such as France, whose experience with immigrant labor dates back 150 years (Spengler, 1938, pp. 194–195).

The politics of pronatalism in the 1980s

In France and Germany, as well as in some other Western European nations, it is not hard to reach consensus on the goal of demographic policy: replacement-level fertility. What is more difficult is agreement on the means to achieve it. As in the 1930s, the political debate over low fertility is strongly influenced by ideologically inspired differences over what conistutes the "good society." It is hardly surprising that political views on an issue of such consequence for society should be shaped in part by the ideological preferences of political parties, and incorporated into their global visions of the ideal society. This was the case in the 1930s and it continues to be true today. Although there is considerable merging of views toward the center of the political spectrum, there are nevertheless distinct left/right differences both in the significance attached to population growth and in the policy instruments the political parties choose to employ.

In Western Europe, both in the 1930s and today, rightist parties have chosen measures that would support the traditional family. An official of the family ministry in Bonn expressed it thus: "For the CDU [Christian Democrats], the starting point of the family is marriage. A family starts when a child is born to or adopted by a couple" (interview, 1985). In terms of reconciling parenthood and work, most right-wing parties would prefer to give women an "education allowance" to remain at home with young children. This type of measure is often justified by conservatives as giving a woman the choice between caring for the child herself or paying someone else to do so. Generally speaking, however, the suggested allowances are too small to compensate for loss of wages.[8] Leftist parties, by contrast, generally dislike education allowances, arguing that they tend to put pressure on women to leave the labor force. Instead, such parties usually attempt to provide sufficient places in daycare facilities for all children who need them. This is a much more expensive proposition that is seldom achieved, although attainment is becoming easier as the number of small children decreases.

Deductions for dependent children from pretax income are another instrument frequently advocated by liberal and conservative parties, whose support often comes mainly from middle and upper income groups. Socialists, on the other hand, regard tax deductions as unfair to low-income families, who derive less advantage from them. Again, in recent years, some of the more extreme elements of the political right have become alarmed at the changes taking place within the family. As in the United States, they would like to limit the right to legal abortion, restrict the access of young people to contraceptives, and, somehow, discourage cohabitation outside of marriage. So far, governments of all political hues have resisted taking such steps; nevertheless, the principal measure introduced by the Conservative/Liberal coalition government in Bonn in its first years in office was the creation of a Mother and Child Foundation with limited funds to assist poor women who would otherwise terminate their pregnancies.

Once elected to office, political parties must compromise, and governments in both France and Germany have deviated significantly from the positions they took while in opposition. During the 1980s, new government coalitions—Socialist/Communist in France, Conservative/Liberal in West Germany—have been forced by economic and political pressures to modify their stance. The result, in both countries, has been a marked convergence toward the policies of the other side. To understand the nature of these shifts and how they came about, we will briefly examine the policy activities of the various governments of France and West Germany.

In France, the first attempt in many years to strengthen the pronatalist impact of family policy was undertaken in the mid-1970s under the center/right administration of President Giscard d'Estaing. Although Giscard spoke often of the importance of population growth for France's international standing, his policy instruments were weak. Simone Veil, his family minister until his last year in office, was a committed feminist who personally disliked the idea of stimulating fertility. It is doubtful whether Veil, whose chief accomplishment was to secure passage of a highly controversial bill to liberalize abortion,[9] gave Giscard's pronatalist initiative more than token support. In fact, a spokesman in her cabinet took pains to stress that the new pronatalist policy was a personal initiative of the president, not of the minister (interview, 1978).

In the mid-1970s, moreover, Giscard had to tread carefully. Public opinion did not support a return to the familiar type of pronatalism. In announcing his "new family policy" before the National Union of Family Associations (UNAF) in 1975, the president denied that it had any pronatalist intent (Giscard d'Estaing, 1975). Steps were taken to remove a number of measures left over from the 1940s that were considered coercive. One of these was an additional allowance payable for babies born within a specified period after their parents' marriage or after the birth of a previous child. In response to their demand for job security, many employed women were given the right to two years of leave after the birth of a baby; however, this leave was not compensated. For most of his term of office, Giscard's policy remained largely in the realm of rhetoric.

Toward the end of the decade, Giscard got a chance to act. A survey conducted by INED (Institut National d'Études Démographiques) showed an upward movement, from two children to three, in "ideal family size," and women stated that poor economic conditions were preventing them from bearing a third child (Girard and Roussel, 1979). As a response, the amounts of several allowances payable for the third child were increased, yet the total still amounted to less than a professional wage. Economic conditions following the oil shock of 1979, and perhaps the president's lack of full commitment to the pronatalist tack, precluded a serious effort to reverse the birth rate.

Arriving in office in 1981, the new socialist government of President Mitterrand attempted to set in place a family policy that would be much broader in scope and more egalitarian. It was intended that family policy would treat all children equally, irrespective of birth order, and efforts were to be made to promote equality between the sexes. The overall aim was to reshape society in ways that would make childrearing less onerous. Within the family ministry, the secretary of state eliminated the most substantial of the special allowances created by Giscard for women having a third child, and simplified the family allowance system. But, as already mentioned, proposals to extend the family allowance to all children equally (including the first) were too expensive and had to be abandoned.

The financial crisis provoked by the Socialists' egalitarian measures marked a turning point in the Mitterrand administration's approach to family policy. Taking the initiative himself, the president returned to the less expensive expedient of placing the emphasis on the third child. The government has also introduced an allowance to cover the previously uncompensated right to leave from work following the birth of a baby. However, the benefit covers only the first 12 months of leave, and is available only to parents having a third or higher order child. In short, the difficulty of making ends meet forced the Mitterrand government into a policy hardly distinguishable from Giscard's.

In West Germany, the first five years of the Christian Democratic/Liberal (CDU/FPD) coalition government brought fewer changes than might have been anticipated from the CDU's position while in opposition. As in France, both political and economic realities tied the government's hands. Compared with France, Germany in the 1970s was an even less favorable place in which to elaborate a population policy. The end of National Socialism had left Germany without demographers and demographic research institutions; with a highly decentralized governmental structure; and with a strong aversion to the idea of population policy. This aversion is said to have been shared by Helmut Schmidt, who succeeded to office in 1974. Although the shortage of expertise is now less acute and population questions have become less sensitive, progress toward enacting a pronatalist policy is inevitably slow and cautious.

For the balance of the 1970s, the Social Democratic/Liberal (SPD/FPD) coalition government concentrated on educating itself on population questions. The Federal Institute for Population Research was created in 1974, and in 1977 an interministerial working group was appointed to synthesize scientific and bureaucratic opinion on the societal implications of declining population growth. Hampered at first by a dearth of information in some critical areas, the group's definitive report did not appear until 1982 (FRG, 1984). After extensive review, the report was accepted virtually unchanged by the conservative government. The working group was then requested to examine whether it would be desirable to draft proposals for policy, but so far the group has not reported.

In terms of policy, the Social Democratic/Liberal government attempted primarily to improve conditions for women: amid intense opposition from the political right, the laws on both abortion and divorce were liberalized. Nevertheless, despite the economic constraints, the child allowance was substantially increased in 1979. In the late 1970s the federal government also underwrote part of the cost of the economic program instituted in West Berlin in an effort to halt the heavy outmigration from that city (McIntosh, 1983, pp. 215–219). This was an exceptional move that reflected West Berlin's symbolic and strategic importance. Beyond this, most pronatalist efforts made during Chancellor Schmidt's term of office were at the state level. Surprisingly, the instrument used by these governments was modeled on the family-formation grants employed by the National Socialists in the 1930s. Low-interest loans were made available to newly married couples to assist them with housing, and their repayment was to be cancelled gradually at the birth of each child, up to the third, born within a stipulated number of years.

In 1979, the opposition Christian Democratic/Christian Socialist parties made population and family a leading issue in their campaign for the federal elections of 1980, attacking the Schmidt government for what the conservatives called its "irresponsibility" in failing to deal with the population decline. There was a strong element of political sophistry in this tactic, however, as the opposition parties were well aware that no money would be available for population policy even if they were elected (interview with the CDU, 1978). In fact, as we have seen, one of the new government's first acts was to reduce the Kindergelt and other allowances for families.

More than five years elapsed before the Christian Democratic/Liberal coalition found it possible to carry out its election promises. As mentioned above, two expensive new pronatalist measures, an allowance to cover the cost of a year of "baby leave" and further tax deductions for dependent children, were announced late in 1984 and were scheduled to take effect in 1986. Within a few months, however, this pronatalist thrust was counterbalanced by the announcement of a new, socially advanced policy for women.

The policy's aim is the achievement of full equality between the sexes, both at home and at work (*German Tribune,* 31 March 1985, p. 3). It was thought by some political elites in West Germany that this was a response to a sharp decline in the number of women's votes going to the government parties in the recent state elections (interviews, 1985).

Irrespective of their ideological preferences, therefore, once in office governments in both France and Germany have adopted a highly pragmatic approach to low fertility. In concrete policy terms, there has been a convergence toward instruments that appeal broadly to the public. Except, possibly, for the new German measures, budgetary appropriations have been relatively modest. An immediate explanation for this low-key approach is the continuing economic weakness that has set a limit on governmental expenditures. A more fundamental explanation, however, is tied to the changes taking place in patterns of family formation: young people—and especially women—no longer want to be tied down by large families. This is one of the reasons behind the West German government's decision to move closer to the position of its center and left wings. As an official of the family ministry told this writer, "The CDU has realized that it must start where the people are" (interview, 1985).

In both France and Germany in 1985, informants spontaneously stated that there no longer exists a political lobby for the traditional family. In both countries, networks of family associations have long played a leading role in articulating the needs and demands of families. This is no longer the case. In Germany, a spokesman for the family ministry, himself a former family association employee, summarized the situation thus: "Remember, there are two sorts of power. There is the kind that comes from being listened to by government, and the kind that brings votes. The family associations only have the first kind." In France, the family associations no longer speak with one voice. In order to survive, these former bastions of tradition have had to open their doors to all comers—single-parent families, divorced and unmarried parents, cohabiting couples—whose interests often differ from those of traditional families. In sum, although they "are useful as critics," family associations are "too divided among themselves to make an effective lobby" (interview, Ministry of Social Affairs, 1985).

Furthermore, advocates of pronatalist policy in France no longer receive the volume of support that used to come from associations whose primary purpose was to lobby for such policy. Today there are only two nationally known pronatalist associations, the century-old and highly respected Alliance Nationale: Population et Avenir, and the newer Association pour la Récherche et l'Information Démographique. Neither of these associations commands widespread support, and both operate on a shoestring budget. More significantly, both associations have been obliged to abandon the strongly pronatalist position characteristic of the past. Neither organization attempts to promote "la famille nombreuse" of former times; nor do they emphasize the third child in a family. Basing their objectives on INED studies that have repeatedly shown that French women bear fewer children than they say they want, both associations now aim only at "removing the obstacles that prevent women from having the number of children they desire" (interviews, 1985). This is a much weaker position.

Concluding remarks

Political leaders in many countries of Western Europe are concerned at the continuation of below-replacement fertility, and many believe that governments should intervene to bring about a recovery in the birth rate. This article illustrated a number of barriers to the formulation of pronatalist policies. At the most practical level there are distinct limits to governments' ability to finance the measures they deem necessary. More profoundly, governments are encountering difficulties in formulating a pronatalist policy. Conscious that traditional family policies have not prevented the decline of fertility, and ignorant of the precise reasons for the fall, political leaders are now considering a more encompassing approach that might bring about a fundamental reshaping of society. As might be expected, policies that touch on numerous aspects of social and economic organization are hard to formulate in a coherent and coordinated manner.

By far the greatest impediment to governmental decisionmaking is that ordinary people do not want a pronatalist policy. Western Europeans have developed a way of life and patterns of family formation that are incompatible with the objectives of pronatalist policy. In the pluralist and democratic nations of Western Europe, governments are unwilling to introduce policies in areas that do not command a broad societal consensus. This is the situation identified decades ago by Gunnar Myrdal and articulated in his Godkin lectures at Harvard University under the title *Population: A Problem for Democracy* (1940). The intervening years have done little to lessen this dilemma of democratic government.

Conceivably, the political climate for population policy might be improved if certain changes were to occur. If public opinion took on once again a more familistic orientation; if researchers identified more precisely how decisions on childbearing are made so that more focused policy instruments could be designed; or if clear evidence were to be adduced that low fertility was visiting serious harm on the economy, the society, or the polity—under such conditions a consensus in favor of pronatalist policy might be achieved. In the absence of one or more of these changes, it is likely that governments in Western Europe will continue to tinker at the edges of family policy, working incrementally and without a clear sense of direction.

Notes

The author thanks Jason Finkle and Gayl Ness for their comments on an earlier draft of this paper.

1 For a discussion of the historical determinants of pronatalist policy see Finkle and McIntosh, 1979, pp. 278–281; and McIntosh, 1983, pp. 27–41.

2 The opinions expressed in this article are based in part on over 100 interviews with politicians, middle and upper level government

officials, and academic and other informed observers in France, West Germany, and Sweden in 1978, in France and Germany in 1985, and less systematically in Great Britain between those two years.

3 Information received in 1985 from informants in the Ministry of Youth, Family, and Health and the Federal Institute for Population Research.

4 The details of family policies are constantly changing, but the main outlines show some stability. Good reviews may be found in Kamerman and Kahn, 1978; and Kamerman, Kahn, and Kingston, 1983.

5 An interesting example of the effect of conflicting objectives presented itself during an interview with an official responsible for French family policy under the socialist government. Asked whether the ministry might consider changing those provisions that result in single-parent and other nontraditional families receiving more assistance than married couples with children, the official replied: "We could do something about it, but it is unlikely. That is an old-fashioned idea. Why should the ministry support only one type of family? *Besides, those are the people who really need the help*" (interview, 1985, my emphasis; see also Sullerot, 1984). For a discussion of the ministry's policy on this point see Laroque, 1984, pp. 50–52.

6 This type of approach was elaborated during the 1970s in Germany, in the family reports prepared periodically for the Ministry of Youth, Family, and Health (FRG, 1975, 1979); in Sweden, where it often came up in interviews in 1978 (see e.g. Liljeström, 1978); and more recently in France (see e.g. Boulaya and Roussille, 1982).

7 See, for example, the remarks of the Minister of Labor and Participation in his introduction to a report on the work of the committee, as well as the minority opinions attached to the report (France, 1980).

8 The education allowance recently introduced in France (starting with the third child) is only FF 1000 a month (approximately US$150), compared with a minimum wage of FF 3500–4000 and an average wage of approximately FF 6000 per month in 1985.

9 Interestingly, although a government bill, both in 1975 when it was adopted for a trial period and in 1979 when it was confirmed, the abortion bill was passed in the National Assembly by the unanimous vote of the opposition left-wing parties. Very few members of the government or parties of the right supported it (*Le Monde*, 1 December 1979, pp. 1, 8).

References

Anton, Thomas J. 1980. *Administered Politics: Elite Political Culture in Sweden*. Hingham, Mass.: Martinus Nijhoff.
Boulaya, Nicole, and Bernadette Roussille. 1982. *L'Enfant dans la Vie: Une Politique pour la Petite Enfance*. Report to the Secretary of State for Family Affairs. Paris: La Documentation Français.
Bulletin (Bonn), 5 January 1985.
Bulletin Quotidien, 25 October 1985. Paris: Journal Officiel.
Calot, Gérard, and Jacqueline Hecht. 1978. "The control of fertility trends," in *Population Decline in Europe*, ed. Council of Europe. New York: St. Martin's Press, pp. 178–196.
Chesnais, Jean-Claude. 1985. "Les conditions d'efficacité d'une politique nataliste: examen théortique et examples historiques," in *International Population Conference, Florence, 1985*, Vol. 3. Liège: IUSSP, pp. 413–425.
Council of Europe. 1978. *Population Decline in Europe*. New York: St. Martin's Press.
Easterlin, Richard A. 1980. *Birth and Fortune: The Impact of Numbers on Personal Welfare*. New York: Basic Books.
Espenshade, Thomas J. 1978. "Zero population growth and the economics of developed nations," *Population and Development Review* 4, no. 4 (December): 645–680.

Eversley, David E. C., and Wolfgang Köllmann (eds.). 1982. *Population Change and Social Planning: Social and Economic Implications of the Recent Decline in Fertility in the United Kingdom and the Federal Republic of Germany.* London: Edward Arnold.

Federal Republic of Germany. 1975. *Zweiter Familienbericht: Familie und Sozialisation-Leistungen und Leistungsgrenzen der Familie hinsichtlich des Erziehungs- und Bildungsprozesses der jungen Generation.* Bonn–Bad Godesberg: Bundesministerium für Jugend, Familie und Gesundheit.

———, Sachverständigen Kommission der Bundesregierung. 1979. "Die Lage der Familien in der Bundesrepublik Deutschland," Dritter Familienbericht. Deutscher Bericht. Drucksache 8/3120. 20 August.

———, Ministry of the Interior. 1984. *Bericht—Über die Befolkerungswicklung in der Bundesrepublik Deutschland,* Part II.

Finkle, Jason L., and Alison McIntosh. 1979. "Policy responses to population stagnation in developed societies," in *Social, Economic and Health Aspects of Low Fertility,* ed. Arthur A. Campbell. NIH Publication No. 80-100. Washington, D.C.: National Institutes of Health, pp. 275–297.

France, Ministry of Labor and Participation. 1980. *Rapport de Synthèse de Travaux du Haut Comité de la Population.* Paris.

German Tribune (Hamburg), 31 March 1985; 13 July 1986.

Girard, Alain, and Louis Roussel. 1979. "Fecondité et conjoncture: une enquête d'opinion sur la politique démographique," *Population* 34, no. 3 (May–June): 567–588.

———, and Louis Roussel. 1982. "Ideal family size, fertility, and population policy in Western Europe," *Population and Development Review* 8, no. 2 (June): 323–345.

Giscard d'Estaing, Valéry. 1975. Speech at La Bourboule, 13 July. Abstracted and reprinted in *Une politique pour la famille,* Actualités-Service, No. 306. Paris: Service d'Information et de Diffusion, n.d.

Glass, David V. 1940. *Population Policies and Movements in Europe.* Oxford: The Clarendon Press.

Hansluwka, Harald. 1980. "Needed research," in *Social, Economic and Health Aspects of Low Fertility,* ed. Arthur A. Campbell. NIH Publication No. 80-100. Washington, D.C.: National Institutes of Health, pp. 299–319.

Hecht, Jacqueline. 1982. "From a third to a second child: Recent changes in French population policy," *Materialien zur Bevolkerungswissenschaft* 32: 141–214.

Kamerman, Sheila B., and Alfred J. Kahn (eds.). 1978. *Family Policy: Government and Families in Fourteen Countries.* New York: Columbia University Press.

———, Alfred J. Kahn, and Paul Kingston. 1983. *Maternity Policies and Working Women.* New York: Columbia University Press.

Kaufmann, Franz-Xaver, and Lutz Leisering. 1983. "Demographic challenges in the welfare state," in *Concern: The Welfare State.* I.B.S.—Materialien, No. 11. University of Bielefeld, Institute for Demographic Research and Social Policy.

Laroque, Michel. 1984. *Les Politiques Sociales dans la France Contemporaine.* Paris: Editions STH.

Laroque, Pierre. Personal communication, February 1985.

Liljeström, Rita. 1978. "Sweden," in Kamerman and Kahn, 1978 pp. 19–48.

McIntosh, C. Alison. 1981. "Low fertility and liberal democracy in Western Europe," *Population and Development Review* 7, no. 2 (June): 181–207.

———. 1983. *Population Policy in Western Europe: Responses to Low Fertility in France, Sweden, and West Germany.* Armonk, N.Y.: M. E. Sharpe.

Myrdal, Alva. 1941. *Nation and Family.* New York: Harper and Brothers.

Myrdal, Gunnar. 1940. *Population: A Problem for Democracy.* Cambridge, Mass.: Harvard University Press.

Reimer, Rita Ann. 1986. "Work and family life in Sweden," *Social Change in Sweden,* No. 34 (April). New York: Swedish Information Service.

Russett, Bruce, and Harvey Starr. 1985. *World Politics: The Menu for Choice.* New York: W. H. Freeman and Co.
Spengler, Joseph J. 1938. *France Faces Depopulation.* Durham, N.C.: Duke University Press.
Sullerot, Evelyne. 1984. *Pour le Meilleur et Sans le Pire.* Paris: Fayard.
Sussmüth, Rita. Personal communication, January 1985.
Tomlinson, Richard. 1984. "The French population debate," *The Public Interest,* No. 76 (Summer): 111–120.
UNAF (National Union of Family Associations). 1981. *Rencontre des Familles à l'Aube du IIIe Millenaire.* Paris.
United Nations, Department of International Economic and Social Affairs, Population Division. 1984. *Population Policy Briefs: Current Situation in Developed Countries, 1983.* ESA/P/WP.72/Rev. 1. 10. September. New York.
Westoff, Charles F. 1978. "Marriage and fertility in the developed countries," *Scientific American* 239, no. 6 (December): 51–57.
Wright, Quincy. 1955. *The Study of International Relations.* New York: Appleton-Century-Crofts.

Pronatalist Policies in Low-Fertility Countries: Patterns, Performance, and Prospects

Paul Demeny

On 18 July 1969, President Richard Nixon transmitted a "Message on Population" to the US Congress. That date is better remembered as marking the day of man's first landing on the Moon, but for today's reader the Message, too, offers a certain degree of fascination. Although American fertility at the time had been steadily declining for over a decade—in 1968 the total fertility rate was 2.43, one-third below its postwar peak 11 years earlier—the passages devoted to domestic issues identified the problem of rapid growth as the focus of policy concern with US population trends:

> ... by the year 2000, or shortly thereafter, there will be more than 300 million Americans.
>
> This growth will produce serious challenges for our society. I believe that many of our present social problems may be related to the fact that we have had only fifty years in which to accommodate the second hundred million Americans. In fact, since 1945 alone some 90 million babies have been born in this country. We have thus had to accommodate in a very few decades an adjustment to population growth which was once spread over centuries. And it now appears that we will have to provide for a third hundred million Americans in a period of just 30 years. . . .
>
> We can be sure that society will not be ready for this growth unless it begins its planning immediately. And adequate planning, in turn, requires that we ask ourselves a number of important questions.[1]

A number of these questions followed. Where will the next hundred million Americans live? How will they be housed? How will this growth affect natural resources and the quality of the environment? How will such a large number of people be educated and employed? How can American families be better assisted so that they will have no more children than they wish to have?

The last of these questions had the distinction that not only did it seem to possess urgency, but it was capable of eliciting a clearcut answer. The Message stated:

> [I]t is clear that the domestic family planning services supported by the Federal Government should be better expanded and integrated. . . . In particular, most of an estimated five million low-income women of childbearing age in this country do not now have adequate access to family planning assistance. . . . I believe, therefore, that we should establish as a national goal the provision of adequate family planning services within the next five years to all those who want them but cannot afford them. . . . In order to achieve this national goal, we will have to increase the amount we are spending on population and family planning.

Thus was an explicit domestic fertility policy articulated for the first time in the United States and translated forthwith into one of the categorical programs of the American welfare state, then in full swing. It was a policy development bound to become controversial, sooner or later. First, it staked out a major role for government in a field that was formerly strictly in the private domain. Just ten years earlier, President Eisenhower summarily dismissed the very notion that the federal government has a role to play in the matter of birth control:

> I cannot imagine anything more emphatically a subject that is not a proper political or governmental activity or function or responsibility. . . . This government will not, as long as I am here, have a positive political doctrine in its program that has to do with the problem of birth control.[2]

Second, by virtue of the context in which it was presented, the new fertility policy was linked to macrodemographic considerations: its effect on population growth. The programs spawned by the policy could have been justified solely as a political decision to make a valued service available to those who otherwise might have had to make do with inferior substitutes. The case for adding another in-kind service to what was already on the government's plate may not have been compelling, but it compared favorably with most existing or would-be competitors among such services. A new array of contraceptive technologies recently had become available: while not particularly expensive, much of it was out of reach to many women and especially to young people. By their characteristics, the new technologies were easily blended in with health services, already increasingly government-financed for the economically less well-off. To imply that in addition to being good in their own right the services would also moderate population growth, and thus yield a presumed extra benefit, was an unnecessary and probably harmful complication. For one, the likely demographic effect was in fact marginal. To assume otherwise not only underestimated the extent to which the new technologies would have spread even without government programs; it also implied, implausibly, that Americans had become less inventive and less competent in applying traditional methods of birth control than their less educated and poorer forebears. Prior to the baby boom, and, of course, prior to the availability of "modern" methods of birth control, US fertility had fallen to below-replacement levels. More to the point, using macrodemographic considerations in justifying the program made the program vulnerable in case that extra prop was found to be no longer valid.

Indeed, the expectation of persistent high fertility born in the baby boom years soon turned out to be quite unfounded in the United States, as it had in a number of instances even earlier in other developed countries. Change, moreover, seemed to be forever faster than demographers' interpretations of it. An outcome of Nixon's Population Message was the creation, by Congress, of the Commission on Population Growth and the American Future. The Commission, chaired by John D. Rockefeller 3rd, submitted its Report in 1972. Perhaps its most quoted recommendation read as follows:

> Recognizing that our population cannot grow indefinitely, and appreciating the advantages of moving now toward the stabilization of population, the Commission recommends that the nation welcome and plan for a stabilized population. (US Commission, 1972a: 110)

But by 1972 US fertility once again had fallen below replacement level, where it has remained ever since. The intrinsic growth rate was, and remains, negative. Population indeed cannot grow at such a rate indefinitely since negative growth leads to eventual extinction. As the growth momentum implicit in the age distribution was transitory, "welcoming and planning for" a stabilized population in effect became a call for *increasing* fertility. The measures recommended by the Commission were not, however, fashioned to serve that end; nor were instruments with an explicitly pronatalist intent added to the armamentarium of US social policies subsequently. Social policies, of course, often have effects that are the opposite of those they were intended to have. Assuming that achieving and maintaining replacement fertility *is* a desirable societal objective, we know by hindsight that neither the recommendations of the Commission that were heeded nor subsequent changes in social policies had such fortuitous consequences, at least not on balance. In the United States and, even more clearly, in much of the rest of the industrialized world, replacement fertility remains not only unrealized but, if present social arrangements and public policies continue, also an increasingly unlikely prospect.

Given that the friendly "welcome" extended to zero population growth was not enough, or rather too much, can purposeful "planning" bring about the hoped-for outcome? Is there a portfolio of pronatalist policies and measures ready to be called into action and offering reasonable promise of success to governments willing to adopt them? The aim of this article is to help answer these questions by examining the patterns of pronatalist policies that have been applied thus far in countries in which too-low fertility has been recognized as a social problem requiring government action; assessing the performance of these policies; and discussing the main public policy options democratic governments face if they wish to approach replacement fertility starting from a below-replacement level. But before turning to these issues, two other topics should be addressed.

First, what is the justification for government intervention aimed at increasing fertility? The absence of explicit pronatalist policies, at least in the United States, suggests that there may be no such role for government: that government's sole proper function in this domain is to help the economy accommodate the macrodemographic results of microdemographic decisions and to ease social problems that might result from such decisions, notably through social policies affecting income distribution. As we shall suggest later, even in democratic countries where a government concern with too-low levels of aggregate fertility has been explicit, and correcting such levels has been acknowledged as a role for government, governments behave as if the justification for bringing about higher birth rates was nonexistent or at best marginal.

Second, since any sound remedial public policy must be based on a correct diagnosis of the disease, the current state of our understanding of the causes and dynamics of fertility decline and, in particular, of below-replacement fertility, will be briefly surveyed and commented upon.

The rationale for pronatalist policy

Any suggestion that in countries with below-replacement fertility concern about that symptom ought to be translated into corrective government policy would seem to be singularly ill-timed and objectionable. This is true not only in the United States of the mid-1980s, but also in most other countries of the West. The reasons for this are not difficult to understand. On a mundane level, virtually everywhere democratic governments find themselves in a state of chronic system-overload. The idea of adding yet another problem awaiting a solution to the already crowded social policy agenda—an item, moreover, that to many observers would seem to possess the unmistakable characteristics of a fiscal time bomb—goes counter to the striving of governments everywhere to trim commitments and balance budgets.

On a more philosophical plane, latent opposition to "social engineering" aimed at tampering with fertility trends remains strong in Western countries, and attempts to legislate active pronatalist policies are likely to generate acrimonious political and ideological conflicts. In a free society relations between individuals ought ideally to rest on mutual consent, and an active role for the state in shaping those relations can be justified only to prevent the use of coercion by individuals or groups of individuals against other individuals or groups (see Knight, 1947: 49). Although this principle has been given an increasingly liberal interpretation in demarcating the permissible limits of government action everywhere in Western societies, in the United States at least state intervention to modify individual fertility decisions with an expressly pronatalist intent has, as yet, never been seriously proposed.

This is not surprising. The kinds of intervention required by pronatalist intent cannot be interpreted as simple extensions, albeit with a changed sign, of the type of antinatalist policies that are routinely considered and are often implemented when society perceives aggregate fertility as excessive. In this latter case, as is illustrated by the US Commission's policy recommendations, the remedy is presumed to be a straightforward extension of a valued freedom. By helping individuals and individual couples to better control their fertility, societal and individual objectives are simultaneously served. Even though the requisite main policy prescription—the subsidized or free provision of family planning services—does require the entry of the redistributive state into an area of activity that was formerly strictly in the private domain, the services now to be collectively provided are "cheap," so that the newly assumed fiscal burdens, as far as such matters go, are minor. This is so not only at the initial stage of the policy but also prospectively: the technological properties of the services in question remove the specter of an open-ended commitment that makes the eventual costs of most redistributive policies so difficult to estimate. Granted, the new policy may be inadequate to reduce fertility to replacement level (as is likely to be the case in many developing countries today, and as was considered to be the case even in the United States by numerous analysts of US population trends at the time of the US Commission's deliberations). Then the most promising extension of policies "beyond family planning" is toward gradual removal of state interference with the spontaneous play of social interaction shaping individual fertility decisions rather than more intrusive interference with such decisions. When the existing policies and institutional structures have a net pronatalist bias, moving toward lower fertility calls for doing less, rather than more: removing counterproductive pronatalist incentives rather than introducing antinatalist incentives through new programs (Blake, 1972; Demeny, 1972). In contrast, if the sum total of individual decisions concerning fertility adds up to a level deemed deficient by society, it is not obvious that any similarly parsimonious policy choices are available. Increasing fertility through government intervention is likely to be far more difficult and costly, politically as well as technically and programmatically, than inducing a fertility decline.[3]

Yet the rationale on which government intervention in fertility decisions may be justified is the same regardless of the sign of deviation of actual fertility from the sought-for replacement level. It is one of market failure.[4] Merely finding that the operation of private markets falls short of perfection is, of course, insufficient to establish a case for collective action. Both in the economic and social domains the argument of market failure has often been pressed into service improperly—to support government programs even when private markets function with reasonable efficiency. Thus it is hardly surprising that calls for government intervention to increase fertility in Western societies tend to be met with skepticism and seen as another, and perhaps more extreme and offensive manifestation of a paternalistic and meddlesome state. But the attitude may be unwarranted: in a large society the spontaneous and voluntary interaction of individual actions can, and often does badly fail to deliver desired macrodemographic patterns. Indeed, the function of the state in seeking to increase persistent below-replacement fertility ultimately comes to resemble that most fundamental function of states anywhere: the provision of national defense. In extreme cases, both have to do with self-preservation; with seeking to assure the very survival of society.

But, again, to establish an abstract rationale for pronatalist policies is not to suggest that once fertility has sunk below replacement, such policies could or even ought to be adopted. Any proposal that might promise a desired effect on fertility must pass the exacting tests of the political decisionmaking process. In a democratic polity, it must command majority support and must satisfy the constitutional rules that protect the rights of a dissenting minority. To anticipate arguments advanced later in this article, at present there may be no significant pronatalist measures that would pass these tests in the United States. The paucity of such measures suggests that the situation elsewhere is not too different. The status quo of fertility policies then can be considered optimal in the sense that substituting a superior alternative is beyond the capacity of the political system to deliver: any remedy offered is certified as worse than the disease.

There are numerous reasons that explain this state of affairs. The longer run negative consequences of a declining population are less than clear in advanced industrial societies. To the extent that there is agreement as to what some of those consequences are, interpretation of their implications for various facets of welfare is often controversial. Adjusting the economy and social institutions to demographic patterns then may be a more logical course than attempting to change fertility. Within fairly broad limits of demographic parameters such adjustments seem eminently feasible. Arguably, after the period of rapid growth experienced in the recent past and indeed over the entire period of modern Western history, there may be some advantage in sustaining a period of retrenchment or even prolonged population shrinkage. Moreover, in many settings, including the United States, declining population is in fact not an immediate prospect. The growth momentum inherent in the age distribution is still strong, and immigration may provide an economically and socially not unwelcome compensation for low domestic fertility. Further, in many cases, including again the United States, fertility is not too far below replacement level, and its decline may have leveled off already. The aim of fine-tuning demographic behavior may be neither feasible nor a strong enough basis for proposing costly policy changes.

Indeed, uncertainty about the future course of fertility is probably the most important factor that counsels caution in entertaining pronatalist proposals. Demographers have become exceedingly wary of making confident predictions. Once bitten, twice shy: they have been bitten more than once. The baby boom came as a nearly total surprise, and the severity and duration of the subsequent downturn was largely unanticipated. The expectation that low fertility will endure, thus bringing long-run demographic decay, could be unwarranted. We may be merely experiencing the trough of a long-term cyclical movement that, kindly obeying "medium" UN projections, may exhibit a net reproduction rate of 1.0 as its central tendency. Even though market-based coordination between micro-level decisions may be faulty concerning fertility, homeostatic mechanisms may be at work that will assure spontaneous corrections if macro trends deviate too far from replacement, thus assuring long-run population growth near the stationary level.

Such considerations notwithstanding, serious and systematic examination of the possible means of inducing an increase in fertility through deliberate policy is overdue. That expert demographic opinion as to spontaneous future trends is both divided and cautious also means that no one is in a position to guarantee a rise of fertility back to replacement level or to exclude the possibility of a continuing downward trend. The extreme situations exhibited by some present-day fertility patterns—such as a total fertility rate of about 1.3 in Central Europe—are the sign of a social pathology that would seem to call for energetic countermeasures. Moreover, the standard practice of looking at fertility trends and levels in national units conceals the fact that significant subpopulations have fertility that is much lower than the national average. Such subpopulations can be identified not only by socioeconomic or ethnic criteria but also by geography, that is, embracing a cross-section of the population. They may be precursors of more generalized patterns of tomorrow. As Charles Westoff observed in discussing the future of Western fertility, "we are moving into largely uncharted territory" (1983: 103). Counting on good luck alone in that excursion would be unwise.

Causes and dynamics of below-replacement fertility

How well do we understand why fertility is what it is, and where it is going and why? Clearly, without an adequate theory of fertility change population policymaking, whether it aims at reducing or increasing fertility, is navigating without a compass. The existing state of affairs, according to many qualified observers, is less than encouraging. In 1980 the Report of the International Review Group of Social Science Research on Population and Development[5] commented:

> Perhaps the most striking aspect of the present state of knowledge on fertility is the absence of an accepted theory of fertility change. The demographic transition has been an object of study for over 25 years, and yet no satisfactory or proven theory is at hand to explain the phenomenon either in now-developed or in presently developing countries. (Miró and Potter, 1980: 94)

This judgment evidently rests on a rather ambitious interpretation of what a proven explanatory theory is: certainly it can be claimed that social scientists have been in possession, and not just in the last few decades, of a broad understanding of what causes fertility to fall, hence could offer cogent recommendations for policymakers. As Malthus (1820) clearly recognized, economic improvement and the opening up of opportunities for upward social mobility is apt to elicit the reinforcing response of reproductive "prudence": the voluntary limitation of fertility by individual action. In the same vein, some decades later the French economist Claude-Frédéric Bastiat commented:

> The means of existence, we cannot repeat too often, are not a fixed quantity: they depend upon one's way of life, on public opinion, on habits. On every rung of the social ladder there is the same repugnance to moving a step down from the position to which one has become accustomed as can be felt by those on the lowest rung. . . . The habit of certain comforts, of a certain dignity in one's way of life, is therefore one of the strongest of incentives for the exercise of foresight; and if the working class once rises to a certain level of satisfactions, it will be unwilling to descend, even though, in order to preserve its position and to maintain a wage scale in keeping with its new habits, it must resort to the infallible means of preventive limitation. (Bastiat, 1964 [1850]: 441)

Although Bastiat's formulation was meant to summarize his understanding of French demographic behavior, this was, like Malthus's before him, a predictive theory: it accurately forecast the generalized decline of fertility experienced a few decades later in virtually all countries of Europe.

Or consider an American interpretation of the causes of fertility decline, that of John Billings, set forth in 1893. Anticipating Ansley Coale (1973: 65) by 80 years, Billings identified three factors that explain the decline of US fertility. The first is that effective methods of fertility control are available. ("[M]arried women are much better informed as to the means by which the number of children may be limited than were those of thirty years ago.") Second, fertility control is considered acceptable. ("[A]bstaining from having children . . . is not only not in itself sinful . . . but it may even be . . . commendable.") Finally, and most importantly, fertility control is advantageous to the individual:

> The third cause of the decreasing birth rate is the great increase in the use of things which were formerly considered as luxuries, but which now have become almost necessities. The greater temptations to expenditure for the purpose of securing or maintaining social position, and the corresponding greater cost of family life in what may be called the lower middle classes, lead to the desire to have fewer children in order that they may be each better provided for, or perhaps, in some cases, from the purely selfish motive of desire to avoid care and trouble and of having more to spend on social pleasures.

> In the struggle for what is deemed a desirable mode of existence at the present day, marriage is being held less desirable, and its bonds less sacred, than they were forty years ago. Young women are gradually being imbued with the idea that marriage and motherhood are not to be their chief objects in life, or the sole methods of obtaining subsistence; that they should aim at being independent of possible or actual husbands, and should fit themselves to earn their own

living in some one of the many ways in which females are beginning to find increasing sources of remunerative employment; that housekeeping is a sort of domestic slavery, and that it is best to remain unmarried until someone offers who has the means to gratify their educated tastes. They desire to take a more active part than women have hitherto done in the management of the affairs of the community, to have wider interests, and to live broader lives than their mothers and grandmothers have done. (Billings, 1893: 281)[6]

Billings's comments seem today extraordinarily perceptive. To the central themes of rising material aspirations and the pressure to improve or maintain one's social position (already present in Malthus's formulation and fully developed in the theory of "social capillarity" by Arsène Dumont, 1890), they add an emphasis on the emancipation of women, increased female education, and increased female labor force participation. They also link the last of these to increasing rewards offered by the workplace relative to home life and hint at the lessened economic security of marriage and at the coming "divorce revolution." They anticipate Philippe Ariès (1980) in suggesting a shift from orientation toward children to orientation toward more self-centered pursuits; a shift in turn rooted in the structural factors, both demographic and economic, identified in the diagnosis. These are the key determinants commonly adduced in explaining contemporary below-replacement fertility levels in the West and in attempting to discern future changes in birth rates.

Mainline modern transition theory (associated with the names of Adolphe Landry (1949) and Alfred Sauvy (1969)—the most prominent representatives of the Continental tradition[7]—and, among Americans, with the names of Warren Thompson, Frank Notestein, Dudley Kirk, and Kingsley Davis[8]) echoed, amplified, and elaborated the themes already present in nineteenth century analyses of fertility change. The theory traces fertility change to the fundamental structural transformation of the economic and social systems generated by the industrial revolution. The linkages it establishes are richly infused with qualifications introduced by historical and cultural peculiarities, and by the interplay of changing values and aspirations that reflect, but also feed back into and shape, socioeconomic change (see, for example, Lesthaeghe, 1983). The distinction between the main causal relationships identified by this theory and the qualifications thereto is, however, crucial. As Davis states, "an interpretation of demographic behavior as a response either to absolute need or to some cultural idiosyncrasy such as a particular 'value system' or 'custom' " represents a failure to recognize the essential character of the nature of the demographic transformation. "When the demographic history of industrialized nations is analyzed comparatively, an amazing similarity of the response syndrome seems to . . . emerge. An explanation of a country's demographic behavior by reference to a peculiarity or accident of its culture fails to cope with this basic similarity of response" (Davis, 1963: 362).

Transition theory has been the dominant influence on the broad lines of policy thinking not only in the developing world but also in the industrial countries. A convincing confirmation of this influence can be found, for example, in the analyses undertaken by the British Royal Commission on Population (United Kingdom, 1949) and by its successor Panel on Population (United Kingdom, 1973) and in much of the scientific supporting work generated by the US Commission on Population. In specific policy proposals, the broader economic analyses offered by transition theory have been complemented by painstaking analyses of the effect of demographic factors on the economic status of the family, and, in particular, the economic costs of children to parents and to society as a whole.[9]

Challenging the traditional approach to fertility analysis, in the 1960s a new school of fertility studies emerged: that of the new household economics.[10] Its practitioners were dissatisfied with and sometimes openly disdainful of the diffuseness and "soft" methodology of extant demographic theorizing; of demographers' often promiscuous flirtations with normative propositions, and their penchant for making pronouncements on policy matters on the basis of presumed causal relationships that were not (and typically could not be) rigorously tested. The promise of successfully applying the refined methodology of standard microeconomic analysis of consumer demand to fertility decision-making was amply fulfilled, as demonstrated by a large and still rapidly growing literature. But this was done at the price of draining virtually all historical, sociological, and institutional insights from the analytic framework: arguably a major flaw in view of the nature of the subject matter. Policy applications of the findings from the new types of analyses were scarce. As Yoram Ben-Porath (whose work within that school is least subject to the charge just made) has noted, the new household economists' steering away from any early attempt to translate findings to policy application was deliberate (Ben-Porath, 1984). But after a quarter century of scientific activity (during which time world population grew by nearly 2 billion and developed country fertility rates dropped by roughly 50 percent), the continuing absence of policy interest is not easily explained or justified. Nor are the findings being translated by others into policy propositions: the practitioners of the new household economics seem to continue talking mostly to each other.

Another important modern development in fertility analysis was Richard Easterlin's theory explaining the American baby boom. Easterlin interprets the baby boom and its low-fertility aftermath as a cyclical phenomenon, reflecting the influence of the relative size of successive generations on expected and realized economic welfare. (For a convenient exposition, see Easterlin, 1980.) There are no obvious direct policy applications flowing from this analysis: aspirations acquired in childhood, which play a key explanatory role in the theory, cannot be modified retroactively. In suggesting a built-in mechanism— a negative association between the size of a generation and its subsequent fertility—shaping fertility trends, Easterlin's theory does, however, hold up the prospect of a spontaneously generated return to higher fertility, thus weakening the force of calls for policy intervention aimed at the same end. But it is unclear how well Easterlin's arguments explaining the baby boom apply also to the present situation. The contrast between postwar prosperity and Depression-time misery was indeed sharp, and the argument that it powerfully shaped American fertility behavior well into the 1950s is persuasive. But any relative deprivation felt by the baby boom cohorts (relative to their parents' status or their childhood expectations) is a less plausible explanation of their low fertility. By virtually all measures of economic status, the swollen cohorts of the baby boom have done exceedingly well compared even with the much less numerous preceding generation (Russell, 1982). The expectations offered by the theory also poorly track recent European fertility trends.

A major effort to understand fertility change, both in the developing world and in the industrialized world, began in the early 1970s. The World Fertility Survey, as the enterprise became known, was, by all odds, the largest social science project ever undertaken. As John Cleland notes, "[t]he WFS programme was not designed to test any particular theory of fertility behaviour, although one of the aims enshrined in its mandate was to help governments to understand the fertility of their populations" (1985: 223). Its results, therefore, were expected to have an important influence on policies affecting fertility.

The completion of the WFS occasioned an assessment of the lessons learned. Taking the authoritative summary provided by Cleland at face value, the lessons, when compared with what was received wisdom among social scientists for perhaps a century and a half, are little short of astonishing:

> [T]aken en masse, the results of WFS are more consistent with an ideational theory of change, based on the spread of new aspirations or new attitudes towards family formation or birth control, than with a structural theory, which emphasizes changes in economic roles of family units, of women or of children. (ibid.: 243)

And further:

> There is little support in [WFS] findings for the central thesis of the National Academy of Sciences work[11] that the driving force of fertility decline is a reduction in parental demand for children, induced by modernization. This diagnosis is surely also true of the low fertility developed countries. Despite the very different divisions of the financial burden of childrearing between parents and the state, the difference in fertility between Eastern and Western bloc countries is minimal. (ibid.: 248)

There seem to be major problems with theorizing of this sort. Surely "new aspirations or new attitudes towards family formation or birth control" are of the nature of intermediate variables, much like the variables of contraceptive practice, duration of lactation, or age at marriage. The issue for policymakers is to discern what determines such aspirations and attitudes and whether and how those underlying determinants can be deliberately affected. To assume that while aspirations and attitudes toward birth control have been changing, other "structural" factors have changed not at all, or did so only at a snail's pace, and hence can be safely ignored as potential underlying explanatory factors, is contrary to overwhelming evidence concerning contemporary socioeconomic change. The point can be confirmed through casual observations by any diligent traveler in the Third World or, more comfortably, by armchair consultation of standard statistical compendia. Along with and before exposure to ideas about and devices for contraception, chances are that there were also more children in schools, more surviving babies, GIs on R&R in the capital, buses running to the nearby town, transistor radios in every hut, television shows in the village square, satellites in the sky, better seeds from the extension workers, girlie magazines on newspaper racks in the city, tiles on rooftops, and possibly a visit by the Pope or Kosygin. If so, the massive "ideational changes" need not be seen as a product of mysterious mutation. Nor can such changes be assumed to center on the use of birth control: that is likely to be the effect, not the fulcrum of change.[12]

As to the present fertility decline in the developed world, characterizing the change as ideational, having to do with attitudes toward birth control, also seems to put the cart before the horse. There was, after all, the massive entry of married women into the labor force, the weakening of economic security provided by marriage for wives, the scramble for upward mobility, the resistance to sliding down the social scale, and the competition for "positional goods" (as chronicled by Hirsch, 1976), and, for every member of the affluent society, the growing scarcity of time (as depicted by Linder, 1970). In coping with the social limits to growth, children increasingly became a liability.

As to the puzzle of similar demographic behavior in East and West, the supposedly very different divisions of the burden of childrearing between parent and state would not hold up under scrutiny, but the point is moot. Whether in Pittsburgh or in Prague, couples contemplating, ex ante, the implications for their living standards of having a first child (or having a second one) would reach very similar conclusions. This is not to say that there are no differences between East and West. When Dörte, the young heroine in Günter Grass's comic novel *Headbirths or The Germans Are Dying Out* (1982), agonized about the "Yes-to-baby No-to-baby" question while on a vacation package tour in Asia with her husband, she might have reflected upon the fact that had she lived in East Germany, her chances for future trips to Bali would not have been weakened materially had she decided to say "yes."

Patterns of pronatalist policies

What, then, can governments do to increase fertility if such an increase, given the right price, appears to be a social desideratum? Clearly, if "language, ethnicity, or region" are the "major independent determinants" of fertility change, as WFS found them to be (Cleland, 1985: 247), they can do precious little; attempting to change peoples' language, ethnicity, or region would represent an awkward undertaking even for the most determined government.

"Parental education"—years of schooling—as a policy lever is not helpful either; parents cannot be easily de-educated.

Placing restrictions on access to contraceptive services (that is, turning on its head the main programmatic approach with which governments try to moderate fertility in developing countries) is at first blush a more promising avenue toward higher birth rates. When in the 1930s European governments first faced the problem of incipient population decline (a false alarm, then, as it turned out), the possibility of making contraceptives less available was routinely raised in discussions of fertility policy options, only to be just as routinely dismissed (Myrdal, 1940; Glass, 1940). The arguments for rejecting this policy option remain as valid today as they were then, or more so. On the principle of parsimony it suffices to point out that even if such measures were politically acceptable (and they are not), substitutes to high-tech contraception are available, hence the likely fertility effects would be minuscule. (For a discussion reaching this conclusion see Andorka, 1978.)

Restriction of access to abortion is in a somewhat different category. In a number of East European countries such restrictions were imposed explicitly to increase the birth rate. They did so with limited and transitory success only, even in Rumania where the ban on abortion introduced in 1966 was backed up by draconian sanctions and was accompanied by a ban on contraceptive devices (Teitelbaum, 1972; Berelson, 1979). In the West, the continuing and increasingly acrimonious debate about access to and limitations on abortion is likely to steer clear of macrodemographic considerations. Indeed, the longer run sensitivity of the birth rate to the availability of any particular method of birth control is likely to be modest, although, at least in France, the issue of low fertility as an argument against a liberal abortion policy is occasionally raised.[13]

Policy measures seeking directly to affect "values" related to fertility are another potential candidate for the attention of governments wishing to increase birth rates. Although values obviously do affect fertility, such an approach (analogous to what passes under the label "population education" in family planning programs in less developed countries, but aiming for an opposite effect on fertility) has little to recommend it in principle and even less in practice. Democratic states are ill-equipped to engage in specialized value education of their citizens: values are embedded in and conveyed by the deeper institutional structures of society. Ministerial exhortations, posters of happy three-child families, and medals to heroine mothers are neither well received nor effective in influencing fertility. Value education as an escape from the prisoner's dilemma situation inherent in lack of congruence between individual and social preferences is not likely to work since individuals realize that their fertility decisions affect their own welfare substantially while exerting only a minuscule influence on aggregate fertility trends.

By a process of exclusion we thus seem to arrive at the one solid proposition that is suggested by standard analyses of fertility determinants: material incentives. In the language of the modern welfare state this translates into the proposition that fertility can be affected by judiciously dispensing public resources so as to relieve parents of some of the costs of childrearing. Modern states, of course, have long made it their policy (albeit not with demographic objectives in mind) to provide much of the cost of children's formal education as a public service. Collective provision of other child-related services appears to be the logical extension of this approach. If children are costly, and parents do not produce voluntarily enough of them to satisfy societal needs for demographic stability, subsidizing parents to raise children should increase parents' willingness to have more of them. If women's participation in the labor force is not compatible with raising children, child care centers may lessen the conflict. If housing is difficult for young parents to find, the state can lend a helping hand. Pronatalist policy thus becomes a specialized function of the redistributive service state. It may take the form of cash grants or services in kind: in either case the key instrument at play is the national budget.

The approach is tersely stated in the main recommendation (Recommendation 35) that addresses the problem of low fertility in the closing document of the International Conference on Population held in Mexico City in 1984:[14]

> Governments that view the level of fertility in their countries as too low may consider financial and other support to families to assist them with their parental responsibilities and to facilitate their access to the necessary services.

The European Population Conference of 1982 considered the matter in more thorough detail. Its concluding document provides a quintessential statement of the policy approach in question:

> [T]he [demographic] situation outlined in the previous paragraphs may lead some governments to take action to influence fertility trends. It is, of course, a matter for individual governments to decide whether or not the demographic and budgetary situation in their countries makes such action desirable, or possible. . . .
>
> It is recognized that parents who bring up children will inevitably be at an economic disadvantage in comparison with those who do not have children. It is widely accepted that it is right for a community to take measures which will at least partly offset the reduction in living standards occasioned by parental obligations. Among such measures, a number deserve specific mention:
>
> a. Tax benefits and cash transfers to families which improve their economic conditions and partially compensate for the loss of income suffered by parents both in the period around the birth of a child, and whilst the child is heavily dependent on parental care;
>
> b. Granting leave to the parent to enable him or her to care for the child, without suffering career disadvantage;
>
> c. Adequate provision of child welfare services, including a safe physical and social environment;

d. To assist families with children in their housing needs. (Council of Europe, 1982: 5)

The list above enumerates the main directions along which pronatalist policies seek to operate but fails to intimate the bewildering variety of specific measures that have in fact been adopted under each rubric by virtually all countries in Europe, and to a lesser extent in low-fertility countries elsewhere. To portray such policies as distinctively serving pronatalist objectives would be, however, incorrect. Many, indeed the majority of these countries, profess no intent to raise fertility rates and have no expectation that the policies in question will in fact result in higher fertility. The policies are pursued because they are considered good in themselves and have been sanctioned as such by the political process. They serve redistributive goals approved by the electorate or respond to the pressure of various interest groups for a slice of the government's social service budget. Social policy and population policy proper thus are inextricably confounded, bearing out Gunnar Myrdal's prediction that, in practice, "population policy will turn out to be simply an intensification of the important part of social policy which bears upon the family and children" (Myrdal, 1940: 205). The absence or presence of pronatalist objectives, and the stridency or tentativeness with which such objectives, if any, are articulated are in fact poor predictors of the scope and generosity of the services made available to the population under each of the above headings. Scandinavian countries, for example, declare themselves satisfied with existing levels of fertility (United Nations, 1982: 40); yet provision there of the types of social services that would be classified in the list above as pronatalist is among the most generous.

There are, of course, exceptions to these generalizations. Providing means-tested entitlements of whatever nature seldom can be characterized as a pronatalist population policy: their dominant objective is to alleviate poverty. In turn, when services are provided that are dependent on some demographic criterion, a primarily pronatalist objective may be clearly revealed. Examples of the latter are frequent in Eastern Europe (see Land, 1979; Klinger, 1984; and Barta et al., 1984 for Hungary, and Frejka, 1980 for Czechoslovakia). In Western Europe (with perhaps the notable exception of France), and even more in the United States and in Japan (see, for example, Kuroda, 1984), speaking of "pronatalist" policies would be, by and large, merely a fancy way of describing social policies that might also have some pronatalist effect. This assertion is clearly borne out by the pertinent literature (see, for example, Berelson, 1974; van de Kaa, 1978; Gendell, 1980; Finkle and McIntosh, 1980; Kirk, 1981; and McIntosh, 1983). It is also confirmed by formal government statements in international forums where, with rare exceptions, representatives of low-fertility countries either declare the neutrality of their governments with respect to aggregate fertility levels (in contrast to professed positive interest in individual and family welfare) or fail entirely to address the matter. (See, for example, the official statements in UNFPA, 1984 and United Nations,

1985.) The concluding document of the European Population Conference of 1982 stated that "almost all delegations indicated . . . that their governments had not formulated explicit population policies" (Council of Europe, 1982: 5).

Performance of pronatalist policies

How well do policies aimed at increasing fertility perform? As suggested above, only a limited number of instances render this question at all meaningful. The modest literature that tries to answer the question is less than unanimous in its conclusions, but the range of variation in the suggested fertility effects is narrow: certainly dwarfed by the amplitude of fertility swings exhibited by the demographic history of the low-fertility countries in the last few decades. We shall only try here to describe the general character of the findings.

The modal finding is that the effects are nil or negligible. An authoritative French analysis in the mid-1970s concluded with the rueful observation that fertility is a reflection of deep underlying currents that are both complex and powerful, leaving only a very narrow margin to the play of voluntaristic intervention (INED, 1976: 44). Earlier analyses either came to the same conclusion or professed agnosticism, which suggests that the effects were too weak to be measurable. Two exceptions are the qualified success of Germany in raising the birth rate in the 1930s and Rumania's temporary but for a while substantial extra birth crop following the ban of abortion in 1966, already noted above.

Assessments published since the INED study just referred to confirm the picture of general impotence attributed to pronatalist measures qua fertility policy. Gérard Calot and Jacqueline Hecht, assessing French population policy (generally considered the most successful in post–World War II Western Europe), suggest that its fertility effect "may have been in the region of 10 per cent, that is 0.2 children per woman" (1978: 191–192). But the methodology underlying this guesstimate is tenuous. Partly it is based on comparing the overall French birth rate with those of neighboring countries. Interpreting evidence of that sort requires massive ceteris paribus assumptions. Somewhat more convincing is their finding that "fertility increased most among the socio-professional categories which benefited most from the pro-family legislative changes made in 1939." Rudolf Andorka and György Vukovich (1985) adduce similar evidence in their relatively sanguine interpretation (compared with those of other Hungarian demographers) of the success of the costly pronatalist population policies introduced in Hungary since 1967. ("Success," of course, is a relative matter: current Hungarian fertility is well below replacement, and the rate of natural increase is negative.) They find that more educated and higher professional categories showed an appreciable relative increase in fertility, as the policy intended. A problem with this evidence is that the groups in question were rapidly growing in size, and, necessarily, their composition by socioeconomic and fertility background also changed. This makes comparisons over time invalid strictly speaking.

Another methodological problem in studies of policy performance concerns reliance on period data. When fertility is low, variations in period fertility need not go hand in hand with variations in cohort fertility. Thus short-term "successes" have poor long-term predictive power. This recurrent qualification removes much of the interest from efforts to study the linkage between a given policy move and its immediate demographic aftermath. Further, disentangling such linkages when policy changes are frequent can be quite hopeless even in a formal statistical sense. In Eastern Europe in particular, during the 1960s and 1970s changes in the structure of family allowances and in other child and family-oriented policies tended to follow each other in such close succession that attempts to describe policies in technical detail were typically out of date by the time they appeared in print. What measure caused what demographic response is then quite impossible to tell.

Finally, secondary effects or unforeseen side effects of pronatalist measures introduce an ambiguity between short-term success and long-term effectiveness that, even with sophisticated data, statistical analysis is ill-equipped to handle. Just being pronatalist by declared intent does not guarantee that the ultimate effect of a given policy measure is either positive or, in case of failure, zero. Appreciation of this ambiguity seems to color skeptical assessments of the effectiveness of conventional pronatalist policy measures (e.g., in David, 1982; Hungary, 1984; and Tomlinson, 1984) and to induce hedging in accounts that are more upbeat (e.g., Vining, 1984 and Chesnais, 1985, commenting on the East German success story). For example, after a new set of benefits is introduced, the novelty tends to wear off quickly and the hoped-for behavioral response soon dissipates. Also, once a benefit is taken for granted, phasing it out or letting its value erode (in terms of constant prices, or at least in comparison with rising incomes) may have a negative effect that outweighs the policy's initial positive yield.

In other instances, even initially, a policy measure may have both negative and positive effects and the sign of the net balance is in doubt to begin with. As an example, consider the comment in the Report of the US Commission on Population on child care. After claiming that subsidized child care programs might enable working women to manage the responsibilities of both employment and childrearing (a claim on the basis of which such programs are sometimes labeled as key pronatalist policy measures), the Commission observed:

> However, it is also possible that child-care programs will have a negative impact on fertility. . . . With child care available, women who want to work will have the opportunity to enter or reenter the labor force much sooner; and the rewards of employment may compete effectively with the satisfactions of additional children. (US Commission, 1972a: 88)

With varying force, similar comments could qualify endorsement of many other components of the standard policy repertoire commonly described as pronatalist. With good reason, the Council of Europe list cited earlier comes with the warning: "there is disagreement about the efficacy of such policies." Not surprisingly, in the extensive literature discussing kindred welfare policies, commentary on the demographic angle, even in book-length treatments, is marginal or entirely absent. (In the recent American literature, see, for example, Anderson, 1978 and Gilbert, 1983. A notable exception in this regard is Fuchs, 1983.)

Prospects and options for pronatalist policies

What of the future? Policy developments will respond to unfolding demographic trends, hence are as unpredictable as the trends themselves. They will also reflect the evolution of the continuing academic and political debate over which policies work and which do not; which are palatable and which are obnoxious. This debate will intensify or wane in relation to the perceived seriousness of the demographic situation of the low-fertility countries, both as viewed in isolation, country by country, and in the context of world demographic trends. There are good reasons to expect, however, that the issue of below-replacement fertility will get far more attention from policymakers and from academics in the coming years than it has received up to now.

One approach that may recommend itself is laisser faire. If the major trends are perceived as beyond human ability to modify, comparable to sea currents, then tampering with surface phenomena is pointless. Depending on mood and temperament, as much as analysis, a declining population may be seen under different lights. To Oswald Spengler, who foresaw "an appalling depopulation" (1928[1922]: 105), it heralded the decline of the West. To John Maynard Keynes, provided that the decline was "slow," it suggested an opportunity to enable us "to raise the standard of life, whilst retaining those parts of our traditional scheme of life which we value" (1937: 17).

Laisser faire is also the right approach if one trusts that reliable homeostatic mechanisms are at work that will bring fertility back to replacement level as a long-run trend bracketed by cyclical ups and downs, resembling Kondratieff-like long swings or short-term fluctuations. Analyses by Easterlin (1980), John Ermisch (1981), William Butz and Michael Ward (1979), and others suggest the plausibility of such an outcome, as do various economic and sociopsychological arguments. As children become scarcer, their attractiveness is likely to increase.

Surprises are also possible. In a Herman Kahn–like exurbanized superaffluent future (Kahn, 1982), the tedium of working at home at one's computer terminal may be relieved by rediscovery of the fun of having children around. Visiting faraway places will no longer be appealing and distracting, since Bali will look much the same as Westchester County. Throw in a pro-family religious revival and rediscovery of "traditional values," and the Nixonian worry of where to put the next hundred million Americans may reassert itself.

Continuation of the present downward fertility trend or stabilization well below replacement are safer bets, however. The arithmetic of the negative growth rates such fertility levels would generate can be daunting. Spengler's "appalling depopulation" was supposed to last for centuries, suggesting a leisurely pace of demographic decline. In the light of what we know now, Spengler seems to have grossly overestimated his countrymen's fondness for children. Present levels of fertility in West Germany imply an intrinsic annual rate of increase of -1.7 percent. If maintained for 200 years, such a rate shrinks a population to one-thirtieth of its original size. As the realization of this sinks in, countermeasures will be put to work.

The most likely initial efforts will be along the lines of past policies, despite their lackluster record. Half-hearted tinkering with family economics—trying to buy children on the cheap—may be replaced by the application of much more heavy and expensive doses of the same medicine. But it is highly likely that such a strategy will amount to destroying the family in order to save it. When parental functions are replaced by the nanny state ("five-days-a-week free child care, optional on weekends"), having a cat might seem preferable to having a child, certainly a second one. Already, as Germaine Greer (1984) charged, Americans and Europeans are not especially keen on children. Her picture, if overdrawn, is not without some validity, as Samuel Preston (1984) has demonstrated with more solid arguments.

Child subsidies going directly to the family in the form of money rather than in kind have more promise because they leave greater scope for the exercise of parental decisionmaking concerning arrangements for childrearing. The income tax offers a flexible mechanism to provide such subsidies without much bureaucracy. Tying increased personal tax exemptions and negative income tax/tax-credit schemes primarily to dependent children (perhaps with further differentiation according to parity) could also avoid some of the incentive drawbacks of the more familiar guaranteed-income schemes (Moynihan, 1973). But for such policies to achieve substantial modification of fertility behavior they could turn out to be very expensive indeed—in the United States, perhaps on the order of the present defense budget. The same can be said of what might be construed as the reverse of an antinatalist measure once proposed by Kenneth Boulding (1964): a scheme offering 20-year annuities against any birth certificate duly presented to the authorities. The value of the annuities that would elicit the socially determined requisite annual aggregate number of bids could be found by trial and error. A nagging problem with such social market solutions is that they recruit clients differentially from different income classes. Singapore-style solutions to this snag—granting richer fertility-stimulating material incentives to families belonging to higher socioeconomic strata—would require a Singapore-style political system.

A radical alternative, also expensive, would be to give up on the family as an institution incompatible with the industrial system, hence, an unreliable guarantor of social reproduction, and, as outlined by Davis (1937), rely upon motherhood practiced as a fully professionalized specialized activity, collectively financed.

But there may exist structural reforms between utopian radicalism and extreme welfare statism that could hold out a realistic expectation of reversing present fertility trends. They would not involve dispensing money (at least not as the exclusive thrust of the policy). Rather, the reforms would seek to change institutional arrangements so as to reinforce parental responsibility and authority over children; strengthen the economic security and the status of women within the family; allow parents to benefit directly in old age from having raised children; and make the political system more responsive to the young generation's interests.

By way of examples, such reforms would:

1 Reassert parental power over children's education. In all low-fertility countries the massive collective subsidies for formal education—in the United States over $130 billion annually for elementary and public schools—are arranged in such a way that parental choice over children's education is greatly restricted and additional spending on children's formal education by the parents themselves is discouraged. Direct allocation of the collective educational support to individual parents in the form of vouchers would help remedy these flaws.

2 Incorporate the nuclear family. Its revenues, however acquired (including wages, salaries, pension rights, and so forth), should accrue to the corporation, hence be equally vested in the spouses. Such an arrangement would enhance women's economic security within the family and provide for greater flexibility of choice between participation in the labor force and specialization in household production and, in particular, in childrearing.

3 Link old-age economic security to prior fertility behavior. Collective systems of social security typical of modern industrial societies assume that the aged, in the aggregate, have raised a succeeding generation of sufficient size to make the system financially viable. Individual parents' contributions to the demographic underpinnings of social security schemes should be recognized by differential allocation related to prior fertility from the collectively managed pool through which such schemes transfer resources from those working to those retired. This could be best carried out by earmarking an appropriately determined portion of individuals' compulsory social security contributions for transfer to their living but retired parents.

4 Strengthen the influence of families with children in the political system. When newcomers are admitted to human society, they should not be left disenfranchised for some 18 years: let custodial parents exercise the children's voting rights until they come of age.

Such institutional reforms, provided that they are effected on a quasi-constitutional level, hence guaranteed on a long-term basis, would tend to be pronatalist, singly and especially in combination, not only because of the nature of the shifts in fertility-affecting material incentives they would engender, but, if more elusively, also because they would induce shifts in values and social rewards favoring responsible parenthood.

Notes

1 *The New York Times*, 19 July 1969, p. 8.

2 Cited in Piotrow (1973: 45). The Foreword to this lucid and detailed, if frankly partisan, account of the early development of US international population policies was written by George Bush, then US Representative to the United Nations. It opens with an observation that rings as true today as when it was written, albeit with an ironic twist: "Few issues in the world have undergone such a rapid shift in public attitudes and government policies over the last decade as the problems of population growth and fertility control."

3 A comment by Carr-Saunders made half a century ago stressed the difficulty of increasing fertility from below-replacement level through policy intervention: "We found reason to believe that, once the voluntary small family habit has gained a foothold, the size of family is likely, if not certain, in time to become so small that the reproduction rate will fall below replacement rate, and that, when this has happened, the restoration of a replacement rate proves to be an exceedingly difficult and obstinate problem" (Carr-Saunders, 1936: 327).

4 For a more detailed discussion of the rationale of policy intervention aimed at affecting fertility, see Demeny (1972, 1975).

5 The work of the International Review Group was a major multiyear enterprise; its contributors, in addition to the principal authors of the Report, included a prestigious array of senior researchers in the field of fertility studies.

6 The page number refers to the reprint in *Population and Development Review*.

7 The first edition of Landry's work appeared in 1934, Sauvy's in 1952.

8 For a convenient source of citations of the most important contributions to this literature, as well as a perceptive discussion of the policy implications and uses of the theories elaborated in it, see Hodgson (1983).

9 Representative examples of such studies are Espenshade (1984), Turchi (1984), and Wander (1984), and studies of the economic costs of children undertaken by the US and British population commissions referred to above.

10 Early landmarks are Becker (1960) and Schultz (1974).

11 The reference is to Bulatao and Lee (1983).

12 See, for example, Oshima (1983) for a discussion of the particularly interesting East Asia case—where fertility change was especially rapid—and Keyfitz (1985) for a portrayal of life in an East Javanese village in 1953 and 1985. The process of "Westernization" as a moving force in the demographic transition is discussed in Caldwell (1976).

13 See, for example, *Population and Development Review* 11 (March 1985): 163–164 concerning Jacques Chirac's views on the subject. A ban on abortion, infringement of which was punishable by death, was part of the pronatalist policy package introduced by the Vichy government in the early 1940s.

14 This document is reprinted in *Population and Development Review* 10 (December 1984): 755–782.

References

Anderson, Martin. 1978. *Welfare: The Political Economy of Welfare Reform in the United States.* Stanford, California: The Hoover Institution.

Andorka, Rudolf. 1978. *Determinants of Fertility in Advanced Societies.* New York: The Free Press.

———, and György Vukovich. 1985. "The impact of population policy on fertility in Hungary," in *International Population Conference, Florence, 1985,* Vol. 3. Liège: International Union for the Scientific Study of Population, pp. 403–412.

Ariès, Philippe. 1980. "Two successive motivations for the declining birth rate in the West," *Population and Development Review* 6 (December): 645–650.

Barta, Barnabás, et al. 1984. *Fertility, Female Employment and Policy Measures in Hungary.* Geneva: International Labour Organization.

Bastiat, Claude-Frédéric. 1964 [1850]. *Economic Harmonies*. Translated by W. Hayden Boyers. New York: D. Van Nostrand.
Becker, Gary S. 1960. "An economic analysis of fertility," in *Demographic and Economic Change in Developed Countries*. Universities-National Bureau Conference Series, no. 11. Princeton: Princeton University Press, pp. 209–231.
Ben-Porath, Yoram. 1984. "On the economic approach to the family," in *Population and Societal Outlook*, ed. Serge Feld and Ron Lesthaeghe. Brussels: Foundation Roi Baudouin, pp. 167–178.
Berelson, Bernard. 1974. *Population Policy in Developed Countries*. New York: McGraw-Hill.
———. 1979. "Romania's 1966 anti-abortion decree: The demographic experience of the first decade," *Population Studies* 33 (July): 209–222.
Billings, John S. 1893. "The diminished birth rate in the United States," *Forum* 15 (June): 467–477. Reprinted in part in *Population and Development Review* 2 (June 1976): 279–282.
Blake, Judith. 1972. "Coercive pronatalism and American population policy," in US Commission on Population Growth and the American Future (1972b), pp. 81–109.
Boulding, Kenneth E. 1964. *The Meaning of the Twentieth Century*. New York: Harper & Row.
Bulatao, Rodolfo A., and Ronald D. Lee (eds.). 1983. *Determinants of Fertility in Developing Countries*. 2 vols. New York: Academic Press.
Butz, William P., and Michael P. Ward. 1979. "The emergence of counter-cyclical US fertility," *American Economic Review* 69 (June): 318–328.
Caldwell, John C. 1976. "Toward a restatement of demographic transition theory," *Population and Development Review* 2 (September/December): 321–366.
Calot, Gérard, and Jacqueline Hecht. 1978. "The control of fertility trends," in Council of Europe (1978), pp. 178–196.
Carr-Saunders, A. M. 1936. *World Population*. Oxford: Oxford University Press.
Chesnais, Jean Claude. 1985. "Les conditions d'efficacité d'une politique nataliste: Examen théorique et exemples historiques," in *International Population Conference, Florence, 1985*, Vol. 3. Liège: IUSSP, pp. 413–425.
Cleland, John. 1985. "Marital fertility decline in developing countries: Theories and the evidence," in *Reproductive Change in Developing Countries: Insights from the World Fertility Survey*, ed. John Cleland and John Hobcraft. London: Oxford University Press, pp. 223–252.
Coale, A. J. 1973. "The demographic transition," in *International Population Conference, Liège, 1973*, Vol. 1. Liège: IUSSP, pp. 53–72.
Council of Europe. 1978. *Population Decline in Europe: Implications of a Declining or Stationary Population*. London: Edward Arnold.
———. 1982. *European Population Conference 1982: Conclusions*. EPC (82) 42, Strasbourg, 27 September.
David, Henry P. 1982. "Eastern Europe: Pronatalist policies and private behavior," *Population Bulletin* 36, no. 6 (February).
Davis, Kingsley. 1937. "Reproductive institutions and the pressure for population," *Sociological Review* 29 (July): 289–306.
———. 1963. "The theory of change and response in modern demographic history," *Population Index* 29 (October): 345–366.
Demeny, Paul. 1972. "Welfare considerations in US population policy," in US Commission on Population Growth and the American Future (1972b), pp. 153–172.
———. 1975. "Population policy: The role of national governments," *Population and Development Review* 1 (September): 147–161.
Dumont, Arsène. 1890. *Dépopulation et civilisation*. Paris: Schleicher Frères.
Easterlin, Richard A. 1980. *Birth and Fortune: The Impact of Numbers on Personal Welfare*. New York: Basic Books.
Ermisch, John. 1981. "An emerging secular rise in the Western world's fertility?" *Population and Development Review* 7 (December): 677–684.

Espenshade, Thomas J. 1984. *Investing in Children: New Estimates of Parental Expenditures.* Washington, D.C.: The Urban Institute.

Festy, Patrick. 1981. "Mesure de l'efficacité des politiques à but nataliste dans les pays industrialisés," *International Population Conference, Manila, 1981,* Vol. 1. Liège: IUSSP, pp. 387–409.

Finkle, Jason L., and Alison McIntosh. 1980. "Policy responses to population stagnation in developed societies," in *Social, Economic and Health Aspects of Low Fertility,* ed. Arthur A. Campbell. (NIH Publication No. 80-100), Washington, D.C.: National Institutes of Health, pp. 275–297.

Frejka, Tomas. 1980. "Fertility trends and policies: Czechoslovakia in the 1970s," *Population and Development Review* 6 (March): 65–93.

Fuchs, Victor R. 1983. *How We Live.* Cambridge, Mass.: Harvard University Press.

Gendell, Murray. 1980. "Sweden faces zero population growth," *Population Bulletin* 35, no. 2 (June).

Gilbert, Neil. 1983. *Capitalism and the Welfare State: Dilemmas of Social Benevolence.* New Haven: Yale University Press.

Glass, D. V. 1940. *Population Policies and Movements in Europe.* Oxford: Oxford University Press.

Grass, Günter. 1982. *Headbirths or The Germans Are Dying Out.* Translated by Ralph Manheim. New York: Harcourt Brace Jovanovich.

Greer, Germaine. 1984. *Sex and Destiny: The Politics of Human Fertility.* New York: Harper & Row.

Hirsch, Fred. 1976. *Social Limits to Growth.* Cambridge, Mass.: Harvard University Press.

Hodgson, Dennis. 1983. "Demography as social science and policy science," *Population and Development Review* 9 (March): 1–34.

Hungary, Central Statistical Office. 1984. *The Impact of Policy Measures Other Than Family Planning Programmes on Fertility.* (Research Reports of the Demographic Research Institute, no. 18.) Budapest.

INED. 1976. *Natalité et politique démographique.* (Travaux et Documents No. 76). Paris: Institut national d'études démographiques.

Kahn, Herman. 1982. *The Coming Boom: Economic, Political, and Social.* New York: Simon & Schuster.

Keyfitz, Nathan. 1985. "An East Javanese village in 1953 and 1985: Observations on development," *Population and Development Review* 11 (December): 695–719.

Keynes, John Maynard. 1937. "Some economic consequences of a declining population," *Eugenics Review* 29 (April): 13–17.

Kirk Maurice. 1981. *Demographic and Social Change in Europe: 1979–2000.* Liverpool: Liverpool University Press.

Klinger, András. 1984. "Fertility and demographic policies," in *Population and Population Policy in Hungary,* ed. Dávid Bíró, Péter Józan, and Károly Miltényi. Budapest: Akadémiai Kiadó, pp. 27–66.

Knight, Frank H. 1947. *Freedom and Reform: Essays in Economics and Social Philosophy.* New York: Harper & Row.

Kuroda, Toshio. 1984. "Population policy," in *Population of Japan* (Country Monograph Series, No. 11). Bangkok: United Nations ESCAP, pp. 269–279.

Land, Hilary. 1979. "The changing place of women in Europe," *Daedalus* (Spring): 73–94.

Landry, Adolphe. 1949. *Traité de démographie,* Second edition. Paris: Payot.

Lesthaeghe, Ron. 1983. "A century of demographic and cultural change in Western Europe: An exploration of underlying dimensions," *Population and Development Review* 9 (September): 411–435.

Linder, Staffan Burenstam. 1970. *The Harried Leisure Class.* New York: Columbia University Press.

Malthus, T. R. 1820. *Principles of Political Economy.* London: John Murray.

McIntosh, C. Alison. 1983. *Population Policy in Western Europe: Responses to Low Fertility in France, Sweden, and West Germany*. Armonk, New York: M. E. Sharpe.

Miró, Carmen, and Joseph E. Potter. 1980. *Population Policy: Research Priorities in the Developing World*. London: Frances Pinter.

Moynihan, Daniel P. 1973. *The Politics of a Guaranteed Income: The Nixon Administration and the Family Assistance Plan*. New York: Random House.

Myrdal, Gunnar. 1940. *Population, A Problem for Democracy*. Cambridge, Mass.: Harvard University Press.

Oshima, Harry T. 1983. "The industrial and demographic transitions in East Asia," *Population and Development Review* 9 (December): 583–607.

Piotrow, Phyllis Tilson. 1973. *World Population Crisis: The United States Response*. New York: Praeger.

Preston, Samuel H. 1984. "Children and the elderly: Divergent paths for America's dependents," *Demography* 21 (November): 435–457.

Russell, Louise B. 1982. *The Baby Boom Generation and the Economy*. Washington, D.C.: The Brookings Institution.

Sauvy, Alfred. 1969. *General Theory of Population*. Translated by Christophe Campos. New York: Basic Books.

Schultz, Theodore W. (ed.). 1974. *Economics of the Family: Marriage, Children, and Human Capital*. Chicago: University of Chicago Press.

Spengler, Oswald. 1928 [1922]. *The Decline of the West*, Vol. 2: *Perspectives of World-History*. Translated by Charles Francis Atkinson. New York: Alfred A. Knopf.

Steinmann, Gunter (ed.). 1984. *Economic Consequences of Population Change in Industrialized Countries*. Berlin: Springer-Verlag.

Teitelbaum, Michael S. 1972. "Fertility effects of the abolition of legal abortion in Romania," *Population Studies* 26 (November): 405–417.

Tomlinson, Richard. 1984. "The French population debate," *The Public Interest*, no. 76 (Summer): 111–120.

Turchi, Boone A. 1984. "The monetary cost of a child," in Steinmann (1984), pp. 258–276.

United Kingdom, Royal Commission on Population. 1949. *Report*. London: His Majesty's Stationery Office.

———. 1973. *Report of the Population Panel*. London: Her Majesty's Stationery Office.

United Nations. 1982. *World Population Trends and Policies, 1981 Monitoring Report*. Vol. II: *Population Policies*. Department of International Economic and Social Affairs. New York.

———. 1985. *The Mexico City Conference: The Debate on the Review and Appraisal of the World Population Plan of Action*. Compiled by the Population Division, Department of International Economic and Social Affairs. New York.

UNFPA. 1984. *Population Perspectives: Statements by World Leaders*. New York: United Nations Fund for Population Activities.

US Commission on Population Growth and the American Future. 1972a. *Population and the American Future*. Washington, D.C.: US Government Printing Office.

———. 1972b. *Aspects of Population Growth Policy*. Vol. VI of Commission Research Reports, ed. Robert Parke, Jr. and Charles F. Westoff. Washington, D.C.: US Government Printing Office.

van de Kaa, Dirk J. 1978. "Towards a population policy for Western Europe," in Council of Europe (1978), pp. 215–230.

Vining, Daniel R., Jr. 1984. "Family salaries and the East German birth rate: A comment," *Population and Development Review* 10 (December): 693–696.

Wander, Hilde. 1984. "What does it cost to support the young and the old generations?," in Steinmann (1984), pp. 238–257.

Westoff, Charles F. 1983. "Fertility decline in the West: Causes and prospects," *Population and Development Review* 9 (March): 99–104.

Authors

Annelise Anderson is Senior Research Fellow, Hoover Institution, Stanford University.

Robert J. Barro is Distinguished Professor of Arts and Science (Economics), University of Rochester.

Gary S. Becker is University Professor of Economics and Sociology, Department of Economics, University of Chicago.

Mikhail S. Bernstam is Senior Research Fellow, Hoover Institution, Stanford University.

Ester Boserup, author and consultant, is an economist based in Brissago, Switzerland.

Jean Bourgeois-Pichat is Président, Comité International de Coopération dans les Recherches Nationales en Démographie (CICRED), Paris.

Barry R. Chiswick is Research Professor, Department of Economics and Survey Research Laboratory, University of Illinois at Chicago.

Carmel U. Chiswick is Associate Professor, Department of Economics, University of Illinois at Chicago.

Ansley J. Coale is Senior Research Demographer, Office of Population Research, and Professor Emeritus of Economics and Public Affairs, Princeton University.

Paul A. David is William Robertson Coe Professor of American Economic History, Department of Economics, Stanford University.

Kingsley Davis is Distinguished Professor of Sociology, University of Southern California, and Senior Research Fellow, Hoover Institution, Stanford University.

Paul Demeny is Vice President and Director, Center for Policy Studies, The Population Council, New York.

Thomas J. Espenshade is Director, Program in Demographic Studies, The Urban Institute, Washington, D.C.

David M. Heer is Professor of Sociology and Associate Director, Population Research Laboratory, University of Southern California.

Nathan Keyfitz is Head, The Population Program, International Institute for Applied Systems Analysis, Laxenburg, Austria.

Shigemi Kono is Director-General, Institute of Population Problems, Ministry of Health and Welfare, Tokyo.

Ronald D. Lee is Professor, Graduate Group in Demography and Department of Economics, University of California, Berkeley.

C. Alison McIntosh is Assistant Professor, Department of Population Planning and International Health, University of Michigan, Ann Arbor.

Geoffrey McNicoll is Senior Associate and Deputy Director, Center for Policy Studies, The Population Council, New York.

Thomas Gale Moore is Member, Council of Economic Advisers, and Senior Fellow, Hoover Institution, Stanford University.

Harriet B. Presser is Professor of Sociology, University of Maryland, and currently Fellow, Center for Advanced Study in the Behavioral Sciences, Stanford, California.

Samuel H. Preston is Director, Population Studies Center, University of Pennsylvania, Philadelphia.

Rita Ricardo-Campbell is Senior Fellow, Hoover Institution, Stanford University.

T. Paul Schultz is Professor of Economics and Director, Economic Growth Center, Yale University.

Carolyn L. Weaver is Senior Research Fellow, Hoover Institution, Stanford University (on leave of absence), and Editor, *Regulation,* Washington, D.C.

Charles F. Westoff is Director, Office of Population Research, Princeton University.